Percutaneous Treatment of Left Side Cardiac Valves

Ferrarotto Hospital

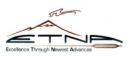
ETNA Foundation

University of Catania

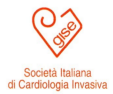
Società Italiana
di Cardiologia Invasiva

Corrado Tamburino • Gian Paolo Ussia

Percutaneous Treatment of Left Side Cardiac Valves

A Practical Guide for the Interventional Cardiologist

In collaboration with
Davide Capodanno
Massimiliano Mulè

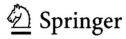

Corrado Tamburino
Full Professor of Cardiology, Director of
Postgraduate School of Cardiology,
Chief Cardiovascular Department,
Director Cardiology Division and
Interventional Cardiology, Ferrarotto
Hospital, University of Catania,
ETNA Foundation, Catania, Italy

Gian Paolo Ussia
Co-Director Interventional Cardiology,
Director Structural Heart Disease Program
Cardiology Division, Ferrarotto Hospital,
Catania, Italy

In collaboration with
Davide Capodanno
Research Fellow, Chair of Cardiology Division, University of Catania, ETNA Foundation, Catania, Italy

Massimiliano Mulè
Research Fellow, Chair of Cardiology Division, University of Catania, ETNA Foundation, Catania, Italy

The authors thank the "Associazione Cuore e Ricerca" of Catania for the technical and scientific support in the realization of this volume

ISBN 978-88-470-1423-7   e-ISBN 978-88-470-1424-4

DOI 10.1007/978-88-470-1424-4

Springer Dordrecht Heidelberg London Milan New York

Library of Congress Control Number: 2010925848

© Springer Verlag Italia 2010

This work is subject to copyright. All rights are reserved, whether the whole or part of the material is concerned, specifically the rights of translation, reprinting, reuse of illustrations, recitation, broadcasting, reproduction on microfilm or in any other way, and storage in data banks. Duplication of this publication or parts thereof is permitted only under the provisions of the Italian Copyright Law in its current version, and permission for use must always be obtained from Springer. Violations are liable to prosecution under the Italian Copyright Law.

The use of general descriptive names, registered names, trademarks, etc. in this publication does not imply, even in the absence of a specific statement, that such names are exempt from the relevant protective laws and regulations and therefore free for general use.

Product liability: The publishers cannot guarantee the accuracy of any information about dosage and application contained in this book. In every individual case the user must check such information by consulting the relevant literature.

9 8 7 6 5 4 3 2 1

Drawings by: Giombattista Barrano
Anatomopathologic pictures by: Giovanni Bartoloni

Typesetting: Compostudio, Cernusco s/N (Milan), Italy
Printing and binding: Arti Grafiche Nidasio, Assago (Milan), Italy
Printed in Italy

Springer-Verlag Italia S.r.l, Via Decembrio 28, I-20137 Milan, Italy
Springer is part of Springer Science+Business Media (www.springer.com)

*This volume is dedicated to the real engine of research,
motivating force of passion and mental vivacity:
my students, young doctors and fellows
to whom I wish to say a sincere "thank you"*

Corrado Tamburino

Preface

Transcatheter therapy of cardiac valve diseases is a rediscovery by interventional cardiologists. Treating cardiac valve diseases with alternative techniques to cardiac surgery using prosthetic devices has rekindled interest in the field of hemo-dynamics, which has been neglected in recent years. Within this framework, two sectors can be distinguished: valvuloplasty techniques using a balloon alone to treat mitral, aortic, and pulmonary stenoses, and those using prosthetic heart valves or repair devices. Valvuloplasty techniques should be considered as palliative, as the duration of their effectiveness varies from just a few weeks, as in the case of aortic valvuloplasty for degenerative stenoses, to years, as in the case of mitral and pulmonary valvuloplasty. By contrast, transcatheter implantation of biological prosthetic valves, or repair techniques using dedicated devices aim to provide a definitive therapeutic solution or at least a solution offering results that are equal to or just as good as those of cardiac surgery. The advent of devices for the percutaneous treatment of left chamber valve diseases is one of the greatest breakthroughs in interventional cardiology. The goal of this handbook is to give interventional cardiologists the means to understand the context of the percutaneous treatment of valve diseases and the state of the art of the techniques and procedures currently available.

Catania, April 2010 **Corrado Tamburino**
Gian Paolo Ussia

Contents

1 Anatomy
1.1	Mitral Valve Anatomy	1
1.1.1	Mitral Leaflets and the Dynamics of Their Movement	2
1.1.2	The Annulus	5
1.1.3	The *Chordae Tendineae* and Papillary Muscles	6
1.2	Aortic Valve Anatomy	7
1.2.1	The Annulus	9
1.2.2	The Leaflets	9
1.2.3	The Commissures	10
1.2.4	The Interleaflet Triangles	10
1.2.5	The Sinuses of Valsalva	11
1.2.6	The Sinotubular Junction	12
	References	12

2 Mitral Valve Disease
2.1	Mitral Stenosis	15
2.1.1	The Pathophysiology of Mitral Stenosis	15
2.1.2	Diagnosis	17
2.1.2.1	Non-invasive Diagnosis	17
2.1.2.2	Invasive Diagnosis	26
2.1.3	Timing of Interventions	28
2.1.4	Patient Selection	30
2.1.5	Percutaneous Therapy	32
2.1.5.1	Procedure and Technical Aspects	35
2.1.5.2	Mitral Valvuloplasty Outcomes	37
2.1.5.3	Complications	39
2.2	Mitral Regurgitation	39
2.2.1	The Pathophysiology of Mitral Regurgitation Physiopathology	39
2.2.2	Diagnosis	42
2.2.2.1	Non-invasive Diagnosis	42

2.2.2.2	Invasive Diagnosis	56
2.2.3	Timing of Interventions	60
2.2.4	Patient Selection	62
2.2.4.1	Anatomical and Functional Assessment of the Mitral Valve	65
2.2.4.2	Assessment of Regurgitation Etiopathogenesis	67
2.2.4.3	Selection of Patients for Implantation	73
2.2.5	Percutaneous Therapy	77
2.2.5.1	Leaflets Repair	78
2.2.5.2	Transcatheter Coronary Sinus Techniques	101
2.2.5.3	Annuloplasty Techniques	108
2.2.5.4	Chamber and Annular Remodeling	111
2.2.5.5	A Glimpse into the Future	113
	References	115

3 Aortic Valve Disease

3.1	Aortic Stenosis	125
3.1.1	The Pathophysiology of Aortic Stenosis	125
3.1.2	Diagnosis	127
3.1.2.1	Non-invasive Diagnosis	127
3.1.2.2	Invasive Diagnosis	135
3.1.3	Timing of Interventions	137
3.1.3.1	Symptomatic Patients	138
3.1.3.2	Asymptomatic Patients	138
3.1.4	Patient Selection	141
3.1.4.1	Valve Annulus	145
3.1.4.2	Sinuses of Valsalva (Width and Height)	147
3.1.4.3	Sinotubular Junction (STJ)	147
3.1.4.4	Left Ventricular Outflow Tract	147
3.1.4.5	Ascending Aorta	148
3.1.4.6	Iliac-femoral Axis and Subclavian Artery	148
3.1.5	Percutaneous Therapy	150
3.1.5.1	Edwards-SAPIEN™ Valve	152
3.1.5.2	CoreValve® ReValving System	168
3.1.5.3	Other Devices	189
3.1.5.4	Procedural Complications	196
3.2	Aortic Regurgitation	197
3.2.1	The Pathophysiology of Aortic Regurgitation	197
3.2.2	Diagnosis	198
3.2.2.1	Non-invasive Diagnosis	198
3.2.2.2	Invasive Diagnosis	204
3.2.3	Timing of Interventions	205
3.2.4	Patient Selection	206

3.2.5		Percutaneous Therapy	207
		References	209

4 Tips and Tricks and Management of Complications in Valvular Interventional Cardiology

4.1	Patient Selection and Work-up	216
4.1.1	Anatomical Typing	216
4.1.2	Valve and Heart Anatomy	217
4.1.3	Vascular Anatomy	218
4.1.3.1	Femoral Arteries	219
4.1.3.2	Iliac Arteries	220
4.1.3.3	Abdominal Aorta	221
4.1.3.4	Thoracic Aorta	222
4.2	Procedure	223
4.2.1	Vascular Access	223
4.2.2	Choosing the Introducer	226
4.2.3	Passing the Aortic Valve	229
4.2.4	Valvuloplasty	234
4.2.5	CoreValve® Revalving System Delivery and Implantation	234
4.2.5.1	Check on Implantation	237
4.2.6	Closing the Arterial Breach with the Prostar™ Device	240
4.2.7	Miscellaneous	241
4.2.7.1	Difficult Navigation of the Delivery Catheter in the Aortic Arch	242
4.2.7.2	Recovery of Catheter Fragments	243
4.2.7.3	Balloon Valvuloplasty Trapping	244
4.2.7.4	Cardiac Perforation	246
4.2.7.5	Introducer Replacement	246
4.3	The MitraClip®	247
4.3.1	Device and Technique	247
4.3.2	Procedure	248
	Reference	254

5 Transcatheter Valve Treatment: Peri-procedural Management

5.1	Pre-procedural Care	257
5.2	Post-procedural Management	258
5.2.1	ICU Care	258
5.2.1.1	Laboratory Tests	259
5.2.1.2	Renal Function and Fluid Balance	260
5.2.1.3	Vascular Access	261
5.2.1.4	Rhythm Control	263

5.2.1.5	Transthoracic Echocardiogram	266
5.2.2	Medical Treatment and Physical Rehabilitation	268
5.2.3	Before Hospital Discharge	269
5.2.4	Medium-term Management (Out of Hospital)	269
	References	271

6 Surgical Treatment of Mitral Regurgitation and Aortic Stenosis

6.1	Treatment of Degenerative Mitral Regurgitation	273
6.1.1	Epidemiology and Natural History	273
6.1.2	Diagnosis and Quantification of Degenerative Mitral Regurgitation	275
6.1.3	Surgical Considerations	276
6.1.3.1	Types of Procedure	276
6.1.3.2	Surgical Indications	277
6.1.3.3	Principles of Mitral Repair Surgery	278
6.1.3.4	Results	287
6.2	Treatment of Functional Mitral Regurgitation	288
6.3	Treatment of Aortic Stenosis	296
6.3.1	Surgical Indications	296
6.3.2	Specific Issues	297
6.3.2.1	Mechanical or Tissue Valves	297
6.3.2.2	Prosthesis–Patient Mismatch	298
6.3.2.3	The Role of Transfemoral or Transapical Aortic Valve Replacement	298
	References	299

List of Authors and Contributors

Corrado Tamburino
Full Professor of Cardiology
Director of Postgraduate School of Cardiology
Chief of Cardiovascular Department
Director of Cardiology Division and Interventional Cardiology
Ferrarotto Hospital
University of Catania
ETNA Foundation
Catania, Italy

Davide Capodanno
Research Fellow
Chair of Cardiology Division
University of Catania
ETNA Foundation
Catania, Italy

Massimiliano Mulè
Research Fellow
Chair of Cardiology Division
University of Catania
ETNA Foundation
Catania, Italy

Gian Paolo Ussia
Co-Director of Interventional Cardiology
Director Structural Heart Disease Program Cardiology Division
Ferrarotto Hospital
Catania, Italy

Ottavio Alfieri
Full Professor of Cardiac Surgery
Director Cardiac Surgery
San Raffaele University Hospital
Milan, Italy

Antonio Maria Calafiore
Full Professor of Cardiac Surgery
Department of Adult Cardiac Surgery
Prince Sultan Cardiac Center
Riyadh, Saudi Arabia

George Dangas
Cardiovascular Research Foundation
New York, USA
Cardiology Department
Onassis Cardiac Surgery Centre
Athens, Greece

Ted Feldman
Division of Cardiology
Evanston Hospital
University of Illinois, US

Patrizia Aruta
Postgraduate School of Cardiology
University of Catania
Catania, Italy

Marco Barbanti
Postgraduate School of Cardiology
University of Catania
Catania, Italy

Gionbattista Barrano
Postgraduate School of Cardiology
University of Catania
Catania, Italy

Giovanni Bartoloni
Professor of Anatomic Pathology
Postgraduate School of Cardiology
University of Catania
Catania, Italy

Michele De Bonis
Cardiac Surgery
San Raffaele Hospital
Milan, Italy

Valeria Cammalleri
Postgraduate School of Cardiology
University of Catania
Catania, Italy

Wanda Deste
Echocardiography Laboratory
Division of Cardiology
Ferrarotto Hospital
Catania, Italy

Lorena Iacò
Department of Adult Cardiac Surgery
Prince Sultan Cardiac Center
Riyadh, Saudi Arabia

Sebastiano Immè
Postgraduate School of Cardiology
University of Catania
Catania, Italy

Sarah Mangiafico
Echocardiography Laboratory
Division of Cardiology
Ferrarotto Hospital
Catania, Italy

Anna Marchese
Postgraduate School of Cardiology
University of Catania
Catania, Italy

Anna Maria Pistritto
Postgraduate School of Cardiology
University of Catania
Catania, Italy

Salvatore Scandura
Director of Echocardiography
Laboratory
Division of Cardiology
Ferrarotto Hospital
Catania, Italy

Marilena Scarabelli
Postgraduate School of Cardiology
University of Catania
Catania, Italy

Konstantinos Spargias
Cardiology Department
Onassis Cardiac Surgery Centre
Athens, Greece

Maurizio Taramasso
Cardiac Surgery
San Raffaele Hospital
Milan, Italy

Adel Tash
Department of Adult Cardiac Surgery
Prince Sultan Cardiac Center
Riyadh, Saudi Arabia

Laura Basile
Executive PA
ETNA Foundation
Catania, Italy

Abbreviations

ACC	American College of Cardiology
ACE	angiotensin-converting enzyme
ACT	activated clotting time
AHA	American Heart Association
AIV	anterior atrioventricular vein
AL-1/AL-2	Amplatz Left-1/2 (catheter)
AMADEUS	Mitral Annuloplasty Device European Study
AR	aortic regurgitation
AS	aortic stenosis
ASA	acetylsalicylic acid
ASD	atrial septal defect
ASS	Amplatz Super Stiff (guidewire)
AVA	aortic valve area
AVB	atrioventricular block
AVR	aortic valve replacement
bpm	beats/min
CABG	coronary artery bypass grafting
CC	intercommisural distance
CD	coaptation distance
CDS	clip delivery system
CI	confidence interval
CIMR	chronic ischemic mitral regurgitation
CIN	contrast-induced nephropathy
CK	creatine kinase
CL	coaptation length
CRS	CoreValve® ReValving System
CT	computed tomography
CVRS	cardiovascular valve repair system
CW	continuous wave (Doppler)

CWP	capillary wedge pressure
2D	two-dimensional
3D	three-dimensional
DCS	delivery catheter system
DT	deceleration E-time
ECG	electrocardiogram
ECMO	extracorporeal membrane oxygenation
EF	ejection fraction
EOA	effective orifice area
ERO	effective regurgitant orifice
EROA	effective regurgitant orifice area
ES	Edwards-SAPIEN™ (heart valve)
ESC	European Society of Cardiology
EuroSCORE	European System for Cardiac Operative Risk Evaluation
EVEREST	Endovascular Edge-to-edge Repair Study Trial
EVOLUTION	EValuation Of the Edwards Lifesciences percUTaneous mItral annulOplasty system for the treatment of mitral regurgitation
FH	Ferrarotto Hospital (Catania)
FIM	First In Man (study)
FMR	functional mitral regurgitation
FSV	forward stroke volume
HIT	heparin-induced thrombocytopenia
IAS	inter-atrial septum
ICU	intensive care unit
IMR	ischemic mitral regurgitation
INR	international normalized ratio
JR	Judkins catheter
IV	intravenous
LA	left atrium
LAA	left atrial appendage
LAP	left atrial pressure
LBBB	left bundle branch block
LDH	lactic dehydrogenase
LIMA	left internal mammary artery
LMCA	left main coronary artery
LMWH	low molecular weight heparin
LV	left ventricle
LVDP	left ventricular diastolic pressure
LVEDP	left ventricular end-diastolic pressure
LVEF	left ventricle ejection fraction
LVESD	left ventricular end-systolic diameter
LVESV	left ventricular end-systolic volume
LVESVI	left ventricular end-systolic volume index

LVOT	left ventricular outflow tract
MACCE	major adverse cardiac and cerebrovascular event
MAE	major adverse event
MI	myocardial infarction
ML	mid-lateral
MP	multipurpose catheter
MR	mitral regurgitation
MRI	magnetic resonance imaging
MSCT	multislice computed tomography
MVA	mitral valve area
NHLBI	National Heart, Lung, and Blood Institute
NYHA	New York Heart Association
OR	odds ratio
OS	opening snap
PAP	pulmonary artery pressure
PCWP	pulmonary capillary wedge pressure
PHT	pressure half-time
PISA	proximal isovelocity surface area
PMC	percutaneous mitral commisurotomy
PMV	percutaneous mitral valvulotomy
PPM	prosthesis–patient mismatch
PTMA	percutaneous transvenous mitral annuloplasty
PTOLEMY	Percutaneous Mitral Annuloplasty (trial)
PVF	pulmonary venous flow
PW	pulsed wave (Doppler)
RBBB	right bundle branch block
RF	regurgitant fraction
RR	risk ratio
RV	regurgitant volume
S_1	first heart sound
S_2	second heart sound
S_3	third heart sound
SAM	systolic anterior motion
SGC	steerable guide catheter
SL	septal–lateral distance
SLE	systemic lupus erythematosus
sPAP	systolic pulmonary artery pressure
SRH	San Raffaele Hospital (Milan)
STJ	sinotubular junction
STS	Society of Thoracic Surgeons
STS-PROM	STS Predicted Risk of Mortality
TA	tenting area
TAVI	transcatheter aortic valve implantation

TEE	transesophageal echocardiogram/echocardiography
TIA	transient ischemic attack
TSV	total stroke volume
TTE	transthoracic echocardiogram/echocardiography
UFH	unfractionated heparin
UGCR	ultrasound-guided compression repair
VC	vena contracta
VKA	vitamin K antagonist

Anatomy 1

1.1 Mitral Valve Anatomy

The mitral valve apparatus comprises the annulus and portion of myocardium located above and below it, the leaflets, the *chordae tendineae*, and the papillary muscles (Fig. 1.1). The mitral valve apparatus and the left ventricle are so interdependent that there is no mitral valve defect that does not affect the left ventricle in some way, and, in turn, there is no morphological or functional alteration of the left ventricle that has no consequence, to a greater or lesser extent, for the mitral valve. Therefore, the mitral valve is not a passive structure that moves solely as a result of the forces generated by cardiac activity, but rather a structure with its own sphinteric activity concentrated mainly in the annulus, which contributes to the ventricle's contractility and, in turn, is heavily affected by it.

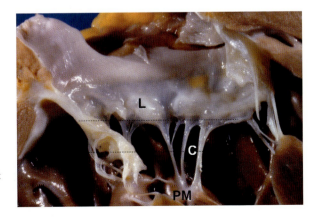

Fig. 1.1 Gross image of the mitral valve apparatus showing the posterior leaflet (*L*), *chordae tendineae* (*C*) and papillary muscles (*PM*)

Percutaneous Treatment of Left Side Cardiac Valves. Corrado Tamburino, Gian Paolo Ussia
© Springer-Verlag Italia 2010

1.1.1
Mitral Leaflets and the Dynamics of Their Movement

The mitral valve has two leaflets: the anterior leaflet, the larger of the two, also called the "large leaflet", and the posterior leaflet, smaller than the other, also called the "small leaflet" (Fig. 1.2).

From a histological viewpoint, the mitral leaflets are formed by a triple layer of tissue (Fig. 1.3):
- *a fibrous layer*, namely the solid collagen core in direct continuity with the *chordae tendineae*
- *a spongy layer*, located on the atrial side and forming the contact margins of the leaflets
- *a fibroelastic layer*, completely covering the leaflets. On the atrial side, this layer is especially rich in elastic fibers, while on the ventricular side it is thinner and located especially on the anterior leaflet.

From a strictly anatomical viewpoint, the mitral valve is a monoleaflet valve. The valve veil encircles the entire circumference of the annulus [1–11]. Two large indentations split the valve veil into an anteromedial leaflet (or aortic, considering its close connection to the aortic root) and a posterolateral leaflet (or mural, considering its connection to the ventricular and atrial wall). These indentations (posteromedial and anterolateral) take the name of "commissures". The anterior leaflet covers about one-third of the area of the annulus, while the posterior leaflet covers the other two-thirds. The anterior leaflet is also longer than the posterior leaflet [1–11]. The posterior leaflet is almost always split into three parts by secondary commissures called "scallops": a lateral scallop (generally defined P1), a central scallop (P2), and a medial scallop (P3) (Fig. 1.4). This

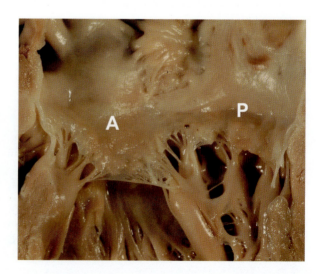

Fig. 1.2 Anterior (*A*) and posterior (*P*) leaflets

division is due to the fact that each scallop may prolapse in the left atrium regardless of the others, requiring different intervention strategies. At times, even more than three scallops can be found. The anterior leaflet is generally a single veil, but alterations involving only a part of it (ruptured *chordae tendineae*, erosion, etc) may also be encountered. Therefore, the anterior leaflet is also divided into three parts (A1, A2, A3), corresponding to the posterior leaflet scallops [1–11].

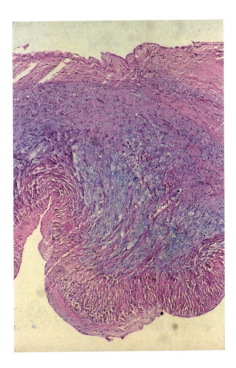

Fig. 1.3 Photomicrograph of a mitral valve leaflet

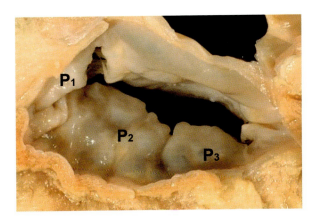

Fig. 1.4 An atrial view of the mitral valve showing the posterior leaflet divided into three scallops (P_1, P_2, P_3)

The two leaflets meet in an area defined as the "apposition zone", which stretches a few millimeters from the free margin of the leaflets towards the body. The mitral tissue is actually redundant compared to the annular area that it must cover. Leaflet coaptation in the apposition zone greatly reduces the pressure that the valve must bear during systole, as it is simultaneously distributed on all the leaflets facing one another, and hence dissipated. The ventricular surface of the leaflets corresponding to the apposition zone is the portion that most of the *chordae tendineae* insert into, hence its name "rough zone" (Fig. 1.5).

During systole, both valve leaflets are concave when observed from the left ventricle, but their shape is actually much more complex. The anterior leaflet is convex towards the ventricle in the regions closest to the free margin, thus giving a sigmoid shape to the leaflets taken as a whole [12, 13]. The valve does not open from the free margin, but from the center of the leaflets, which, starting from a concave configuration, first flatten out and then become convex towards the left ventricle. All this takes place while the extremities are still in contact with one another [12, 14, 15]. Then the free margins separate and move inside the left ventricle. Once they reach their maximum degree of opening, the leaflets show a slow "back-and-forth" movement like that of a flag blowing in the wind. Then there is another slight opening pulse triggered by atrial systole. The valve closes, starting with the movements of the leaflets towards the left atrium. The speed at which both leaflets move is different, as the anterior leaflet is about twice the size of the posterior one. This allows the free margin of both leaflets to reach the closing point at the same time [16].

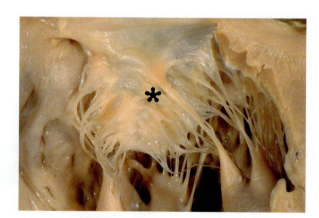

Fig. 1.5 Ventricular side of the anterior mitral leaflet. Note the "rough zone" (*)

1.1.2
The Annulus

In the human heart, the mitral annulus has a mean area of about 7.6 cm^2, ranging between 5 and 11 cm^2 [17]. As already described, the annular perimeter of the posterior leaflet is larger than that of the anterior leaflet by a ratio of about 2 to 1. The annular area varies physiologically during the cardiac cycle, depending on atrial and ventricular contraction, cavity dimensions and pressure [4, 18]. The variation in the size of the mitral annulus during the cardiac cycle is estimated to be of the order of 20–40% [4, 8, 9, 18]. The dimensions of the annulus start to increase during telesystole, reaching maximum breadth during the late diastolic phase [3, 4, 8, 17, 18]. Two-thirds of the reduction in annulus dimensions occurs during atrial systole, i.e. during ventricular presystole, and it is less when the PR interval is reduced, while it is absent in the presence of atrial fibrillation or ventricular pacing. The mitral annulus area is at its smallest in the initial systolic phases [4, 7, 8, 17, 18]. In a healthy heart the annulus has an almost elliptical shape, which becomes more eccentric during systole compared to diastole [3, 4, 8, 17, 18]. In this elliptical configuration, the ratio between the smaller and larger diameters of the annulus amounts to about 0.75 [3, 4, 8].

The mitral annulus moves vertically inside the cardiac chambers, according to the phase of the cardiac cycle. During diastole, the annulus moves towards the left atrium, while during systole it moves towards the apex of the heart. The duration and extent of the vertical movement are directly correlated with the state of filling of the left atrium [4, 8, 19, 20]. The systolic motion towards the apex is extremely important for atrial filling; it is also present in cases of atrial fibrillation and it is correlated with the degree of end-systolic ventricular emptying [4, 8, 20]. During diastole, the mitral annulus moves back towards the left atrium, increasing the velocity of transmitral flow during diastole by about 20% [9, 20].

From an interventional cardiology perspective, it was clear from early on that intervention in the mitral annulus was easy to perform in an aggressive manner, because of its anatomical interface with the coronary sinus (Fig. 1.6). The coronary sinus runs behind the posterior region of the mitral annulus at an average of 10 mm above the mitral annulus. In subjects affected by dilated cardiopathy associated with moderate or severe mitral regurgitation, it has been reported that it runs at about 8 mm above the annulus [21]. The circumflex artery also interacts with the coronary sinus, as it is located right below it (Fig. 1.6). In 80% of the population, the two vessels cross at an average distance of 78 mm from the coronary sinus ostium, and the mean distance between the circumflex artery and coronary sinus at the point of intersection is about 8 mm [21]. This favorable anatomical picture has allowed for the creation of metal devices for transjugular placement, which, once inside the coronary sinus, exert a force capable of remodeling the mitral annulus and reducing the antero-posterior diameter, and subsequently the degree of mitral failure.

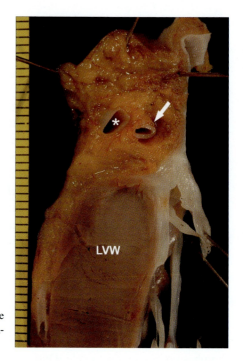

Fig. 1.6 Lateral left ventricular wall (*LVW*): the coronary sinus (*) is very close to the circumflex coronary artery (*white arrow*)

1.1.3
The *Chordae Tendineae* and Papillary Muscles

The papillary muscles originate in the distal third of the ventricular wall and have a variable morphology, although the posteromedial papillary muscle is generally smaller than the anterolateral one. The epicardial fibers in the left ventricle run from the base of the heart to the apex, where they contribute to forming the two papillary muscles, which are marked by a vertical arrangement of the myocardial fibers [11, 12]. The mitral fibers join the papillary muscles by means of *chordae tendineae*, which also run inside the mitral leaflets. These, in turn, are in continuity with the mitral annulus. The vascularization of the papillary muscles differs though: the posteromedial papillary muscle is usually supplied with blood by the right coronary artery, while the anterolateral papillary muscle is supplied by the left anterior descending and the circumflex arteries [11, 22, 23]. The anterolateral and posteromedial papillary muscles contract simultaneously and are innervated by both the parasympathetic and sympathetic systems [24, 25].

Functionally speaking, the *chordae tendineae* are divided into three groups [11, 26] (Fig. 1.7):
- *the primary chordae tendinae* originate near the extremity of the papillary muscles, progressively split, and insert on the extremities of the valve

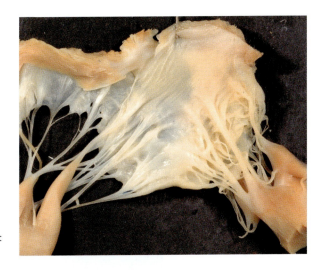

Fig. 1.7 Ventricular surface of the anterior mitral leaflet: the *chordae tendineae*

leaflets; their purpose is to prevent prolapse of the valve leaflets during systole
- *the secondary chordae tendineae* originate in the same area as the primary ones, are thinner and less numerous, and fit into the junction between the rough zone and the smooth zone; their job is to anchor the valve. They are more present in the anterior leaflet and play a key role in the systolic function of the left ventricle
- *the tertiary chordae tendineae*, also called the *basal chordae*, directly originate from the ventricular wall and head to the posterior leaflet near the annulus.

The papillary muscles have a major hemodynamic function during the cardiac cycle. During diastole they form a groove allowing inflow into the left ventricle, and during systole they create a route favoring systolic ejection. The shortening and thickening of the papillary muscles with the subsequent increase in volume are associated with a smaller blood content in the left ventricle at the end of systole, and hence an increase in the ejection fraction. The shortening of the papillary muscle during isovolumetric relaxation seems to play a major role in the mechanism that opens the mitral valve, while the stretching in the late diastolic phase seems to favor optimal closing [27].

1.2 Aortic Valve Anatomy

The aortic valve should be considered within the wider context of its anatomical and functional unit, namely the *aortic root*. The latter is the connection between the left ventricle and the ascending aorta, and it is located on the right, posteriorly to the subpulmonary infundibulum; its posterior margin is wedged between the mitral valve orifice and the muscular portion of the interventricular septum. The aortic root goes from the basal plane where the aortic valve leaflets enter the left ventricle, to the peripheral point where they enter the sinotubular junction (Fig. 1.8) [28]. About two-thirds of the circumference of the lower part of the aortic root are connected to the muscular portion of the interventricular septum. The remaining one-third is in continuity with the aortic leaflet of the mitral valve (Fig. 1.9). Its components include: the annulus, valve leaflets, commissures, sinuses of Valsalva, sinotubular junction, and interleaflet triangles.

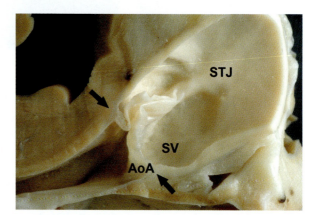

Fig. 1.8 Long axis showing the aortic root between the aortic annulus (*AoA*) and the sinotubular junction (*STJ*). *SV*, sinus of Valsalva; *black arrows*, margins of aortic annulus

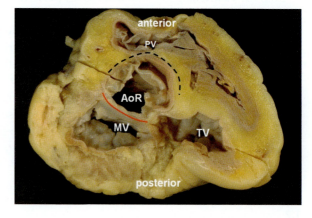

Fig. 1.9 Short-axis view of the cardiac basis: about two-thirds of the circumference of the lower part of the aortic root are connected to the muscular portion of the interventricular septum (*black dotted line*). The remaining one-third is in continuity with the anterior aortic leaflet (*red line*). *AoR*, aortic root; *MV*, mitral valve; *PV*, pulmonary valve; *TV*, tricuspid valve

1.2.1
The Annulus

The annulus is a crown-shaped fibrous semilunar structure marked off by the attachments of the aortic leaflets. The attachment of each leaflet is the area where the leaflet enters the aortic root. The aortic root has at least three circular rings and one crown-shaped ring [29]. The three-dimensional arrangement of the leaflets takes the form of a three-pointed crown. The crown's base is a virtual ring formed by the plane joining the basal points where the leaflets enter the left ventricle. The crown's upper part is a true ring called the sinotubular junction, forming the point where the aortic root opens into the ascending aorta. The semilunar lines of attachment cross another true ring, the anatomic ventriculo-aortic junction. Even though an annulus is traditionally described, in the aortic valve it can be said that the annulus takes on the cylindrical shape of the aortic root in which the valve leaflets are supported by a crown-shaped structure [28]. The diameter of the aortic annulus in a normal adult usually ranges between 21 and 24 mm [30].

1.2.2
The Leaflets

The aortic valve is normally tricuspid. The valve's proper functioning depends on the correct relationship between the leaflets inside the aortic root. The leaflets consist of a core of fibrous tissue inside an endothelial sheath on both the arterial and ventricular side. The locus where they originate from the supporting ventricular structures gives way to the fibroelastic walls of the aortic valvar sinuses and marks off the anatomic ventriculo-aortic junction.

Each leaflet is composed of an attachment, body, coaptation surface, and lunule with the nodules of Arantii. The nodules of Arantii are located halfway on the free margin of the coaptation surface. On both sides of this nodule, there is a thin portion called a "lunule"; it consists of a margin, which is thin at its free end and continues into the coaptation area where the three leaflets meet and allow for complete valve closing. The lunules are attached to the wall of the aortic root in the area of the commissures. The main part of each leaflet is called the "body". As specified above, the attachment is the area where the leaflet joins the aortic root [31]. Considering the size of the leaflets, it can be said that the non-coronary leaflet tends to be larger, followed by the left coronary leaflet and then the right coronary leaflet, although these differences are not significant (Fig. 1.10) [30, 32, 33].

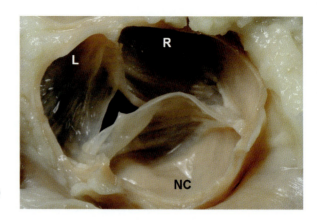

Fig. 1.10 Aortic view showing the left (*L*), right (*R*), and non-coronary (*NC*) cusps

1.2.3
The Commissures

The top of the crown-shaped structure in the area where the lunules of two leaflets are attached to the aortic wall at the sinotubular junctions is called the commissure. There are three commissures. The commissure between the right and left leaflets is located anteriorly, more or less in front of the matching commissure of the pulmonary valve. The one between the right and non-coronary leaflets is located anteriorly to the right, and the one between the left and non-coronary leaflets is usually located on the posterior face of the aortic root. The commissures have a fibrous structure and support the valvular leaflets located above the three triangular areas called interleaflet triangles.

1.2.4
The Interleaflet Triangles

These are extensions of the ventricular outflow tract and reach the sinotubular junction in the area of the commissures. They are not formed by ventricular myocardium, but rather by the thinned fibrous tissue of the aortic walls between the sinuses of Valsalva.

The triangle between the right and left sinuses is located in front of the pulmonary valve. The triangle between the right and non-coronary sinuses is located in front of the right atrium and is proximally in continuity with the membranous septum. This is the area where the conduction system is closely linked to the aortic root. This has major implications allowing for the induction of alterations in conduction following percutaneous aortic valve replacement. The bundle of His is an anterior extension of the atrioventricular node, and

1.2 Aortic Valve Anatomy

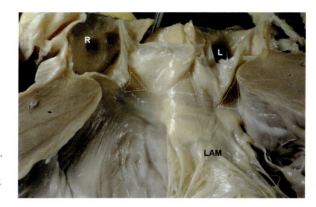

Fig.1.11 Interleaflet triangles. *L*, left coronary ostium; *LAM*, anterior mitral leaflet; *R*, right coronary ostium

penetrates through the central fibrous portion just below the lower margin of the membranous ventricular septum at the ridge of the muscular ventricular septum right below this triangle, which is closely interconnected with the septal leaflet of the tricuspid valve.

Finally, the triangle between the left and non-coronary sinuses is inferiorly in direct continuity with the aortic or anterior leaflet of the mitral valve. These triangles separate and mark off the three sinuses in a normal valve (Fig. 1.11) [34, 35].

1.2.5
The Sinuses of Valsalva

The sinuses of Valsalva are defined as expanses separating the ventricle and aorta (Fig. 1.8). They border superiorly or distally with the sinotubular junction, and inferiorly or proximally with the valvar leaflet attachments. Each sinus takes its name from the coronary cusp it originates from (right, left or non-coronary) [36] (Fig. 1.10).

The coronary orifices normally originate from the two anterior right and left sinuses of Valsalva, usually right below the sinotubular junction. Their origin may vary from patient to patient. The distance from the annular plane may vary greatly and there are some congenital anatomic variants, which are very often associated with the bicuspid aortic valve [37]. Knowledge of the precise position of the coronary ostia and accurate measurement of the distance from the annulus is of the utmost importance during the screening of patients undergoing percutaneous aortic valve replacement. If this distance is too small, there is a risk of coronary occlusion by the aortic leaflets displaced by the device.

1.2.6
The Sinotubular Junction

The sinotubular junction marks the transition from the aortic root to the ascending aorta, and also the upper part of the attachment of each valve leaflet (Fig. 1.8). The mean diameter of the sinotubular junction ranges between 22 and 26 mm [30]. Dilation of the aortic root at this point has been associated with the onset of aortic failure.

References

1. Van Gils FA. The fibrous skeleton in the human heart: embryological and pathogenetic considerations. Virchows Arch A Pathol Anat Histol 1981;393:61–73.
2. Davila JC, Palmer TE. The mitral valve: anatomy and pathology for the surgeon. Arch Surg 1962;84:174–198.
3. Silverman ME, Hurst JW. The mitral complex: interaction of the anatomy, physiology, and pathology of the mitral annulus, mitral valve leaflets, *chordae tendineae*, and papillary muscles. Am Heart J 1968;76:399–418.
4. Tsakiris AG, Von Bernuth G, Rastelli GC et al. Size and motion of the mitral valve annulus in anesthetized intact dogs. J Appl Physiol 1971;30:611–618.
5. Perloff JK, Roberts WC. The mitral apparatus: functional anatomy of mitral regurgitation. Circulation 1972;46:227–239.
6. Fenoglio J Jr, Tuan DP, Wit AL et al. Canine mitral complex: ultrastructure and electro-mechanical properties. Circ Res 1972;31:417–430.
7. Walmsley R. Anatomy of human mitral valve in adult cadaver and comparative anatomy of the valve. Br Heart J 1978;40:351–366.
8. Ormiston JA, Shah PM, Tei C et al. Size and motion of the mitral valve annulus in man: I. A two-dimensional echocardiographic method and findings in normal subjects. Circulation 1981;64:113–120.
9. Toumanidis ST, Sideris DA, Papamichael CM et al. The role of mitral annulus motion in left ventricular function. Acta Cardiol 1992;47:331–348.
10. Anderson RH, Wilcox BR. The anatomy of the mitral valve. In: Wells FC, Shapiro LM (eds) Mitral valve disease. Oxford: Butterworth-Heinemann, 1996.
11. Fenster MS, Feldman MD. Mitral regurgitation: an overview. Curr Probl Cardiol 1995;20:193–230.
12. Karlsson MO, Glasson JR, Bolger AF et al. Mitral valve opening in the ovine heart. Am J Physiol Heart Circ Physiol 1998;274:H552–563.
13. Levine RA, Triulzi MO, Harrigan P, Weyman AE. The relationship of mitral annular shape to the diagnosis of mitral valve prolapse. Circulation 1987;75:756–767.
14. Sovak M, Lynch PR, Stewart GH. Movement of the mitral valve and its correlation with the first heart sound: selective valvular visualization and high-speed cineradiography in intact dogs. Invest Radiol 1973;8:150–155.
15. Pohost GM, Dinsmore RE, Rubenstein JJ et al. The echocardiogram of the anterior leaflet of the mitral valve: Correlation with hemodynamic and cineroentgenographic studies in dogs. Circulation 1975;51:88–97.
16. Tsakiris AG, Gordon DA, Mathieu Y et al. Motion of both mitral valve leaflets: a cineroentgenographic study in intact dogs. J Appl Physiol 1975;39:359–366.

17. Pollick C, Pittman M, Filly K et al. Mitral and aortic valve orifice area in normal subjects and in patients with congestive cardiomyopathy: determination by two-dimensional echocardiography. Am J Cardiol 1982;49:1191–1196.
18. Tsakiris AG, Sturm RE, Wood EH. Experimental studies on the mechanisms of closure of cardiac valves with use of roentgen videodensitometry. Am J Cardiol 1973;32:136–143.
19. Davis PKB, Kinmonth JB. The movements of the annulus of the mitral valve. J Cardiovasc Surg 1963;4:427–431.
20. Keren G, Sonnenblick EH, LeJemtel TH. Mitral annulus motion: relation to pulmonary venous and transmitral flows in normal subjects and in patients with dilated cardiomyopathy. Circulation 1988;78:621–629.
21. Choure AJ, Garcia MJ, Hesse B et al. In vivo analysis of the anatomical relationship of coronary sinus to mitral annulus and left circumflex coronary artery using cardiac multidetector computed tomography: implications for percutaneous coronary sinus mitral annuloplasty. J Am Coll Cardiol 2006;48:1938–1945.
22. Luther RR, Meyers SN. Acute mitral insufficiency secondary to ruptured *chordae tendineae*. Arch Intern Med 1974;134:568.
23. Voci P, Bilotta F, Caretta Q et al. Papillary muscle perfusion pattern: a hypothesis for ischemic papillary muscle dysfunction. Circulation 1995;91:1714–1718.
24. Armour JA, Randall WC. Electrical and mechanical activity of papillary muscle. Am J Physiol 1978;218:1710–1717.
25. Cronin R, Armour JA, Randall WC. Function of the in-situ papillary muscle in the canine left ventricle. Circ Res 1969;25:67–75.
26. Lam JHC, Ranganathan N, Wigle ED et al. Morphology of the human mitral valve: I. *Chordae tendineae*: a new classification. Circulation 1970;41:449–458.
27. Marzilli M, Sabbah HN, Lee T et al. Role of the papillary muscle in opening and closure of the mitral valve. Am J Physiol Heart Circ Physiol 1980;238:H348–354.
28. Hokken RB, Bartelings MM, Bogers AJ, Gittenberger-DeGroot AC. Morphology of the pulmonary and aortic roots with regard to the pulmonary autograft procedure. J Thorac Cardiovasc Surg 1997;113:453–461.
29. Cheng A, Dagum P, Miller DC. Aortic root dynamics and surgery: from craft to science. Philos Trans R Soc Lond B Biol Sci 2007;362:1407–1419.
30. Silver MA, Roberts WC. Detailed anatomy of the normally functioning aortic valve in hearts of normal and increased weight. Am J Cardiol 1985;55:454–461.
31. Misfeld M and Sievers H. Heart valve macro- and microstructure. Philos Trans R Soc Lond B Biol Sci 2007;362:1421–1436.
32. Vollebergh FE, Becker AE. Minor congenital variations of cusp size in tricuspid aortic valves. Possible link with isolated aortic stenosis. Br Heart J 1977;39:1006–1011.
33. Kunzelman KS, Grande KJ, David TE et al. Aortic root and valve relationships. Impact on surgical repair. J Thorac Cardiovasc Surg 1994;107:162–170.
34. Anderson RH. Clinical anatomy of the aortic root. Heart 2000;84:670–673.
35. Piazza N, De Jaegere P, Schultz et al. Anatomy of the aortic valvar complex and its implications for transcatheter implantation of the aortic valve. Circulation Cardiovasc Interv 2008;1:74–81.
36. Mihaljevic T, Sayeed MR, Stamou SC, Paul S. Pathophysiology of aortic valve disease. In: Cohn LH (ed) Cardiac surgery in the adult. New York: McGraw-Hill, 2008.
37. Roberts WC. The congenitally bicuspid aortic valve. A study of 85 autopsy cases. Am J Cardiol 1970;26:72–83.

Mitral Valve Disease

2.1 Mitral Stenosis

2.1.1 The Pathophysiology of Mitral Stenosis

Mitral stenosis is an obstruction of blood flow from the left atrium to the left ventricle. It is generally caused by rheumatic heart disease [1, 2]. Other causes of mitral stenosis are: severe calcification of the valve leaflets, congenital defects of the mitral valve, systemic lupus erythematosus (SLE), tumors, left atrial thrombi, vegetations due to endocarditis, and causes linked to prior device implants.

A history of rheumatic disease is generally present in about 60% of mitral stenosis patients. Women are affected more frequently than men, with a ratio ranging between 2:1 and 3:1 [3]. The pathology develops slowly and takes about 20 years before it becomes clinically manifest. Today the incidence of rheumatic disease, and hence of mitral stenosis, has decreased in industrialized countries, while in developing countries the incidence of both diseases is still very high. The cause of rheumatic fever is beta-hemolytic group A streptococcus. Streptococcal antigens react with the human immune system and lead to the formation of antibodies, which, besides destroying the bacterial cells, attack valve tissues as well due to cross-reactivity with some heart valve components. The bacterial components involved are hyaluronic acid in the bacterial capsule, and the streptococcus M antigen and its peptides [4, 5]. During the chronic phase of rheumatic disease, markers typical of inflammation can be found and it has been observed that their levels have a direct correlation with the severity of valve involvement and the quantity of valve scars [6]. Besides affecting the mitral valve, rheumatic disease can potentially cause pancarditis, leading to myocardial, endocardial and pericardial damage [1, 7]. In most cases (60%), only the mitral valve is affected, followed by involvement of both the aortic and mitral valves (30%); the involvement of the aortic valve alone is less frequent (10%).

The pathognomonic lesions of rheumatic disease consist of commissural fusion, valve leaflet fibrosis and retraction, and shortening and fusion of the *chordae tendineae* [8] (Fig. 2.1). The *chordae tendineae* can suffer from such a serious shortening that the valve leaflets merge with the papillary muscles. Calcifications are much more common and severe in males, elderly patients, and subjects with a higher transvalvular gradient [7]. Calcifications of the mitral annulus may lead to valve sclerosis and stenosis. The anterior mitral leaflet can thicken and become stiff, but the obstruction of ventricular filling is also the result of calcification of the posterior leaflet.

In patients affected by mitral stenosis, the diastolic pressure gradient between the left atrium (LA) and left ventricle (LV) typically rises as mitral stenosis worsens [9–12]. In patients with mitral stenosis alone, the size of the LV is either normal or reduced, the end-diastolic pressure is typically reduced [9, 13, 14], and hence the maximum filling flow is reduced as well. Cardiac output is reduced due to the narrowing of the flow into the LV, while the mass of the LV is normal in most patients [13].

Since the mitral transvalvular flow depends on the cardiac output and heart rate, if the latter is high, there is a reduction in ventricular filling time during diastole, leading to an increase in the transvalvular gradient and consequently in LA pressure [11, 15]. Hence it is important to monitor heart rhythm in mitral stenosis patients. Patients with a normal sinus rhythm have, on average, lower atrial pressures than patients with atrial fibrillation [16, 17]. Sinus rhythm increases the flow through the stenotic valve and helps maintain an adequate cardiac output. The onset of atrial fibrillation is associated with a 20% reduction in cardiac output and, if there is rapid ventricular response, it leads to a sharp

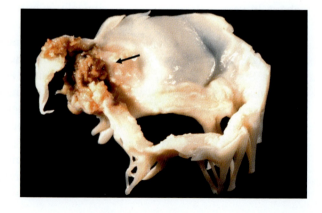

Fig. 2.1 Surgically resected mitral valve. Note leaflets' retraction, *chordae* shortening, and calcific ulceration of the anterolateral commissure (*arrow*)

rise in left atrial pressure and hence dyspnea and pulmonary edema [1, 16, 17].

The chronic rise in LA pressure leads to atrial dilation and fibrillation and, along with this, the formation of atrial thrombi. Atrial muscle fiber disarray, abnormal conduction velocity, and inhomogeneous refractory periods are the causes leading to the onset of atrial fibrillation, which is present in about half of patients affected by mitral stenosis [7, 14, 18].

In patients with mild and moderate mitral stenosis, pulmonary arterial pressure is normal or slightly elevated, with normal pulmonary vascular resistance at rest, only increasing during exercise. In severe mitral stenosis, there is a rise in pulmonary arterial pressure due to elevated left atrial pressure ("passive" postcapillary pulmonary hypertension).

When left atrial pressure exceeds 30 mmHg, plasma oncotic pressure cannot ensure effective elimination of trasudate, and this leads to extravasation of fluids in the interstitial and alveolar spaces (pulmonary edema). However, a long-standing increase in left atrial pressure may cause major changes in pulmonary vascular resistance, which results in pulmonary arterial vasoconstriction and remodeling ("reactive" postcapillary pulmonary hypertension). The increase in right ventricular afterload due to pulmonary hypertension leads to right ventricular failure and peripheral congestion [13]. Therefore, the changes occurring in the pulmonary circulation in the early phases of mitral stenosis are aimed at protecting it against pulmonary edema, but, in the long run, they damage the right ventricle causing congestive heart failure. Finally, if untreated, mitral stenosis leads to irreversible changes in the pulmonary vascular bed.

2.1.2
Diagnosis

2.1.2.1
Non-invasive Diagnosis

The first diagnostic approach to patients with mitral stenosis includes the clinical history, physical examination, electrocardiogram (ECG), chest x-ray and echocardiogram [19, 20].

The symptoms can have varying degrees of severity and may be multiple: dyspnea, palpitation, asthenia, abdominal tension, chest pain, and hemoptysis. These are matched by other important circulatory consequences like the redistribution of pulmonary blood flow (increase in flow in the upper lobes compared to the lower ones) and systemic blood flow (reduction in renal flow) [21]. Patients in an advanced phase of disease, often with concurrent pulmonary hypertension and right ventricular overload, typically have cyanosis of the lips, nose, and cheekbones (malar flush, mitral facies) and cold and cyanotic hands. In severe forms, the arterial pulse is small.

The most important auscultation findings for diagnosis are accentuated first heart sound (S_1), opening snap (OS), low-pitched mid-diastolic rumble, and a presystolic murmur. These signs are perceived in the mitral auscultation area and, better still, if the patient is resting on his left side. These findings, however, may also be present in patients with non-rheumatic mitral valve obstruction (e.g. left atrial myxoma), and may be absent in the presence of severe pulmonary hypertension, low cardiac output, and a heavily calcified immobile mitral valve. A shorter second heart sound (S_2)–OS interval and longer duration of diastolic rumble indicates more severe mitral stenosis. An S_2–OS interval of less than 0.08 s implies severe mitral stenosis [21].

The ECG is usually completely normal in mild forms. In more severe mitral stenosis, signs of left atrial overload ("mitralic P") (Fig. 2.2) and of hypertrophy and right ventricular overload can be seen when mitral stenosis is associated with pulmonary hypertension. Evidence of atrial fibrillation is also frequent.

In the anteroposterior and laterolateral views, the chest x-ray can be entirely normal, or at times show aspecific and indirect signs both in the cardiac silhouette and in the pulmonary fields. In the anteroposterior view, the heart may have a roughly triangular shape resulting from an increase in the volume of the atrium and left atrial appendage (LAA), the pulmonary artery, and the right ventricle and atrium. The radiological picture of the lungs varies with the progression of the mitral disease and hemodynamic impairment (Fig. 2.3).

The gold standard for diagnosis of mitral stenosis is two-dimensional (2D) echocardiography with Doppler [19–22]. In mitral stenosis, echocardiography must define:
- the morphology of the valve leaflets and subvalvular apparatus
- the severity of the stenosis
- the dimensions of the LA
- the presence of thrombi in the LA and/or LAA
- pulmonary artery pressure
- associated valve defects
- left and right ventricular function
- the therapeutic indication.

The morphological alterations of the leaflets and subvalvular apparatus can be assessed by 2D echocardiography in the parasternal and apical regions. The echocardiography elements characterizing mitral stenosis are thickening, reduced leaflet mobility, and calcification. Narrowing of the diastolic leaflet opening due to "doming" (Fig. 2.4) of the anterior leaflet and reduced or no mobility of the posterior leaflet [22] can be visualized on the parasternal long-axis view, while reduced valve opening with the resulting reduction in the relative valve area can be seen on the parasternal short-axis view (Fig. 2.5). In M-mode, reduced valve opening is indicated by a reduced "E-F slope" of the

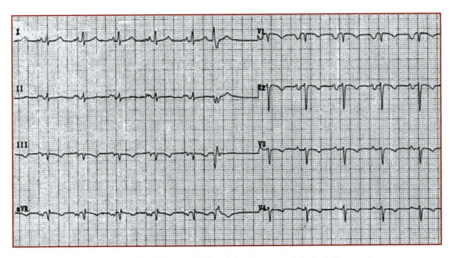

Fig. 2.2 ECG showing the typical signs of left atrial enlargement (mitral P waves)

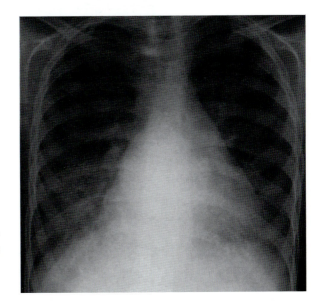

Fig. 2.3 Chest x-ray in anteroposterior view. Modification of cardiac silhouette, increased in volume and with a coarsely triangular shape, with signs of pulmonary venous congestion in both lower lobes

anterior mitral value leaflet and by movement of the posterior leaflet in accordance with the anterior leaflet. The sensitivity and specificity of 2D echocardiography in assessing mitral valve anatomy are 70% and 100% respectively, if compared to anatomical and pathological findings. The sensitivity rises to 90% if the examination is integrated with transesophageal echocardiogram or real-time 3D ultrasound [23, 24].

The description of the morphological alterations in the valvular apparatus in

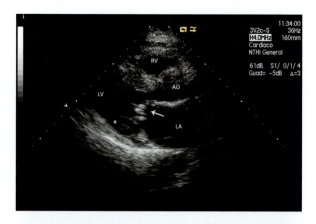

Fig. 2.4 Transthoracic echocardiogram, parasternal long-axis view; stenotic mitral valve with reduced diastolic excursion and typical diastolic doming shape (*arrow*) and clear fusion of the subvalvular apparatus (*). *AO*, aorta; *LA*, left atrium; *LV*, left ventricle; *RV*, right ventricle

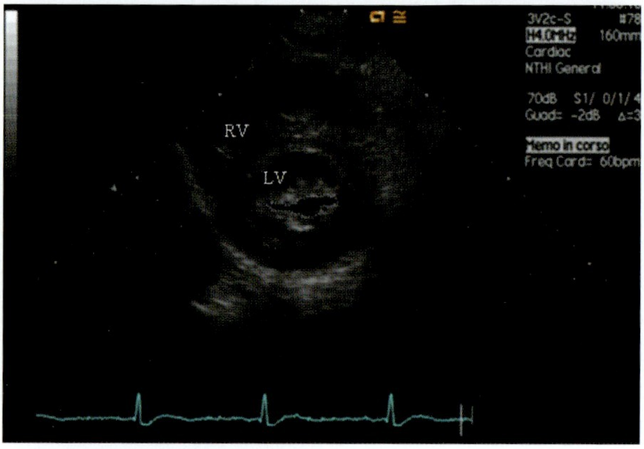

Fig. 2.5 Transthoracic echocardiogram, parasternal short-axis view; stenotic mitral valve orifice (*dotted line*) with typical "fish-mouth" shape. The area was measured manually. *LV*, left ventricle; *RV*, right ventricle

mitral stenosis is codified in the Wilkins score [25]. It takes into account four parameters (leaflet mobility, leaflet thickening, remodeling of the subvalvular apparatus, calcifications), and each is given a score of 1 to 4 (Table 2.1). The single values are summed together to get a score reflecting the severity of valve damage. These characteristics are important for the timing and type of intervention to be performed [25–27]. While not being the only one, the Wilkins score is the one most frequently used to assess the degree of damage to the valve apparatus. Other scores used are Cormier's score [28] (Table 2.2) and Reid's score [29] (Table 2.3).

The severity of mitral stenosis is defined based on the value of the mean transvalvular gradient and mitral valve area (MVA).

The mean transvalvular gradient can be measured accurately and with a high degree of reproducibility by continuous wave (CW) Doppler through the mitral valve using the simplified Bernoulli equation, $\Delta P = 4v^2$ [23, 30, 31], where ΔP is the mean transvalvular gradient and v is the mitral inflow velocity. If pulsed wave (PW) Doppler is used, the sample volume should be applied at or right

Table 2.1 The Wilkins score

Degree	Mobility	Subvalvular thickening	Leaflet thickening	Calcifications
1	Extremely mobile valves with reduction in excursions only at the tips of the leaflets	Minimal thickening below the mitral leaflets	Leaflets with almost normal thickness (4–5 mm)	Single hyperechogenic zone
2	Middle and basal portions of the leaflets have normal structure and mobility	Thickening of the *chordae* stretching up to one-third of their length	Normal leaflets in central portions, considerable thickening of margins (5–8 mm)	Hyperechogenic multiple areas limited to leaflet margins
3	Valve continues to move forward during diastole, mainly at its base	Thickening extending up to the distal third of the *chordae*	Thickening extending through the entire leaflet (5–8 mm)	Hyperechogenicity extending in the medial portion of the leaflets
4	No or minimal forward motion of the leaflets during diastole	Massive thickening and shortening of the *chordae* extending below the papillary muscles	Major thickening of the entire tissue of the leaflets (>8–10 mm)	Intense hyperechogenicity covering most of the leaflet tissue

Table 2.2 Cormier's anatomical score

Echocardiography group	Anatomy of the mitral valve
1	Non-calcified mobile anterior leaflet Mild subvalvular disease (thin *chordae* ≥10 mm long)
2	Non-calcified mobile anterior leaflet Severe subvalvular disease (thickened *chordae* <10 mm long)
3	Calcification of mitral valve of any extent, as assessed by fluoroscopy, whatever the state of the subvalvular apparatus

after the tip of the leaflets [23]. The mean gradient has a greater correlation with the hemodynamic findings, while the maximum gradient, being derived from the peak mitral inflow velocity, is affected by LA compliance and left ventricular diastolic function [13], and plays a minor role in determining the severity of mitral stenosis. Based on the mean values of the gradient, mitral stenosis is mild when the gradient is <5 mmHg, moderate when it ranges between 5 and 10 mmHg, and severe when it is >10 mmHg [23] (Fig. 2.6; Table 2.4). The limitations imposed by the transmitral gradient in determining the severity of stenosis lie in the fact that it depends on MVA and is affected by heart rate and by concurrent mitral regurgitation, if present [27].

Table 2.3 Reid's score

	Degree	Score
Leaflet motion: H/L ratio[a]		
≥ 0.45	Mild	0
0.26–0.44	Moderate	1
≤ 0.25	Severe	2
Leaflet thickening: mitral valve/aortic wall		
1.5–2	Mild	0
2.1–4.9	Moderate	1
≥5	Severe	2
Subvalvular disease		
Thin, faintly visible *chordae tendineae*	–	0
Areas of increased density equal to endocardium	–	1
Areas denser than the endocardium with thickened *chordae tendineae*	–	2
Commissural calcium		
Homogeneous density of mitral valve orifice	–	0
Increased density of anterior/posterior commissure	–	1
Increased density of both commissures	–	2

[a]H (height)/L (length) = anterior leaflet excursion

Table 2.4 Criteria for the assessment of mitral stenosis severity

Severity of mitral stenosis	Mean gradient (mmHg)	Mitral valve area (cm^2)	Systolic pulmonary artery pressure (mmHg)
Mild	<5	>1.5	<30
Moderate	5–10	1.5–1.0	30–50
Severe	>10	<1.0	>50

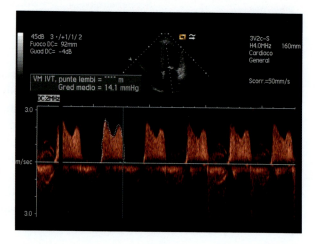

Fig. 2.6 Transmitral diastolic flow. Continuous wave Doppler gives a mean transvalvular gradient of 14.1 mmHg

2.1 Mitral Stenosis

MVA can be calculated with various methods, each of which offers advantages and disadvantages. Two-dimensional planimetry of the mitral orifice offers the benefit of being a direct measurement of MVA and, unlike other methods, it is not affected by conditions related to the flow, compliance of the heart chambers, or presence of other associated valve diseases. Two-dimensional planimetric study of MVA has shown to be better correlated with the anatomical valve area calculated on explanted valves [32]. The planimetric measurements are obtained directly on the mitral orifice in mid-diastole, including the open commissures, in the parasternal short-axis view (Fig. 2.5). However, this method is negatively affected by the quality of the image and it cannot be performed accurately in patients with a scarce acoustic window or in the presence of a severely distorted valve anatomy, often due to the presence of calcifications [23]. Recent studies suggest that 3D real-time echocardiography and 2D-guided biplane imaging are useful in optimizing measurements improving reproducibility [24]. Based on MVA values, mitral stenosis is defined as mild when the area is >1.5 cm^2, moderate when the area ranges between 1.5 and 1 cm^2, and severe when it is <1 cm^2 [23] (Table 2.4).

Another way to determine valve area is the diastolic pressure half-time (PHT) method, which is based on the hemodynamic principle that the reduction in the gradient between the atrium and ventricle is inversely proportional to the extent of valve stenosis and hence to valve area (Fig. 2.7). MVA is obtained from the following empirical formula [23, 33]:

$$MVA = 220/PHT$$

PHT is easy to obtain, but it is affected by other factors such as the presence of aortic regurgitation, LA compliance, left ventricular diastolic function [34], or prior mitral valvotomy [35].

MVA can still be calculated with the continuity equation [23, 36] based on the principle of mass conservation by which the transmitral flow volume should

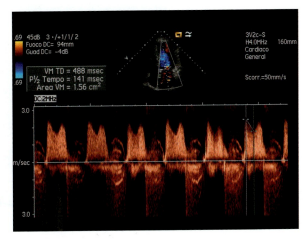

Fig. 2.7 Transmitral diastolic flow. Mitral valve area (*Area VM*) measured using the PHT method

be equal to the systolic output, i.e. the flow through the aorta. By measuring aortic area, the aortic flow velocity integral, and the integral of the velocity through the mitral valve, the mitral area can be caluclated. The continuity equation cannot be used in the case of atrial fibrillation or major mitral or aortic valve regurgitation [23].

Another method for calculating MVA is the proximal isovelocity surface area (PISA). The velocities of a flow approaching a stenotic or diseased orifice gradually rise and spread in a concentric fashion with an almost hemispherical shape, as shown by color-Doppler on the atrial side of the mitral valve. According to this method, MVA is obtained from the following formula:

$$MVA = \pi(r^2) \, (V_{aliasing}) \text{ peak } V_{mitral} * \alpha/180°$$

where r is the hemispherical convergence radius (cm), $V_{aliasing}$ is the aliasing velocity (cm/s), peak V_{mitral} is the peak CW Doppler of mitral flow velocity (cm/s), and α is the opening angle of the mitral leaflets compared to the flow direction [37]. This method can also be used in the presence of major mitral regurgitation.

Doppler echocardiography is needed to assess mitral stenosis patients to determine systolic pulmonary artery pressure (sPAP) from the maximum tricuspid regurgitation velocity [23, 38] (Fig. 2.8). The increase in sPAP is an indicator of hemodynamic impairment. Mitral stenosis classification based on the estimated sPAP values defines mitral stenosis as mild when sPAP is <30 mmHg, moderate when sPAP is between 30 and 50 mmHg, and severe when sPAP is >50 mmHg [23] (Table 2.4).

Ultimately, the severity of mitral stenosis should be determined by echocardiogram, quantifying both the mean gradient and MVA, and pulmonary artery pressure should be estimated when possible to complete the diagnostic picture and determine the timing and choice of the type of treatment.

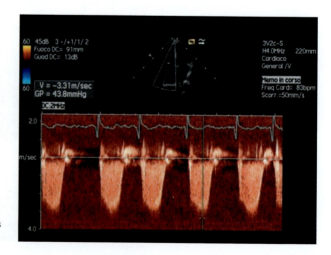

Fig. 2.8 Measurement of systolic pulmonary artery pressure using continuous wave Doppler

Transesophageal echocardiogram (TEE) is not a routine examination unless the quality of the transthoracic echocardiogram (TTE) is not satisfactory [19]. TEE is also recommended before mitral valvuloplasty for [19, 20]:
- detailed assessment of morphological alterations in the valvular and subvalvular apparatus
- search for thrombi, particularly in the interatrial septum (trans-septal puncture site) or on the LA roof, as they are an absolute contraindication to percutaneous mitral commissurotomy (PMC), while the presence of thrombi in the left atrial appendage is considered by some authors as a relative contraindication (Figs. 2.9 and 2.10)
- morphological characterization of the left atrial appendage, which typically has a "bull's horn" shape, although it can be bilobate or trilobate with lobes located on different planes. Therefore, the search for thrombi must be performed with multiplane probes
- assessment of the Doppler velocities in the left atrial appendage; if values are <40 cm/s, there is a correlation with an increased risk of thromboembolism
- identification of spontaneous echo contrast, a predictor of an increased risk of thromboembolism (Fig. 2.11)
- more accurate assessment of the severity of the associated MR.

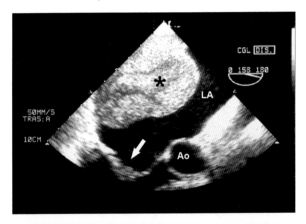

Fig. 2.9 Transesophageal echocardiogram, showing a thrombotic formation in the left atrium (*LA*). *, the thrombus; *arrow*, mitral leaflet; *Ao*, aorta

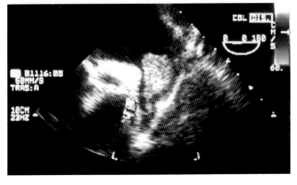

Fig. 2.10 Transesophageal echocardiogram, thrombotic formation in the left atrial appendage

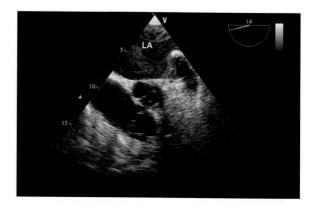

Fig. 2.11 Intense smoke-like effect in the left atrium (*LA*)

2.1.2.2
Invasive Diagnosis

Left and right cardiac catheterization plays a major role in determining the severity of mitral stenosis and assessing a patient's degree of hemodynamic impairment. Unlike echocardiography, catheterization gives direct measurements of pressure in the atrium and LV, which are necessary to obtain the transmitral gradient [39], pulmonary artery pressure, and an estimate of pulmonary vascular resistance values, which give an idea of the impact of mitral stenosis on pulmonary circulation. The Gorlin equation, by which the severity of an obstruction depends on the flow and gradient, allows calculation of the valve area (A) [40]:

$$A = F/k*(\Delta P)^{(1/2)}$$

where F is flow during the valve opening period, k a constant = 38 for the mitral valve, and ΔP is the transmitral gradient.

The cardiac catheterization protocol in patients with mitral stenosis includes the following measurements and calculations:
- simultaneous left ventricular diastolic pressure, left atrial (or pulmonary capillary wedge) diastolic pressure, heart rate, diastolic filling period, and cardiac output (Fig. 2.12)
- if the transmitral pressure gradient is <5 mmHg, it can present a significant error in calculation of the mitral valve orifice. The circulatory measurements should be repeated under circumstances of stress (exercise, reversible increase in preload resulting from passive elevation of the patient's legs, tachycardia induced by pacing) to increase the pressure gradient across the mitral valve
- simultaneously, or in close sequence, pulmonary arterial mean pressure, left atrial (or pulmonary capillary wedge) mean pressure, and cardiac output for the calculation of pulmonary vascular resistance

2.1 Mitral Stenosis

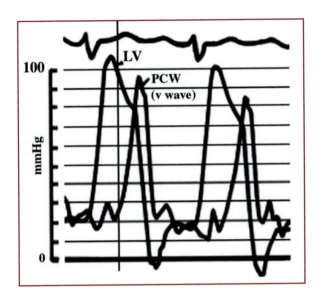

Fig. 2.12 Simultaneous left ventricular (*LV*) pressure and pulmonary capillary wedge (*PCW*) pressure traces in mitral stenosis

- right ventricular systolic and diastolic pressures for assessment of right ventricular function
- if other lesions are suspected (e.g. MR, aortic valve disease, tricuspid stenosis, left atrial myxoma, atrial septal defect), they too must be evaluated. In this regard, it should be pointed out that certain lesions tend to occur in combination with mitral stenosis.

According to the current guidelines [19], cardiac catheterization is indicated when non-invasive tests are insufficient or when there is a discrepancy between the hemodynamic data obtained from Doppler echocardiogram and the clinical conditions of a symptomatic patient. It is also indicated to determine the causes of severe pulmonary hypertension observed in the echocardiogram when there is a discrepancy with other severity criteria (mean gradient and MVA) and to define the hemodynamic response to exercise when the symptoms and hemodynamics at rest contrast. If there are any doubts about the the accuracy of the pulmonary capillary wedge pressure (PCWP), trans-septal catheterization can be performed to directly measure left atrial pressure [19].

Invasive tests for the hemodynamic assessment of mitral stenosis patients also include ventriculography to determine the size of mitral regurgitation (MR) when there is a difference between the mean gradient obtained with Doppler and the valve area, and aortic root angiography to determine the severity of the associated aortic failure, if any. Moreover, a selective coronary angiography is required to assess the site, severity, and extension of a concurrent coronary artery disease. It should be performed in patients with angina, reduced systolic function of the LV, a history of coronary artery disease, and the presence of risk factors, including age [19].

2.1.3
Timing of Interventions

The drop in the incidence of rheumatic disease has greatly changed the time of the appearance of the onset symptoms of mitral stenosis in the general population, and the pathology's natural history. The latency between the episode of acute rheumatic fever and the appearance of symptoms varies greatly and is correlated with the presence of recurrent episodes of streptococcal infection. Transition from the asymptomatic to the symptomatic stage depends on the progression of the mitral stenosis. The onset of dyspnea on effort is generally associated with a one-third reduction in valve area compared to the normal value [41]. Further reductions in area are associated with major hemodynamic impairment, and hence a progressive worsening of dyspnea symptoms, which become apparent with minimal effort or even at rest.

Several studies were carried out in the 1950s and 1960s on the natural history of untreated mitral stenosis patients [1, 42, 43]. These showed that mitral stenosis is a disease with a slow and progressive course, with a first phase, possibly lasting for several years, during which the patient is clinically stable and has no or very few symptoms. This phase is followed by a rapid decline with debilitating symptoms [1, 42–44]. In industrialized countries, a long latency of 20 to 40 years ranging from the first episode of rheumatic fever to the outbreak of symptoms has been observed. It is followed by another long period of about 10 years from the outbreak of the first mild symptoms to the worsening of dyspnea and the functional class [1]. Overall, the 10-year survival of untreated patients presenting with mitral stenosis is 50% to 60%, depending on the symptoms at presentation [1, 42]. In the asymptomatic or minimally symptomatic patient, survival is greater than 80% at 10 years, with 60% of patients having no progression of symptoms [42–44]. Patients with an advanced New York Heart Association (NYHA) class have a survival at 10 years ranging from 0% to 15% [1, 42–45]. The onset of severe pulmonary hypertension reduces the survival of untreated mitral stenosis patients by 3 years on average [46].

Considering the poor prognosis of symptomatic mitral stenosis patients, a therapeutic strategy for these patients should be considered as soon as the symptoms appear. Therefore, the choice of the type of treatment and the timing of intervention basically depend on two factors: the patient's clinical characteristics and the anatomical and functional appearance of the valve affected by the pathology [19, 20, 47, 48].

The management strategy for mitral stenosis patients varies depending on whether or not they are symptomatic. Once the diagnosis of mitral stenosis has been confirmed by echocardiography, and the degree of stenosis and the morphology of the diseased valve have been determined, asymptomatic patients with mild mitral stenosis do not need further diagnostic examinations except for clinical and instrumental checks on an annual basis (physical exam, chest x-ray,

ECG). Evidence shows that valve disease remains stable for years in these patients [1, 42, 43]. In the case of asymptomatic patients with moderate or severe mitral stenosis, percutaneous mitral valvulotomy (PMV) should be considered. In patients with pliable, non-calcified valves with no or little subvalvular fusion, no calcification in the commissures, and no left atrial thrombus, PMV can be performed with a low complication rate [19, 20, 47]. High pulmonary artery pressures and pulmonary vascular resistance play a major role in the timing of intervention in asymptomatic patients with moderate/severe mitral stenosis, as these parameters are significantly correlated with greater hemodynamic impairment. In a patient with moderate pulmonary hypertension (systolic pulmonary artery pressure greater than 50 mmHg) and a valve anatomy favorable to PMV, percutaneous treatment is recommended by current guidelines, even without symptoms [19, 20, 47]. In asymptomatic patients leading a sedentary lifestyle, a hemodynamic exercise test with Doppler echocardiography is useful [47, 48–51]. Objective limitation of exercise tolerance with a rise in transmitral gradient greater than 15 mmHg and a rise in pulmonary artery systolic pressure greater than 60 mmHg may be an indication for percutaneous valvotomy if the mitral valve morphology is suitable [47]. In asymptomatic patients, intervention is also indicated in cases of increased risk of thromboembolism (prior history of embolism, recent episode of paroxysmal atrial fibrillation, left atrial spontaneous echo contrast) [47]. With regard to the subgroup of asymptomatic patients with severe mitral stenosis and severe pulmonary hypertension (pulmonary artery systolic pressure greater than 75% of systemic pressure either at rest or with exercise), if these patients do not have a valve morphology favorable for PMV or surgical valve repair, it is controversial whether mitral valve replacement should be performed in the absence of symptoms to prevent right ventricular failure, but surgery is generally recommended in such patients [47].

Symptomatic NYHA class II patients with moderate or severe mitral stenosis must be directly referred to PMV, if valve morphology allows for it and if there are no thrombi in the LA. NYHA class III or IV patients should be considered for intervention with either PMV or surgery [47].

Patients with significantly limiting symptoms but not severe mitral stenosis should undergo exercise testing or dobutamine stress to distinguish between the symptoms due to valve disease and those due to other causes. Patients who are symptomatic with a pulmonary artery pressure >60 mmHg, mean transmitral gradient >15 mmHg, or pulmonary artery wedge pressure >25 mmHg during exercise have hemodynamically significant mitral stenosis and should be considered for further intervention. On the other hand, patients who do not manifest elevation in either pulmonary artery, pulmonary capillary wedge, or transmitral pressures coincident with development of exertional symptoms would probably not benefit from intervention on the mitral valve [47].

Therefore, it can be concluded that according to current guidelines, in centers

Table 2.5 Classes of indications for percutaneous mitral commissurotomy in patients with mitral stenosis and mitral valve area <1.5 cm^2, according to the 2007 European Guidelines on the Treatment of Valve Diseases

	Class
Symptomatic patients with favourable characteristics for percutaneous mitral valvulotomy (PMV)[a]	IB
Symptomatic patients with contraindication or high risk for surgery	IC
As initial treatment in symptomatic patients with unfavorable anatomy but otherwise favorable clinical characteristics[a]	IIaC
Asymptomatic patients with favourable characteristics[a] and high thromboembolic risk or high risk of hemodynamic decompensation:	
Previous history of embolism	IIaC
Dense spontaneous contrast in the left atrium	IIaC
Recent or paroxysmal atrial fibrillation	IIaC
Systolic pulmonary pressure >50 mmHg at rest	IIaC
Need for major non-cardiac surgery	IIaC
Desire of pregnancy	IIaC

[a]Favorable characteristics for PMV can be defined by the absence of several of the following: *clinical characteristics* – old age, history of commissurotomy, NYHA class IV, atrial fibrillation, severe pulmonary hypertension; *anatomic characteristics*: Wilkins score >8, Cormier score 3, very small mitral valve area, severe tricuspid regurgitation

with expert operators, PMV (Table 2.5) is the procedure of choice for symptomatic patients with moderate-to-severe mitral stenosis with a favorable valve anatomy and without significant MR or thrombi in the LA. There is also controversy related to the role played by PMV in patients with debilitating symptoms and a less favorable valve morphology. In this patient subgroup, the rationale for PMV is possibly linked to the clinical and hemodynamic stabilization offered by the percutaneous approach before the patient undergoes surgery [52]. In patients with severe calcifications and a completely altered valve morphology, surgical mitral valve replacement is to be preferred [47]. As regards asymptomatic or NHYA class II patients, given the lesser degree of invasiveness, and lower morbidity and mortality of PMV compared to surgery, percutaneous therapy should be considered [47].

2.1.4
Patient Selection

The determining factors for the short and long-term results of PMV are proper patient selection and the possibility of performing PMV in a center with good experience and procedure skills.

As already mentioned, PMV is currently the procedure of choice for symptomatic patients with moderate-to-severe mitral stenosis with a favorable valve anatomy and without significant MR or thrombi in the LA. In asymptomatic patients with a favorable valve morphology, PMV is to be considered only in the presence of proven hemodynamic impairment [19, 20, 47].

This does not exclude the possibility of performing PMV on patients with low cardiac output or who have undergone prior cardiac surgery, including surgical mitral commissurotomy, who have subsequently developed restenosis due to commissural refusion [53]. In rare cases, PMV can also be performed on stenotic biological prostheses [54–58]. PMV is also an important therapeutic strategy in pregnant women, as the procedure has few complications and low fetal mortality thanks to lead shielding of the abdomen [19, 20, 47, 59, 60]. Pregnant women with severe cardiac failure due to mitral stenosis have a high morbidity rate and there is an unfavorable effect on the fetus [61]. Compared to surgical open commissurotomy, PMV has shown fewer fetal complications, with a lower neonatal and fetal mortality rate and excellent long-term results [60, 62]. The procedure can also be performed as a bridge to surgery in patients in extremely poor clinical conditions, with an unfavorable valve anatomy, to allow for clinical and hemodynamic stabilization and better functional recovery in the run-up to intervention [52].

When screening mitral stenosis patients to undergo PMV, special attention must be paid to possible contraindications (Box 2.1) [20, 63]. Absolute contraindications to PMV include floating thrombus in the LA or interatrial septum, while a left atrial appendage thrombus is not an absolute contraindication. In these cases, PMV can be preceded by adequate anticoagulation therapy and monitoring by TEE [64, 65]. Atriomegaly and atrial fibrillation are not a contraindication to PMV.

Another critical factor in patient selection is echocardiographic assessment aimed, in particular, at studying the anatomy and functions of the mitral apparatus and quantifying alterations using the Wilkins score, as described earlier (Table 2.1). Values ≤8 indicate a favorable anatomy and are generally associated with excellent post-PMV final results. However, patients with a Wilkins score >8, and hence an unfavorable anatomy, in whom results will be partial and temporary, cannot a priori be excluded as candidates for percutaneous treatment. In these cases, comorbidities and the presence of any other valve diseases or multiple significant coronary stenoses should be assessed in order to choose between surgical treatment or palliative PMV [66].

Other score-based models have been proposed, among which are the Reid's score [67] (Table 2.3) and Fatkin's score [66], by which post-PMV commissural splitting, examined by echocardiography in parasternal short-axis view, is the major determinant of procedural success.

> **Box 2.1 Contraindications (absolute/relative) to percutaneous mitral valvuloplasty**
>
> **Related to valve**
> - Mitral valve area ≥1.5 cm^2
> - Left atrial thrombus
> - Mitral regurgitation ≥2+
> - Severe or bicommissural calcification
> - Absence of commissural fusion
> - Mild mitral stenosis
>
> **Related to medical center**
> - Lack of appropriate procedural skill and experience
>
> **Concomitant valvulopathy and need for open heart surgery**
> - Severe concomitant aortic valve disease
> - Severe concomitant tricuspid regurgitation or tricuspid stenosis
> - Concomitant coronary artery disease requiring bypass surgery
> - Concomitant aorta disease requiring surgery
>
> **Procedural difficulties related to transseptal puncture**
> - Severe tricuspid regurgitation
> - Huge right atrium
> - Distorted/displaced atrial septum
> - Femoral-iliac veins obstructed or thrombosed
> - Inferior vena cava, obstructed or thrombosed; drainage into azygous vein
> - Severe kyphoscoliosis (thoracic/abdominal)

2.1.5
Percutaneous Therapy

Before the advent of percutaneous therapy, the treatment of mitral stenosis consisted solely in the surgical option, and the range of techniques included open or closed commissurotomy and replacement with biological or mechanical prostheses [68]. Later on, the development of percutaneous devices has allowed PMV to become, since the 1980s, not only a valid alternative to surgery, but also the procedure of choice for all mitral stenosis patients with a favorable valve anatomy [19, 20, 69, 70].

PMV is a low-risk and low-cost replicable procedure, which does not require general anesthesia, is not a contraindication for subsequent surgical valvuloplasty or valve replacement, and does not require permanent anticoagulant therapy, with the exception of few cases, such as atrial fibrillation, major dilation of the LA, and prior episodes of embolism [71].

2.1 Mitral Stenosis

The main objective of PMV is to separate fused commissures, thus reducing the transmitral pressure gradient (ΔP), left atrial pressure (LAP), and systolic pulmonary artery pressure (sPAP), and increasing mitral valve area (MVA) and cardiac output.

In the past, several techniques were used to perform PMV. The major difference between the various techniques described by the various authors lies in the route of access (antegrade or retrograde) and in the number of balloon catheters used (single balloon, double balloon; elastic, stiff, or metal material) (Figs. 2.13 and 2.14) [66, 72–76]. Today PMV is universally performed using the antegrade route via trans-septal catheterization [72, 77] and placement of the balloon catheter through the mitral valve following the blood flow [74]. In some rare cases, Cribier's metallic valvulotome is used [78].

Currently, the technique of choice in most centers performing PMV uses the Inoue catheter (Toray Industries, Japan). It is a special device with a balloon at one end, which is anchored on the valve plane and then inflated. The catheter has a 12 Fr diameter with a length of 70 cm; the length of each balloon is 2.5 cm (unstretched). Two proximally positioned stopcocks accomplish balloon inflation and catheter venting. A stainless steel tube is used to stretch and slenderize the balloon prior to insertion, and a 14 Fr tapered dilator enlarges the interatrial opening. The stainless steel stylet and guidewire are employed to guide the catheter inside the heart and blood vessels. The Inoue balloon is made of nylon and a rubber micromesh and has three different degrees of elasticity, which give sequential expansion, thus allowing optimal and stable placement on the mitral valve [72]. As mentioned earlier, the mechanism by which valve area

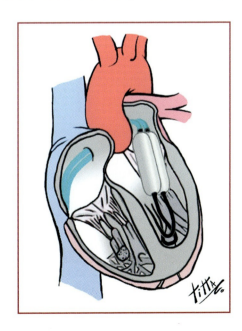

Fig. 2.13 Percutaneous mitral valvulotomy: catheter positions for double-balloon valvuloplasty

is increased consists in "splitting" the fused commissures and mobilizing the valve leaflets. The presence of paracommissural calcifications requires that the technique be performed gradually, namely by means of progressive inflations using balloons with smaller diameters compared to those normally used based on the body surface. The Inoue catheter ensures stability during inflation thanks to its hourglass shape, with the narrower portion placed on the valve and the wider portions located upstream and downstream of it. It also ensures minimal trauma and, above all, it offers various inflation diameters without any need for changing catheter [73, 74, 79]. The reference diameters for the Inoue balloon are normally chosen based on the patient's weight and height, surface area, degree of valve apparatus damage, and mitral valve area, as measured by cardiac catheterization and/or with non-invasive methods, and vary between 22 and 30 mm (Table 2.6). Patient age and sex may also be factors affecting the choice of the balloon.

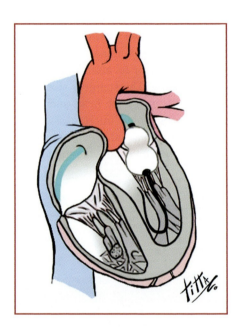

Fig. 2.14 Mitral balloon valvuloplasty: single-balloon technique

Table 2.6 Reference diameters for Inoue balloon

Catalogue number	Balloon dilation available range (mm)	Diameter maximum (mm)	Patient weight (kg)	Patient height (cm)	Surface area (m^2)
PTMC-30	26–30	30	≥70	≥180	≥1.9
PTMC-28	24–28	28	45–70	160–180	1.6–1.9
PTMC-26	22–26	26	≤45	≤160	≤1.6

2.1.5.1
Procedure and Technical Aspects

The procedure is performed using the antegrade approach and requires access through the femoral vein and trans-septal puncture with a Brockenbrough needle. A Mullins dilator is then placed and a catheter is inserted through it into the LA. A small quantity of contrast medium is injected to confirm that the catheter is in the right position. The operator then measures the pressure in the LA and LV to confirm the hemodynamic gradient generated by the stenosis. A 0.6 mm guidewire is then inserted up to the LA, and the Mullins dilator is removed (Fig. 2.15). The next step consists in dilating the orifice in the femoral vein and the inter-atrial septum using a special 14 Fr dilator; the dilator is then run through the guidewire previously placed. At this point, the Inoue balloon is prepared, tested, and inserted through the guidewire up to the LA. After advancing the Inoue balloon inside the LV and making sure that it does not interfere with the *chordae tendineae*, the distal end of the balloon is inflated (Fig. 2.16). The catheter is pulled back to position the device on the stenotic valve, and the balloon is sequentially expanded from the distal to the proximal portion (Fig. 2.17). Each time it is expanded, the transmitral gradient and any damage generated is assessed. Dilations will be continued until the desired result is achieved (Fig. 2.18).

If an acceptable transvalvular gradient is not reached, dilation can be continued using Inoue devices that are 1 or 2 mm larger [80].

The technique also envisages right and left catheterization with cine-angiography both before and after the procedure, ventriculography in a 30° right anterior oblique projection, and, in the case of MR, also in laterolateral projection. Cardiac output and MVA are also measured using the Gorlin formula. If effective, there is an increase in MVA by at least 25%, and a sudden drop in

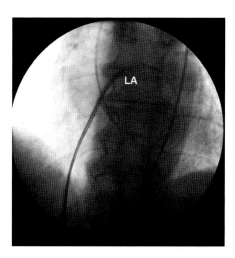

Fig. 2.15 Trans-septal placement of 14 Fr dilator on guidewire positioned in the left atrium (*LA*)

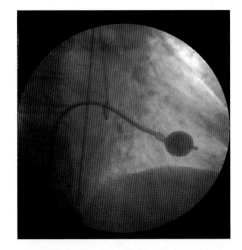

Fig. 2.16 Distal end of the balloon inflated in the LV. The partially inflated balloon is pulled back toward the left atrium and anchored to the stenotic valve orifice

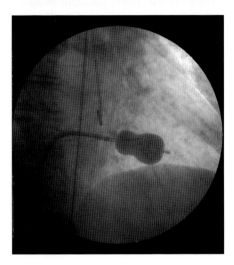

Fig. 2.17 Inflation of the proximal portion of the balloon, which takes the shape of a "dog-bone"; the incision corresponds to the mitral valve plane

LAP, sPAP, and ΔP. There can also be an increase in left ventricular telediastolic pressure due to the greater transmitral diastolic flow and an increase in cardiac output. Pulmonary resistance values may behave inconsistently. The rise in resistance is, above all, the result of the increased difference between the mean pulmonary artery pressure and left atrial pressure following the sudden drop in the latter, which is greater than the concurrent drop in sPAP. In the case of pulmonary hypertension, the return to normal pulmonary vessel pressures and resistance values can be either immediate or slow and gradual.

PMV performed in patients with a Wilkins score ≤8 has a success rate of 85–90% [25]. In patients with a score of 9–12, the procedure is successful in 80–85% of cases [25, 71]. An optimal result is an area of ≥1.5 cm^2, an increase

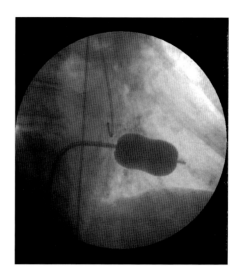

Fig. 2.18 Completion of balloon inflation with opening of the commissures

by at least 25% compared to the initial area in the absence of MR ≥2/4+; a suboptimal result is an MVA increase of less than 25% or a final area of <1.5 cm^2; the procedure fails when there is no increase in MVA or the onset of MR ≥3/4+. Mortality is very low (<1%) [71].

Echocardiographic guidance in the catheterization lab is useful for transseptal puncture, placement of the balloon at the commissures, assessment of the immediate result, and early detection of any complication. Echocardiographic guidance is usually performed by TTE, while TEE is seldom used during PMV, as it may not be easily tolerated by the conscious patient lying on the catheterization laboratory table for the entire duration of the procedure. TEE is especially useful in pregnant women, as it reduces exposure to x-rays. Echocardiography allows for real-time measurement of MVA, ΔP, commissure opening, leaflet mobility, leaflet tears and the degree of residual MR. Area calculation by PHT is not reliable in the catheterization laboratory, as this method cannot be applied due to sudden changes in compliance such as those occurring during valve dilation.

2.1.5.2
Mitral Valvuloplasty Outcomes

Many studies have shown the short- and long-term efficacy of PMV [26, 28, 81–84] (Table 2.7). These studies show quite satisfactory results for this technique. A study by Iung et al [26] on 528 patients who successfully underwent percutaneous mitral commissurotomy (dilation was performed using a single balloon in 13 patients, a double balloon in 349, and the Inoue balloon in 166)

Table 2.7 Long-term follow-up in patients that underwent balloon mitral valvuloplasty

Author [reference]	Patients	Mean age (years)	Follow-up (months)	Survival (%)	Freedom from surgery (%)
Palacios et al [82]	327	54	48	90	79
Cohen [63]	146	59	60	76	51
Pan et al [83]	350	46	60	94	91
Iung et al [26, 28]	606	46	60	94	74
NHLBI [81]	736	54	48	84	66

reports a survival rate for patients in NYHA functional class I or II, with no cardiac-related deaths or need for mitral surgery or repeat dilation in 76 ± 6% at 5 years. By multivariate analysis, the independent predictors of good functional results were echocardiography group, functional class, and cardiothoracic index before the procedure, and valve area after the procedure.

The National Heart, Lung, and Blood Institute (NHLBI) Balloon Valvuloplasty Registry reported multicenter results in 736 patients older than 18 years of age who were monitored for 4 years [81]. The actuarial survival rates at 1, 2, 3, and 4 years were 93%, 90%, 87%, and 84%, respectively. The rates of event-free survival (freedom from death, mitral valve surgery, or repeat balloon valvuloplasty) at 1, 2, 3, and 4 years were 80%, 71%, 66%, and 62%, respectively. Multivariate predictions of mortality were NYHA functional class IV, Wilkins score >12, post-procedure sPAP >40 mmHg, and left ventricular end-diastolic pressure >15 mmHg.

Restenosis is defined as a loss of 50% of the result obtained and a reduction of MVA to <1.5 cm^2. Post-PMV mitral restenosis has been seen in younger populations in 2–10% of cases with a 37-month follow-up, and among older patients in about 22% of cases with a follow-up of 13 months [84, 85]. The main index associated with restenosis, as reported by Thomas et al [86], is a high Wilkins score; differents results are probably obtained using the same technique: commissural splitting is most common in patients with low Wilkins score and carries a low risk of restenosis, whereas valve stretching is frequent in those patients with high Wilkins score and high restenosis rate. However, re-PMV can be performed in the case of restenosis. Encouraging results have been obtained by Iung et al [87] in 53 cases of restenosis, with a doubling of the mitral area and a 5-year survival of 69% in NYHA class I or II.

2.1.5.3
Complications

The most frequent complication in PMV is an increase and/or new-onset of significant MR (2–3%) [28, 75, 80]. MR is the result of tearing of the valve leaflets or placement of the balloon at too short a distance between the fused *chordae tendineae*, thus tearing them. By contrast, mild and transient MR or a slight worsening of it is due to the temporary dysfunction of the mitral subvalvular apparatus immediately after balloon inflations. It is normally solved within the next 24 hours. However, the new onset of mild MR or worsening in the degree of pre-existing MR is usually well tolerated in patients with enlarged atrial chambers and pulmonary vessels that are used to high venous pressures. Another complication is the onset of a major atrial septal defect (ASD) with a left–right shunt volume of >1.5 (<5% of cases if PMV is performed using the Inoue technique). The frequency of iatrogenic ASD caused by trans-septal puncture and catheter placement varies between 30% and 53%. However, in most cases, the ratio between pulmonary output and systemic output is <1.5 and thus negligible; in any event, ASD tends to close spontaneously over time. Its persistence is usually linked to a sharp drop in LAP, which is almost always a sign of inadequate valve dilation. Other complications are rather rare and almost always reported during the early phases of application of the procedure; these include peripheral embolism (0.3–1%), left ventricular perforation followed by cardiac tamponade (2–5%), interventricular septum perforation, or severe MR requiring emergency surgery (2–6%) [28, 71, 88]. A study of several case histories has nonetheless shown that the procedure-related complications are directly related to operator experience; it has been noted that at the centers with the highest number of procedures, complications are much fewer than those at centers with a low number of procedures [80].

2.2
Mitral Regurgitation

2.2.1
The Pathophysiology of Mitral Regurgitation Physiopathology

The pathophysiology of MR differs depending on whether valve damage is acute or the result of a chronic process. The causes that generally elicit acute MR are myocardial infarction (MI), spontaneous rupture of the *chordae tendineae*, acute endocarditis, or chest trauma [89–92].

In severe acute MR, the LA and ventricle receive a sudden volume overload, which, in turn, leads to a rise in ventricular preload, thus allowing for a moderate increase in systolic output. However, being an acute form, eccentric hypertrophy, a compensatory mechanism maintaing CO constant, cannot take place. The consequences of the failure of the left heart chambers to adapt to volume overload are large "V" waves in the LA, and pulmonary edema. This serious condition of hemodynamic decompensation requires urgent mitral valve repair or replacement.

In the case of chronic MR, the LA and ventricle have all the time needed to make compensatory changes allowing for increased atrial and pulmonary vein compliance. Therefore, patients do not usually report the symptoms of pulmonary edema for many years.

During systole, in the presence of MR, blood is not entirely directed along the outflow tract into the aorta and is pushed in part into the LA. The quantity of blood reflowing into the atrium takes the name of regurgitant volume; the volume is strictly correlated with the square root of the systolic gradient between the left ventricle and atrium, the duration of regurgitation, and effective regurgitant orifice (ERO) [89, 93–95]. Regurgitation in the LA leads to an increase in atrial pressure, while reducing antegrade output. In cases of major regurgitation, left atrial pressure remains high even during the late diastolic phase.

At a ventricular level, MR is the cause of major preload, while afterload is normal or reduced due to the regurgitant volume returning to a low-pressure chamber, thus allowing the ventricle to spend most of its energy in shortening the fibers, rather than generating tension [89, 96]. These reduced wall stress conditions resulting from low afterload, associated with high preload, lead to left ventricular remodeling with an increase in chamber volume, thus allowing an increase in end-diastolic volume and preserved antegrade output. As stated above, this type of compensation allows MR to remain asymptomatic for a long period of time [89, 97, 98]. The type of hypertrophy generated is given by the serial replication of sarcomeres, namely the opposite of what happens with the increase in afterload in which sarcomeres replicate in parallel.

After an initial compensation phase, the LV's contractility progressively reduces [99, 100]. In this case, if the left ventricular ejection fraction (LVEF) is taken as an index of left ventricular contractility, it can remain within normal range, despite a drop in systolic function [101–103], because of the impact of the regurgitant volume in the measurement of LVEF. Therefore, a LVEF less than 60% in the presence of severe MR is a sign of left ventricular dysfunction [102].

Another index for the assessment of LV function is the end-systolic diameter (LVESD) or end-systolic volume (LVESV), both of which are more independent factors compared to ventricular preload conditions [104–108]. The greater the LVESV, the worse left ventricular contractility is. It has been noted that preoperative measurements of LVESV and the left ventricular end-systolic volume index (LVESVI) are the best predictors of postoperative left ventricular systolic function [108].

2.2 Mitral Regurgitation

The mitral valve's functional competence is ensured by the coordinated and adequate interaction of the mitral annulus and cusps, *chordae tendineae*, papillary muscles, and left atrium and ventricle. Therefore, dysfunction of one or more of these components can lead to MR during ventricular systole. If there is damage or an alteration primarily affecting the mitral annulus, and especially its diameter, functional MR develops. If damage affects the leaflets, *chordae tendineae*, or papillary muscles, MR is degenerative.

Carpentier and colleagues classified MR into three main types based on the movement of the leaflets and *chordae tendineae* [109, 110]:

- *type I*: normal leaflet motion
- *type II*: leaflet prolapse or excessive motion
- *type III*: restricted leaflet motion. Type III is further divided into IIIa and IIIb depending on whether the restriction occurs during ventricular diastole or systole.

Type I is often the result of mitral annulus dilation secondary to left ventricular dilation (thus comprising patients with dilated cardiomyopathy or ischemic heart disease); this group also includes patients with leaflet perforation secondary to endocarditis.

Type II, instead, occurs following the stretching or rupture of the *chordae tendineae*, but it can also be observed in patients with coronaropathy, as they may suffer rupture or stretching of the papillary muscles.

Finally, type III is associated with rheumatic disease, ischemic heart disease, and dilated cardiomyopathy [110,111].

Functional mitral regurgitation (FMR) is the result of incomplete mitral leaflet closing due to left ventricular dysfunction and dilation, as it has been observed in patients with dilated cardiomyopathy or ischemic heart disease [112]. Although left ventricular dilation and dysfunction are less marked in forms of infarction of the inferior myocardium compared to those affecting the anterior ventricular wall, the incidence and severity of MR are greater if infarction affects the inferior wall [96]. FMR affects 40% of patients with infarction due to dilated cardiomyopathy [113]. The incidence of ischemic mitral regurgitation (IMR) is spreading, as increasing numbers of patients survive acute MI. IMR occurs in about 15% of patients with infarction affecting the anterior wall and in more than 40% of patients with inferior infarction [96]. The severity of MR is generally correlated with the dimensions of the akinetic or dyskinetic area of the LV.

2.2.2
Diagnosis

2.2.2.1
Non-invasive Diagnosis

Patients affected by chronic MR are often asymptomatic, even in the presence of severe regurgitation. When mitral valve disease is symptomatic, the symptoms most commonly reported by patients are fatigue and dyspnea on effort, which, at times, may develop into orthopnea, paroxysmal nocturnal dyspnea, and peripheral edemas, leading even to acute pulmonary edema. An accurate clinical history is often an essential instrument providing information of the valvulopathy's etiology (e.g. prior MI, episodes of angina pectoris, rheumatic carditis, infectious endocarditis) [114].

At *physical examination*, arterial pressure is normal, arterial pulse is rapid, and heart auscultation directs us towards MR in the presence of systolic murmur, often holosystolic, including the first and second heart sound. In cases of prolapse, the murmur is often telesystolic, while it is protosystolic in cases of functional MR. The murmur is typically very load and blowing, but it can even be harsh, especially in cases of mitral prolapse. The first sound (S_1) is included in the murmur and is usually normal, but it may also be loud in the case of a rheumatic valvulopathy; the second sound (S_2), too, is generally normal, but it may be split if the LV's ejection time is very short. There can also be a third sound (S_3), which is directly correlated with the regurgitant volume, typically becomes louder with exhalation and, in the case of functional or ischemic MR, is often associated with a restrictive ventricular filling pattern. A gallop rhythm (S_4) can be detected in the case of MR with a recent onset and functional and/or ischemic MR. MR is often associated with a protodiastolic murmur generated by the increase in mitralic flow in diastole. A mid-diastolic click can be heard in cases of prolapse [114].

In cases of chronic MR, the *ECG* shows signs of enlarged left heart chambers with increased P waves and QRS complexes. When MR is ischemic, there can be ECG signs of recent or prior ischemic damage.

In chronic MR, the *chest x-ray* usually shows a dilation of the left chambers, and calcifications can be seen in the mitral annulus in degenerative valvulopathy, or near the mitral leaflets in rheumatic valvulopathy.

Echocardiography is still today the method of choice for diagnosing MR. Both TTE and TEE make it possible not only to assess the magnitude of regurgitation, but also to obtain information on the valve's morphofunctional characteristics, define the pathogenic mechanisms, and assess left ventricular function, and, when necessary, are useful for planning the best possible therapeutic strategy [19, 20, 47]. To date, one of the main obstacles to MR diagnosis is still the lack of a single "gold standard" method, and this is probably due to the great individual variability of regurgitation, which is heavily affected by the hemodynamic conditions at the moment of assessment. A rise or reduction in preload and/or afterload, changes in heart rate, myocardial contractility, and atrial compliance are all factors that may cause relatively major changes in regurgitant volume. Therefore, a multiparameter echocardiography assessment is necessary to quantify the extent of regurgitation as reliably as possible [115].

Echocardiographic 2D assessment allows anatomical and morphological description of the mitral valve in all its features and of the effects of the valve defect on the heart chambers. MR can be surmised in the presence of:
- altered morphology of the valve apparatus (valve prolapse, flail, valvular annulus calcifications, papillary muscle dysfunction, or rupture) (Fig. 2.19)
- enlarged LA (Fig. 2.20)
- atrial septal aneurysm with convex shape toward the right atrium (atrial pressure and/or volume overload)
- enlargement of the LV (Fig. 2.21)
- hyperkinesia of the left ventricular wall
- visualization of akinetic zones/aneurysms of some ventricular segments in IMR (Fig. 2.22)
- clear signs of right ventricular overload.

In general, flail motion of a leaflet or of a part of it, associated with ruptured *chordae tendineae*, can lead to the suspicion of significant regurgitation (Fig. 2.23). Severe MR can also be suspected when there is a coaptation gap between the leaflets (Fig. 2.24). In this case, an eccentric jet moving in the direction opposite to that of the prolapsing leaflet should be expected (Fig. 2.25). In the case of rheumatic carditis causing mitral valve disease, signs of fibrosis on the leaflets, reduced leaflet motion due to shortening of the *chordae tendineae*, and, generally, associated mitral stenosis can be observed.

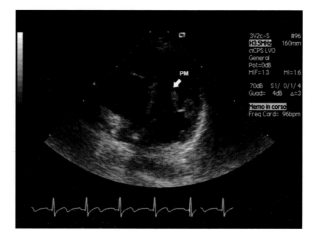

Fig. 2.19 Transthoracic echocardiogram. Apical four-chamber view. Rupture of the posterolateral papillary muscle (*PM*), *arrow*

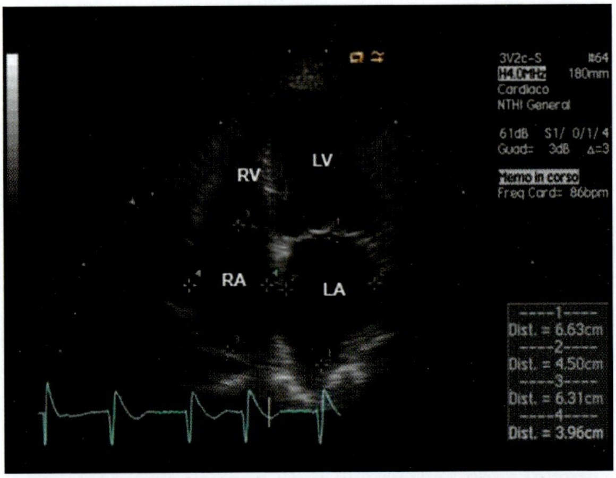

Fig. 2.20 Transthoracic echocardiogram. Apical four-chamber view. Superoinferior and lateromedial dilation of the left and right atrium. *LA*, left atrium; *LV*, left ventricle; *RA*, right atrium; *RV*, right ventricle

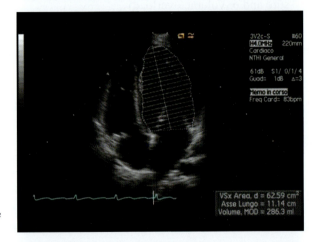

Fig. 2.21 Transthoracic echocardiogram. Apical four-chamber view. Increase in left ventricular volume

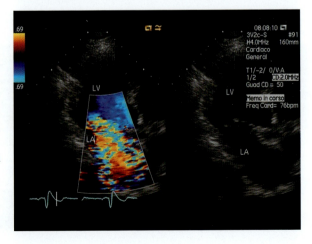

Fig. 2.22 Transthoracic echocardiogram. Apical two-chamber view. Anterior leaflet tethering, with MR, in a patient with previous myocardial infarction. *LA*, left atrium; *LV*, left ventricle; *RA*, right atrium; *RV*, right ventricle

2.2 Mitral Regurgitation

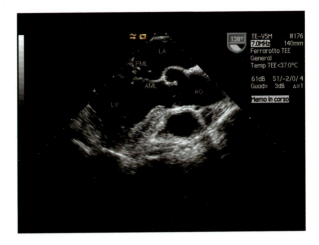

Fig. 2.23 Transesophageal echocardiogram at 138°. Posterior leaflet prolapse (P2) with rupture of the chorda tendinea. *AO*, aorta; *LA*, left atrium; *AML*, anterior mitral leaflet; *PML*, posterior mitral leaflet; *LV*, left ventricle; *RA*, right atrium; *RV*, right ventricle

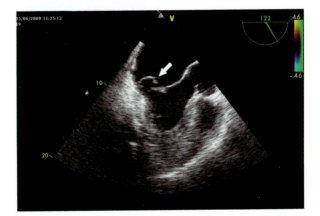

Fig. 2.24 Transesophageal echocardiogram at 132°. Coaptation gap, posterior leaflet prolapse (*arrow*) (P2)

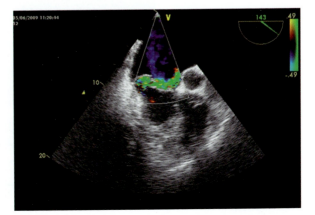

Fig. 2.25 Transesophageal echocardiogram at 143°. Coaptation gap, with severe eccentric MR

Echocardiography can also provide useful information on the extent of endocarditis by identifying the sessile or pedunculated masses (Figs. 2.26 and 2.27), valve tissue damage, and any associated valve regurgitation (Figs. 2.28 and 2.29).

The echocardiographic assessment of MR requires, nonetheless, M-mode examination, which can be useful to detect the presence of MR in the case of an enlarged LA or LV (Fig. 2.30). In addition, M-mode color echocardiography is useful to study MR with a better time resolution (Fig. 2.31).

Doppler echocardiography is the technique most commonly used to detect and assess the extent of regurgitation. A review of literature and clinical practice makes it possible to distinguish the Doppler parameters into parameters derived from regurgitant jet and parameters not derived from regurgitant jet sampling. These are summarized in Table 2.8.

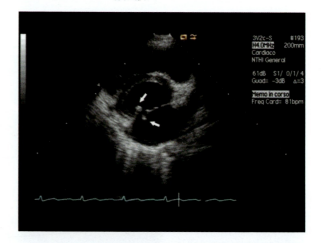

Fig. 2.26 Transthoracic echocardiogram. Short-axis view (off-axis) showing vegetation due to endocarditis (*arrows*)

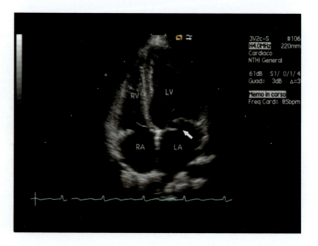

Fig. 2.27 Transthoracic echocardiogram. Endocarditis on the anterior leaflet (*arrow*). *LA*, left atrium; *LV*, left ventricle; *RA*, right atrium; *RV*, right ventricle

2.2 Mitral Regurgitation

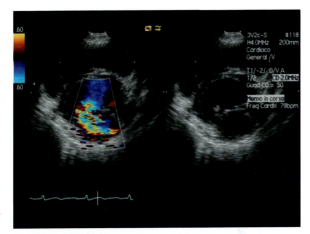

Fig. 2.28 Transthoracic echocardiogram. Short-axis view (off axis). Severe mitral regurgitation

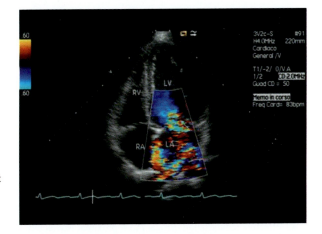

Fig. 2.29 Transthoracic echocardiogram. Apical four-chamber view. Severe mitral regurgitation. *LA*, left atrium; *LV*, left ventricle; *RA*, right atrium; *RV*, right ventricle

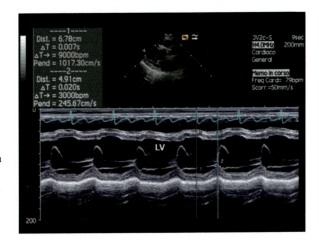

Fig. 2.30 Transthoracic echocardiogram. M-mode in parasternal long-axis view, left ventricular dilation with preserved septal and posterior wall kinesis. *LV*, left ventricle

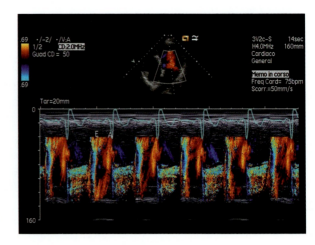

Fig. 2.31 Transthoracic echocardiogram. Color M-mode, apical four-chamber view. Holosystolic mitral regurgitation

Table 2.8 Color-Doppler parameters to assess the extent of mitral regurgitation

Parameters	Extent of mitral regurgitation			
	Mild	**Moderate**	**Medium**	**Severe**
Extension of regurgitant jet/LA (%)	< 20	Variable	Variable	>40
Vena contracta (mm)	<3	Variable	Variable	>7
PISA radius	Variable	Variable	Variable	> 1 cm
ERO (cm^2)	<0.20	0.20–0.29	0.30–0.39	>0.40
Regurgitant volume (ml)	<30	30–44	45–59	>60
Regurgitant fraction	<30	30–39	40–49	>50
Pulmonary venous flow	Normal	Normal	Monolateral systolic inversion	Bilateral systolic inversion
Transmitral diastolic flow	E/A <1			E/A >2

ERO, effective regurgitation orifice; *PISA*, proximal isovelocity surface area; *LA*, left atrium

2.2.2.1.1
Parameters Derived from the Regurgitation Jet

There are three areas in the regurgitant jet:
- the *pre-orifice* convergence area of the velocities (area in the near vicinity of the valve where the flow converges and accelerates before entering the regurgitant orifice)
- the vena contracta (zone where the flow is smallest *after the regurgitant orifice*)
- distribution of the regurgitant jet in the LA (*post-orifice* turbulence area).

These three areas identify just as many methods to quantify MR: PISA method, vena contrata quantification, and regurgitant jet analysis.

2.2.2.1.2
Proximal Isovelocity Surface Area (PISA) Method

The flow convergence region proximal to a circular orifice is a laminar field of converging flow lines associated with a family of concentric and hemispherical isovelocity surfaces with decreasing area and increasing velocity (Fig. 2.32). Based on the principle of continuity, the flow (Q) is constant on all isovelocity surfaces and it is equal to the flow to the orifice. This way, the effective regurgitant orifice (ERO) area can be calculated by dividing the flow peak (obtained from the flow convergence region and aliasing velocity) by the maximum velocity through the orifice (obtained by continuous wave Doppler) [116].

$$\text{Regurgitant flow} = (2\pi r^2 \times V_a)$$
$$\text{ERO} = \text{regurgitant flow}/V_{reg}$$
$$\text{Regurgitant volume} = \text{ERO} \times (\text{MR–VTI})$$

where r is the hemispherical convergence radius (cm), V_a is the velocity at which aliasing occurs in the flow convergence towards the regurgitant orifice, V_{reg} is the peak velocity of the regurgitant jet, and MR–VTI the velocity–time integral of the regurgitant jet, determined by continuous wave Doppler.

The PISA method, though, has four major limitations, which need to be taken into account [117]:
- flattening of the isovelocity profile and hence the loss of its hemispherical shape, which leads to significant underestimation of regurgitation (this occurs especially when the aliasing velocity exceeds 10% of the flow velocity through the orifice)
- containment of the convergence area by adjacent structures, hindering its free spatial development (typical of mitral prolapse)
- difficulty in precisely identifying the orifice site, as the hemisphere's radius is determined based on the orifice's location and the radius is squared

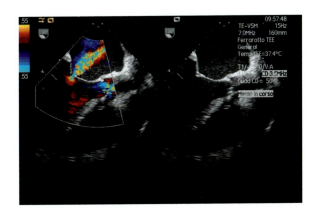

Fig. 2.32 Transthoracic echocardiogram at 130°. Severe mitral regurgitation with proximal convergence area

- in many patients, regurgitation is not constant throughout systole and assessment of the degree of regurgitation based on the maximum area of the regurgitant orifice can be misleading.

The PISA method cannot be considered as an absolute quantitative parameter and independent from MR quantization. Therefore, it needs to be integrated with other approaches to estimate regurgitation. 3D echo can be useful in the case of PISA with an elliptical or dome-shaped morphology, although the issue is still being studied.

2.2.2.1.3
Vena Contracta

Vena contracta (VC), namely the narrowest portion of the jet at or immediately below the orifice, is the zone of maximum transformation of the pressure energy of the regurgitant flow into kinetic energy. It is characterized by a laminar flow with the highest velocity [115]. Using VC as a parameter to assess the extent of MR is based on the assumption that its width is correlated with the regurgitant area: a VC width of >7 mm indicates severe MR; a width of VC <3 mm indicates mild MR; VC values of 3–7 mm indicate moderate MR (Table 2.8).

VC is measured perpendicularly to the intercommissural coaptation line of the leaflets (parasternal long-axis view or apical long-axis) and it gives the anteroposterior dimension of the effective regurgitation area. According to some authors, this quantification method is independent from the hemodynamic variables and orifice geometry and it appears to be associated with a low interobserver variability [118]. It can be used for single jets, while it poses limits for multiple jets. Sections in which the commissural fissure runs parallel to the scanning plane are to be avoided (as is the case for the two apical chambers, for instance). In these cases, small regurgitations can have a very wide VC. In searching for the VC, a zoom with maximum time resolution, and hence with a color-Doppler angle as narrow as possible, can be useful. Since the measurement is in millimeters, minor assessment errors lead to great variations in the grading of severity.

2.2.2.1.4
Regurgitant Jet Analysis

Turbulence visualized in the LA by color Doppler is not the regurgitant volume, but is the chromatic representation of the flow direction (red/blue), its velocity (more or less bright color), and type of flow (laminar or turbulent). The spatial dispersion of the regurgitant jet is proportional to the flow's kinetic energy, which is the product of the mass by the velocity, which, in turn, depends on the pressure gradient. The dimensions of the turbulence area due to MR are hence only partially influenced by regurgitant volume, as they are affected by the conditions modifying the transmitral gradient in systole as well as by technical aspects more specifically linked to the type of equipment used [119].

The most commonly adopted criterion is the maximum disturbed flow area, either as an absolute value or related to LA area [115]. The cross-sections studied as a routine are: parasternal long axis, four-chamber apical view, and two-chamber apical view; the study envisages a thorough assessment of changes throughout systole. Jet dimensions are not always representative of regurgitation severity; one example is given by extremely eccentric regurgitation (Fig. 2.33), in which the jet is directed against the atrial walls, thus transferring a part of its kinetic energy (Coanda effect) and leading to underestimated Doppler exam results. Despite its evident limits, regurgitant jet analysis is the most widely used method in the semi-quantitative study of MR severity.

Regurgitation is considered *mild* when:
- the LA color jet is visible only on the valvular plane and if the wavefront is thin (Fig. 2.34)
- the regurgitant jet area is <4 cm^2 (absolute value)
- the jet area/LA area ratio is <20%.

Regurgitation is considered *moderate* when:
- the color jet is visible up to the middle of the LA (moderately wide jet)
- the absolute area is between 4 and 8 cm^2 (Fig. 2.35)
- the jet area/LA area ratio varies, but it is generally <20–40%.

Regurgitation is considered *severe* when:
- the color jet propagates in all directions filling the atrial cavity
- the absolute area is >8 cm^2 (Fig. 2.36)
- the jet area/LA area ratio is >40%.

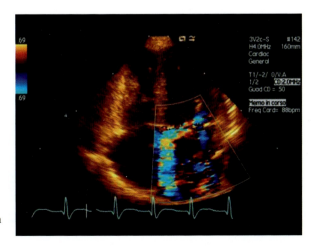

Fig. 2.33 Transthoracic echocardiogram. Apical four-chamber view. Severe eccentric mitral regurgitation (Coanda effect)

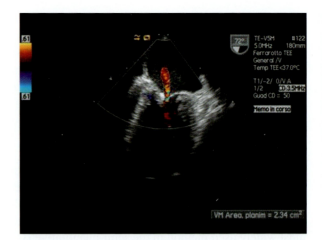

Fig. 2.34 Transesophageal echocardiogram at 72°. Mild mitral regurgitation (planimetric jet area 2.34 cm^2)

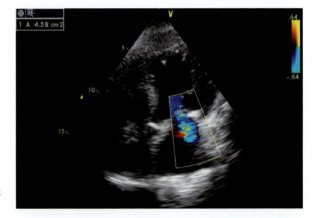

Fig. 2.35 Transthoracic echocardiogram. Apical four-chamber view. Moderate mitral regurgitation (planimetric jet area of 4.58 cm^2)

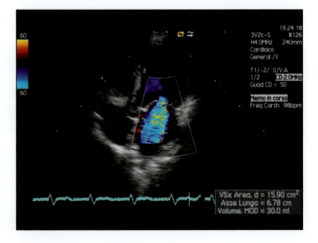

Fig. 2.36 Transthoracic echocardiogram. Apical four-chamber view. Severe mitral regurgitation (planimetric jet area of 15.90 cm^2)

2.2 Mitral Regurgitation

MR assessment correlated with the jet study also includes its spectrum analysis by means of CW Doppler [115]. The velocity does not provide useful data on the severity of the regurgitation, unlike the profile and density of the jet at CW Doppler. A truncated, triangular jet contour with early peaking of the maximal velocity indicates elevated LA pressure or a prominent regurgitant pressure wave in the LA. Jet density, too, is correlated with MR severity. An intense signal indicates severe MR, while an incomplete or faint signal is a sign of mild MR. In the case of eccentric jets, though of some relevance, it can be difficult to fully capture the regurgitation's CW Doppler signal, due to the eccentric direction of the flow.

2.2.2.1.5
Parameters Not Derived from the Regurgitation Jet

The ideal approach to assessing MR comprises other parameters as well:
- regurgitant fraction (RF)
- pulmonary venous flow (PVF)
- transmitral diastolic flow.

Regurgitant Fraction

The relationship between regurgitant volume and LVEF is called regurgitant fraction (RF). It is calculated by dividing the difference between the mitral output and the aortic valve output by the transmitral output [115]. This method can be used also with multiple and eccentric jets, providing information on jet severity and volume overload. However, this method is not widely used, as it is difficult and has limitations [115]:
- small variations in heart rate or small errors in measuring ventricular diameters and volumes can lead to errors in output calculation
- there is no standardization based on the body mass index
- it cannot used if there is aortic failure or atrial fibrillation
- technical difficulties due to annulus calcifications.

Recourse to the 3D approach, by improving accuracy in quantifying volumes, can increase the reliability of the systolic jet calculated, but its clinical validation is still in progress.

The quantification of the degree of MR based on the RF is as follows:
- RF <30%, mild MR
- RF 30–50%, moderate MR
- RF >50%, severe MR.

Pulmonary Venous Flow

Pulsed wave (PW) Doppler assessment of PVF is useful to determine the hemodynamic consequences of MR. Normal PVF typically has two velocity peaks, a systolic one and a diastolic one (the systolic peak is higher than the diastolic one), and a small inverted wave corresponding to atrial contraction. In MR, there is an increase in left atrial pressure matched by a decrease in systolic velocity. In severe MR, there is total systolic wave inversion (Fig. 2.37) [115]. Due to the anatomical position of the pulmonary veins, this sign is searched for in clinical practice, primarily by using TEE and directing the sample volume at 1–2 cm inside the outlet of the pulmonary veins to the LA by means of PW Doppler (Fig. 2.38).

Since the regurgitant jet is generally directed towards a pulmonary vein and

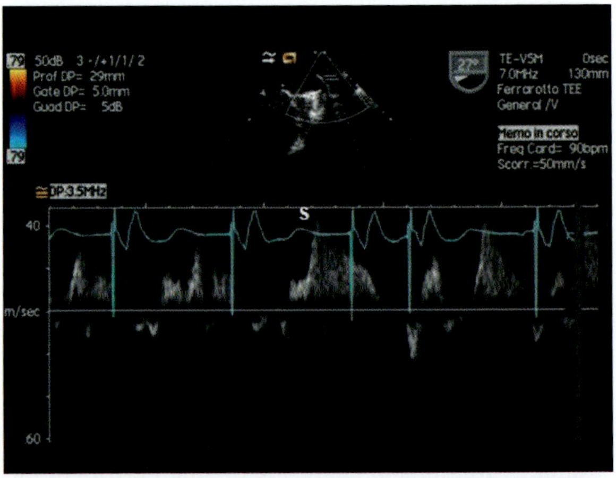

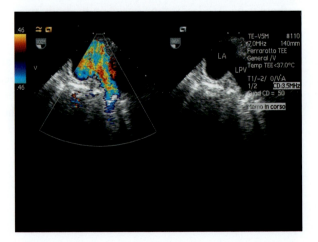

Fig. 2.37 Pulmonary venous flow profile in case of severe mitral regurgitation, pulsed wave Doppler in 90° transesophageal two-chamber view. The curve shows a clearly defined inversion of the systolic wave (*S*)

Fig. 2.38 Transesophageal echocardiogram at 96°. Severe mitral regurgitation flow, recorded in the left superior pulmonary vein (*LPV*). *LA*, left atrium

the systolic flow of that vein is negative while the others have positive systolic waves, all four pulmonary vessels need to be examined.

This type of assessment of MR is affected by several factors, such as patient age, heart rhythm, jet direction and LA distensibility. A flow inversion may also occur without any significant MR, in patients with high LA pressures or with an eccentric jet [120]. This sign is often unreliable in patients with left ventricular dysfunction with a reduced systolic component.

Transmitral Diastolic Flow

Diastolic mitral flow by PW Doppler, though indicating a prevalence of the atrial component over the protodiastolic one, can be an easy, immediate and very useful parameter to exclude a diagnosis of severe MR [121]. However, this method depends on the LA pressure and can hence be used if there is no mitral stenosis or other causes leading to an increase in LA pressure. This type of study is recommended for the apical portions. Color Doppler allows for a better analysis of the nature and direction of the flow. In the four-chamber apical view, by applying the sample volume at the apex of the opening valve leaflets, the rapid filling protodiastolic wave (E) and the wave secondary to atrial contraction (A) are recorded in patients with normal sinus rhythm. Once the velocity peak is reached, the E wave progressively returns to the baseline value in a period defined as "deceleration E-time" (DT). A normal transmitral flow pattern in a middle-aged subject with sinus rhythm is given by a prevalent E wave with a DT of about 200 ms.

An E/A ratio of <1 indicates MR without hemodynamic relevance, while, by contrast, an E/A ratio of >2 is an indicator of severe MR (Table 2.8).

Table 2.9 summarizes the various echocardiography methods that are useful for multiparameter assessment of MR and any resulting hemodynamic impairment.

Table 2.9 Echocardiography methods to assess the degree of regurgitation

2D Echo	Color	Pulsed wave Doppler	Continuous wave Doppler
Mitral valve morphology	Jet area	Regurgitant volume	Jet spectral analysis
Left atrium volume	Vena contracta	Regurgitant fraction	Systolic pulmonary artery pressure
Left ventricle dimension	Convergence area PISA-EROA	EROA A wave, E wave Pulmonary venous flow	

PISA, proximal isovelocity surface area; *EROA*, effective regurgitation orifice area

2.2.2.1.6
Transesophageal Echocardiography in Assessing Mitral Regurgitation Severity

According to current guidelines [19, 20, 47], TEE is indicated to assess MR severity when TTE does not provide adequate information on MR severity, or when TTE is technically limited. Moreover, TEE is needed to study the mechanisms behind MR and schedule valve surgery. All of the MR quantification criteria mentioned above can be used during TEE, and the greater resolution, greater anatomical vicinity to the mitral valve, and the use of multiplane probes make VC and PISA the most easily obtainable and accurate criteria. TEE also allows for an easier sampling of the flow of all of the pulmonary veins.

2.2.2.2
Invasive Diagnosis

The invasive diagnostic examinations are TEE, already discussed in the previous paragraph, and cardiac catheterization.

The current guidelines recommend hemodynamic and angiographic assessment when there is a major difference between the patient's clinical status and the data resulting from the non-invasive approach. They are recommended if the non-invasive examinations have provided incomplete data and left doubts about MR severity, LV contractility, and the indication for treatment [19, 20, 47].

The information being sought and that is obtainable from cardiac catheterization is MR severity, pulmonary and systemic hemodynamic impairment, and LV dimensions and contractility. Coronarography should always be performed to search for and rule out the presence of coronary artery disease in patients with risk factors for atherosclerosis [19, 20, 47].

2.2.2.2.1
Hemodynamic Assessment

The hemodynamic parameters that are useful to assess MR severity and hemodynamic impairment are: pulmonary artery pressure (PAP), PCWP, left ventricular end-diastolic pressure (LVEDP) and oxygen saturation in the pulmonary artery and aorta, which allow calculation of cardiac output using the Fick method [80].

When the V wave in the PCWP tracing gives a value more than double that of the mean PCWP, MR is severe (Fig. 2.39). There are other situations with a high V wave without severe MR; these include, for instance, left ventricular

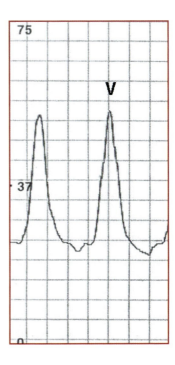

Fig. 2.39 Pulmonary capillary wedge pressure tracing; *V*, wave

failure of any etiology with a small and non-compliant LA, or, in the case of acute pulmonary hyperflow, post-infarction interventricular defect. By contrast, severe MR does not always have a high V wave, as in the case of chronic forms with marked LA dilation, since the atrium can receive large regurgitant volumes without increasing the mean PCWP or height of the V wave [80, 122]. Severe MR with concurrent left ventricular dysfunction often has a V wave inscribed in the dicrotic phase of the pulmonary pressure curve (Fig. 2.40), often with a maximum pressure value equal to the pulmonary systolic pressure. An increased afterload in the presence of MR can increase the regurgitant volume and/or the V wave height (e.g. aortic stenosis or systemic blood hypertension).

Dynamic exercise test with a supine cycloergometer can sometimes be useful for assessing the severity of MR with normal cardiac output at rest, especially when the patient's symptoms occur with exertion. In this case the increase in cardiac output is less than 80% of predicted [80].

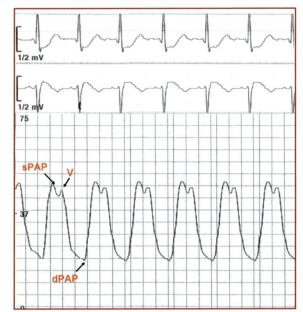

Fig. 2.40 Pulmonary capillary wedge pressure tracing; *V*, wave inscribed in the dicrotic phase of the pulmonary pressure curve. *dPAP*, diastolic pulmonary artery pressure; *sPAP*, systolic pulmonary artery pressure

2.2.2.2.2
Angiographic Assessment

Left ventriculography is very useful to assess MR, as it provides important information on MR severity using the qualitative method (Table 2.10), LV, dimensions and ejection fraction (EF) (Fig. 2.41). Angiographic assessment of the severity of MR consists also of a quantitative evaluation of the RF, measuring the total left ventricular stroke volume (TSV) from the left ventriculogram and the cardiac output (the forward stroke volume, FSV) by Fick or thermodilution technique (Table 2.11).

The accuracy of the calculations is affected by various factors. Since FSV is obtained by dividing the cardiac output by the heart rate at the time of Fick, or other, it will give a mean stroke volume. Therefore, the beat chosen for left ventriculography to determine the volume must be an "average" or representative beat; alternatively, volumes from multiple beats may be calculated and averaged. In patients with atrial fibrillation and ectopic beats during ventriculography, RSV and RF calculation using this method is not recommended due to the great inaccuracy.

FSV quantification should be carried out simultaneously with cardiac output calculation, since, as mentioned above, an increase in arterial pressure can lead to an increase in the degree of MR with a reduction of forward output. Therefore, if the blood pressure or other hemodynamic variables change significantly

2.2 Mitral Regurgitation

Table 2.10 Examinination of any systolic leakage of contrast from the left ventricle back into the left atrium and the opacification of the left atrium relative to the left ventricle during ventriculography

Grade	Qualitative assessment criteria
1+ (mild)	Regurgitation clears with each beat and never opacifies the entire left atrium
2+ (moderate)	Regurgitation does not clear with one beat and generally does opacify the entire left atrium (albeit faintly) after several beats; however, opacification of the left atrium does not equal that of the left ventricle
3+ (moderately severe)	Left atrium completely opacified and equal opacification with the left ventricle
4+ (severe)	Opacification of the entire left atrium within one beat, opacification becomes progressively more dense with each beat, and contrast material can be seen refluxing into the pulmonary veins during left ventricular systole

Table 2.11 Quantitative estimate of regurgitant fraction by angiographic assessment

Angiographic measurement	Formula
Ventricular stroke volume (VSV)	EDV − ESV
Regurgitant stroke volume (RSV)	VSV − FSV
Regurgitant fraction (RF)	RSV/VSV

EDV, end-diastolic left ventricular volume; *ESV*, end-systolic left ventricular volume; *FSV*, forward stroke volume

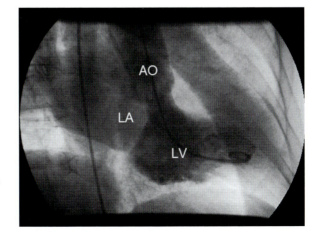

Fig. 2.41 Left ventriculography. Opacification of the entire left atrium (*LA*) during the systolic phase of the cardiac cycle; this is indicative of severe mitral regurgitation. *AO*, aorta, *LV*, left ventricle

between the time of cardiac output determination and left ventriculography, it is useless to calculate RF. Finally, the RF quantifies, at best, the total amount of regurgitation. Therefore, if a patient has both mitral and aortic regurgitation, the RF gives an assessment of the regurgitation resulting from both lesions combined [80].

2.2.3
Timing of Interventions

Due to greater life expectancy, MR is currently the most frequent valve defect after aortic stenosis. The often advanced age of patients with valve disease, and the development of percutaneous techniques and more conservative surgical approaches make the decision-making process rather complex with regard to both the right timing of intervention and the choice of the most appropriate therapeutic strategy. In addition, it must be considered that today there are no randomized clinical studies on such a complex population, taking into account recent therapeutic options. Therefore, the decision to intervene on a patient with valve disease is based on the individual risk–benefit analysis considering the fact that the improvement of the prognosis compared to the pathology's natural history should exceed the risk associated with the intervention and the possible late complications related to it.

The elements to be considered in the risk–benefit analysis are multiple and associated with:
- pathophysiological and prognostic characteristics of the specific valvulopathy
- the patient's clinical characteristics, especially with regard to comorbidities.

Recourse to an "evidence-based" approach to treat heart valve diseases has been hindered by the lack of rigorous data on clinical outcome predictors. Determining the right timing of surgical intervention in MR patients is controversial for two reasons: the different causes of valve dysfunction and the lack of a precise estimate of disease severity.

The natural history of MR is marked by its different forms:
- *chronic organic MR* is a progressive disease, with an estimated risk at 5 years of cardiac events (death due to cardiac causes, heart failure, new-onset atrial fibrillation) of $33 \pm 3\%$ [95]; besides the symptoms, the risk factors are age, atrial fibrillation, degree of regurgitation, left atrial dilation, left ventricular dilation, pulmonary hypertension, and low EF
- *chronic ischemic MR* is a dynamic condition with an unfavorable prognosis [94]; its severity can vary from time to time due to the onset of arrhythmias, ischemia, and hypertension, or to exercise
- *significant functional MR* is an independent prognostic factor in patients with chronic heart failure [123].

Clinical outcomes and therapeutic approaches depend on the causes of valve dysfunction. For instance, in patients with MR secondary to dilated cardiomyopathy or ischemic heart disease, the prognosis mainly depends on the baseline disease, and valve surgery is still controversial. On the other hand, in patients with primary regurgitation, the clinical outcomes are mostly the consequence of regurgitation through the valve, and the recovery of valve competence is hence the therapeutic rationale. In these patients, the main clinical question is to determine when in the course of the disease's natural history the benefits of valve surgery exceed the related risks. Of course, treatment must be performed in patients with severe MR before the onset of irreversible left ventricular dysfunction.

Clinically speaking, the best indices for the worsening of heart function are the development of symptoms and the presence of echocardiographic signs of ventricular failure. Therefore, it is widely accepted that patients with limiting symptoms should be treated [19, 20, 47].

The management of asymptomatic patients is still debated due to the lack of randomized clinical trials. On the one hand, the good results of conservative surgery and the preliminary results of percutaneous treatment, associated with the potential risk of postoperative ventricular dysfunction, vouch for early treatment. On the other hand, though based on a small number of case histories, there is a clear risk of surgical mortality, and percutaneous techniques are not yet supported by large trials.

Treatment is recommended in asymptomatic patients with severe MR and signs of left ventricular dysfunction, atrial fibrillation, or pulmonary hypertension [19, 20, 47]. The indications to treatment depend, in turn, on the stratified risk, the possibility of conservative surgery on the valve, and the possibility of percutaneous treatment.

In patients with MR, echocardiography is an important diagnostic instrument to determine the correct timing for intervention. Since the postoperative results are worse when LVEF is <60% or when the left ventricular telesystolic diameter is ≥45 mm, these indices are believed to be predictors of the onset of heart disease [124, 125].

Recently, the physiological effects of valve competence recovery have been assessed. Up to about two decades ago, in most cases there was a reduction in EF following valve replacement due to mitral MR. It had been hypothesized that this event was the inevitable consequence of elimination of the favorable hemodynamic conditions created by MR. It was believed that restoring valve competence would reduce the preload and increase the afterload, leading to a reduction in EF. Therefore, if EF was already reduced, surgery would further reduce it. For this reason, it had to be ruled out in the presence of advanced left ventricular dysfunction. There is anatomical and functional evidence showing that this concept is false [125]. Two decades ago mitral valve surgery consisted of replacing the valve by removing the entire valve apparatus. There was still a lack of understanding of the fact that the mitral valve and its apparatus were an important functional component of the LV, contributing to maintaining its shape and contractility. Today it is known that destruction of the subvalvular apparatus, and not the hemodynamic changes following intervention, is the cause for the reduction in EF after mitral surgery [126–128]. This has been proven by the fact that in cases of mitral repair with recovery of valve competence without destroying the apparatus, there has been no or only a slight reduction in EF. If you consider Laplace's law, as a result of valve repair, the afterload drops instead of rising, as the radius is reduced. Therefore, there are almost no cases of MR that cannot be operated by an expert, in the absence of other comorbidities, and it makes no difference whether the EF is reduced and what the left ventricular telesystolic diameter is, provided that the valve apparatus is preserved during surgery. On the other hand, if the valve and its apparatus cannot be preserved, valve replacement for patients with an EF of <35% is not recommended [123]. These considerations relate to non-ischemic MR.

The treatment of ischemic MR gives less satisfactory results in any type of left ventricular dysfunction, partly because, by definition, it is matched by another potentially fatal heart disease [94]. Nonetheless, the revascularization of the vital myocardium during valve surgery can improve cardiac performance [129]. The complexity of ischemic MR makes the recommendations on the inoperability of this condition rather problematic. Unlike non-ischemic MR, in which surgical valve repair is clearly the treatment of choice, in ischemic disease, repair seems to benefit only patients with better preoperative ventricular performance and fewer comorbidities. It is assumed that in patients with a higher risk the prognosis is so bad that the type of surgical procedure performed would have little impact on the clinical outcome.

2.2.4
Patient Selection

As already discussed above, the treatment of severe MR is recommended according to current guidelines for symptomatic patients, even without signs of left ventricular dysfunction, and in asymptomatic patients with left ventricular dysfunction, atrial fibrillation, or pulmonary hypertension [19, 20, 47]. The indications for treatment and the choice of the most appropriate treatment between repair and replacement or the possibility of percutaneous treatment depend on thorough patient assessment and risk stratification for each type of procedure.

In this regard, setting up a multidisciplinary team comprising a cardiologist, cardiac surgeon, and anesthesiologist working together is essential for the proper selection of candidates for the percutaneous approach.

This is done in four steps:
- confirmation of the severity of MR
- assessment of symptoms
- analysis of surgical risk, life expectancy, and quality of life
- assessment of the procedure feasibility and any contraindications to percutaneous treatment.

While the first three items have been discussed when dealing with the timing of intervention and diagnosis, we will now focus our attention mainly on the clinical and anatomical indications and contraindications to percutaneous valve repair using the MitraClip® system (Abbott Vascular Devices, California, USA), to date the only available device for percutaneous mitral valve repair to have the CE mark.

Possible candidates for this procedure are MR patients who meet the criteria of the current guidelines described above [19, 20, 47], namely symptomatic patients with moderate-to-severe (3+) or severe (4+) MR, overall contractile function (LVEF) >25%, telediastolic diameter (LVESD) ≤55 mm; or asymptomatic patients with one or more of the following: LVEF between 25% and 60%; LVESD ≥40 mm; new-onset atrial fibrillation; pulmonary hypertension defined as systolic pulmonary artery pressure (sPAP) >50 mmHg at rest or >60 mmHg on effort. In addition to meeting guidelines criteria, patients should be high-risk candidates for mitral valve surgery including cardiopulmonary bypass. High risk should be established on a consensus between a local independent cardiologist and a cardiac surgeon that conventional surgery would be associated with excessive morbidity and mortality. Criteria of high risk include European System for Cardiac Operative Risk Evaluation (EuroSCORE) >20% [130], hepatic cirrhosis, autoimmune disease, chronic degenerative disease of the central nervous system, severe renal failure requiring hemodialysis, or any contraindication to extracorporeal circulation. Preinterventional screening of patients includes TTE and TEE, chest x-ray, and invasive cardiac evaluation with coronary angiogram, left ventriculography, and right catheterization. Key inclusion and exclusion criteria are listed in Box 2.2.

Therefore, along with accurate patient clinical assessment based mainly on the identification of high surgical risk, usually due to old age and associated comorbidities, it is important to assess some anatomical and morphological parameters that may not just rule out MitraClip® implantation, but also prejudice the success and duration of the result over time [131]. According to data in the literature, percutaneous mitral valve repair using the MitraClip® system requires that patients undergo specific TTE and TEE assessment [131, 132] to identify the anatomical and functional state of the mitral valve and the etiopathogenesis of the regurgitation, and to select patients for whom percutaneous mitral valve repair can achieve an optimal result.

Box 2.2 Major inclusion and exclusion criteria for valve repair using the MitraClip®

Inclusion criteria
> Age 18 years or older
> Moderate to severe (3+) or severe (4+) chronic mitral valve regurgitation with symptoms or without symptoms but LVEF <60% or LVESD >45 mm
> High-risk candidate for mitral valve surgery including cardiopulmonary bypass
> Primary regurgitant jet originating from malcoaptation of the A2 and P2 scallops of the mitral valve. If a secondary jet exists, it must be considered clinically insignificant
> Presence of sufficient leaflet tissue for a mechanical coaptation
> Non-rheumatic/endocarditic valve morphology
> Trans-septal catheterization determined to be feasible by the treating physician

Exclusion criteria
> Evidence of an acute myocardial infarction in the 12 weeks before the intended treatment
> Need for any other cardiac surgery including surgery for coronary artery disease, atrial fibrillation, pulmonic, aortic, or tricuspid valve disease
> Mitral valve orifice area <4.0 cm^2
> If leaflet flail[a] is present:
  – flail width[b] ≥15 mm
  – flail gap[c] ≥10 mm
> If leaflet tethering is present:
  – coaptation depth[d] ≥11 mm
  – coaptation length[e] <2 mm
> Severe mitral annular calcification
> Any leaflet anatomy that may preclude clip implantation, proper clip positioning on the leaflets, or sufficient reduction in MR
> Hemodynamic instability defined as systolic pressure <90 mmHg without afterload reduction or cardiogenic shock or the need for inotropic support or intra-aortic balloon pump
> Need for emergency surgery for any reason
> Systolic anterior motion of the mitral valve leaflet
> Hypertrophic cardiomyopathy
> Echocardiographic evidence of intracardiac mass, thrombus, or vegetation
> History of, or active, endocarditis
> History of, or active, rheumatic heart disease
> History of atrial septal defect, whether repaired or not
> History of patent foramen ovale associated with clinical symptoms (e.g. cerebral ischemia) or previously repaired or when, in the judgment of the investigator, an atrial septal aneurysm is present that may interfere with trans-septal crossing

(cont. →)

Box 2.2 *(continued)*

> History of a stroke or documented transient ischemic attack (TIA) within the prior 6 months
> Patients in whom TEE is contraindicated.

^aFlail is defined as when a leaflet has both ruptured *chordae* and a free edge that extends above the opposing leaflet or above the plane of the annulus during systole.
^bFlail width is defined as the width of flail leaflet segment as measured along the line of coaptation in the short-axis view.
^cFlail gap is defined as the greatest distance between the ventricular side of the flail leaflet segment and the atrial side of the opposing leaflet edge.
^dCoaptation depth is defined as the shortest distance between the coaptation of the leaflets and the annular plane.
^eCoaptation length is defined as the vertical length of leaflets that is in contact, or is available for contact, during mid-systole in the atrial-to-ventricular direction in the four-chamber view.

2.2.4.1
Anatomical and Functional Assessment of the Mitral Valve

The procedure cannot be performed in the presence of a rheumatic valve; therefore, the criteria for exclusion are fibrotic or calcified leaflets, retracted leaflets, severe calcification of the subvalvular apparatus or annulus [133].

In addition, careful assessment of the subvalvular apparatus is needed and the presence of chordal tissue in excess or the implantation of abnormal *chordae*, especially in the rough zone of the leaflets, is to be sought, as it may render orientation, recovery, and clip stability cumbersome. This assessment should be performed solely by TEE in intercommissural view (Fig. 2.42), and, if necessary, the zoom should also be used to avoid amplifying the error. TEE is also needed to exclude any endocarditis processes (Fig. 2.43), including pre-existing ones, with splitting of the leaflet or a part of it. Special attention must be paid to the middle scallops (A2–P2), as they are the implantation site.

After careful anatomical assessment of the mitral valve apparatus, functional assessment of the valve has to be performed. The anatomical and flow area value must be >4.0 cm^2 without any significant transvalvular gradient [134] (Figs. 2.44–2.46).

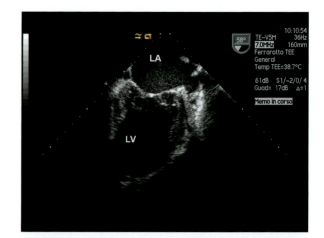

Fig. 2.42 Transesophageal echocardiogram ~60°, intercommissural view. *LA*, left atrium; *LV*, left ventricle

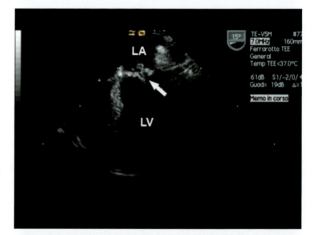

Fig. 2.43 Transesophageal echocardiogram ~0°, apical four-chamber view, presence of vegetation due to endocarditis on both leaflets (*arrow*). *LA*, left atrium; *LV*, left ventricle

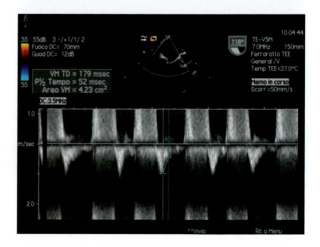

Fig. 2.44 Transesophageal echocardiogram ~120°. Continuous wave Doppler examination, flow area >4 cm^2

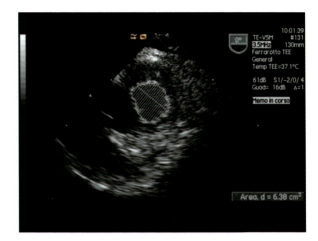

Fig. 2.45 Transesophageal echocardiogram ~0°. Transgastric view: anatomical view >4 cm^2

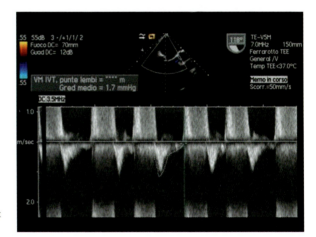

Fig. 2.46 Transesophageal echocardiogram ~120°. Continuous wave Doppler examination, non-significant transmitral gradient

2.2.4.2
Assessment of Regurgitation Etiopathogenesis

As already described, MR can either be organic or functional. The former is caused almost uniquely by a degenerative valve disease (Fig. 2.47) or by endocarditis or congenital defects (cleft), as rheumatic disease has greatly decreased today. Functional MR is secondary to coronary artery disease or dilated cardiomyopathy (Fig. 2.48) and is mainly due to local or global remodeling of the LV with a prevalence of tethering forces and apical displacement of the coaptation point in the mitral valve tissue [135].

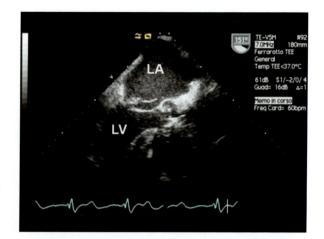

Fig. 2.47 Transesophageal echocardiogram at 151°. Mitral valve with prolapsed body of the posterior leaflet (flail). *LA*, left atrium; *LV*, left ventricle

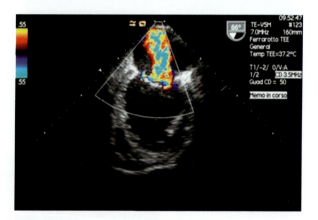

Fig. 2.48 Transesophageal electrocardiogram at 75°. Color-Doppler ultrasound: severe functional mitral regurgitation in dilated cardiomyopathy

An important feature of functional MR is its dependence on remodeling and on the degree of LV systolic dysfunction. Therefore, echocardiography is absolutely necessary to assess the "tethering and annular deformation indices" [136, 137]. The parameters conventionally used to assess the degree of functional MR are:
- *CL – coaptation length* (normal value >2 mm), defined as the vertical stretch of the effective length of coaptation of the leaflets (or part available for contact), at mid-systole on the atrioventricular side. It is usually measured at TTE in apical three-chamber view or at about 120° with TEE (Fig. 2.49)
- *CD – coaptation distance* (normal value <5 mm), defined as the distance between the mitral valve annulus and the first point where coaptation of the two leaflets occurs during mid-systole on the atrioventricular side. It is

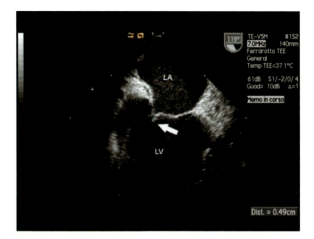

Fig. 2.49 Transesophageal echocardiogram at ~120°. Coaptation length: 0.49 cm. *LA*, left atrium; *LV*, left ventricle; *arrow*, line of coaptation

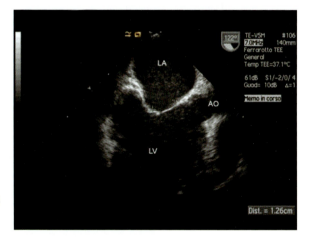

Fig. 2.50 Transesophageal echocardiogram at ~120°; coaptation distance: 1.26 cm. *Ao*, aorta; *LA*, left atrium; *LV*, left ventricle

usually measured at TTE in apical three-chamber view or at about 120° with TEE (Fig. 2.50)
- *TA – tenting area* (normal value <1 cm^2), defined as the area of leaflet malapposition below the annular plane, expressed in cm^2 (Fig. 2.51)
- *mitral annulus dimensions*:
  - CC, which measures the intercommissural distance both during systole and diastole (Fig. 2.52)
  - SL, which measures the septal–lateral distance both during systole and diastole (Fig. 2.53); CC is physiologically larger than SL.

The anterior and posterior leaflets should also be measured, remembering not to include the leaflet's rough zone (Fig. 2.54). The leaflets are measured to assess whether grasping is impossible because one or both leaflets are too short.

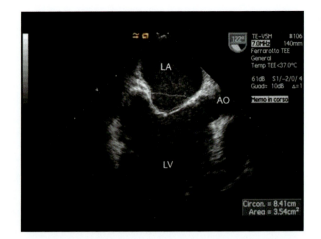

Fig. 2.51 Transesophageal echocardiogram at ~120°; tenting area: 3.54 cm^2

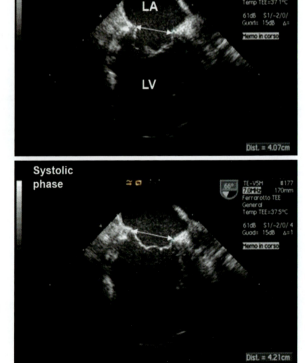

Fig. 2.52 Transesophageal echocardiogram at ~60°; left – right intercommisural distance (LCC – RCC): 4.07 – 4.21 cm. *LA*, left atrium; *LV*, left ventricle

2.2 Mitral Regurgitation

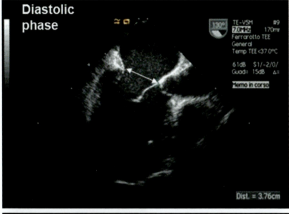

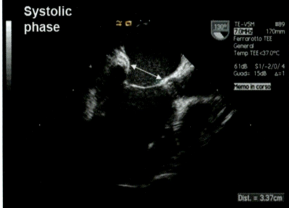

Fig. 2.53 Transesophageal echocardiogram at ~120°; right – left septal lateral distance: 3.76 – 3.37 cm

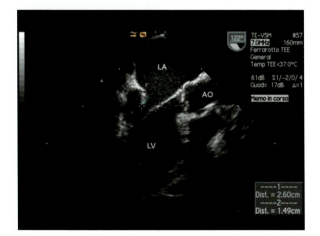

Fig. 2.54 Transesophageal echocardiogram at ~120°; anterior mitral leaflet: 2.60 cm; posterior mitral leaflet: 1.49 cm. *Ao*, aorta; *LA*, left atrium; *LV*, left ventricle

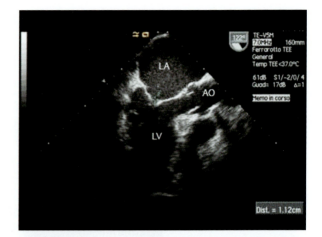

Fig. 2.55 Transesophageal echocardiogram at ~120°; coaptation distance: ~1 cm. *Ao*, aorta; *LA*, left atrium; *LV*, left ventricle

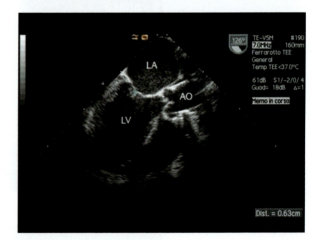

Fig. 2.56 Transesophageal echocardiogram at ~120°; coaptation length: 0.63 cm. *Ao*, aorta; *LA*, left atrium; *LV*, left ventricle

As regards MitraClip® implantation more specifically, if there is tethering the following exclusion criteria are considered:
- CD ≥11 mm (Fig. 2.55)
- CL <2 mm (Fig. 2.56).

In the case of MR due to coaptation alteration as a result of excess leaflet mobility (leaflet prolapse/flail), the parameters that need measuring are flail gap and flail width, [131, 138], with *flail* being a leaflet with a free tip, which passes the opposite leaflet during systole; *flail gap*, the maximum distance between the edge of the floating leaflet on the ventricular side and the tip of the opposite leaflet on the atrial side (measurement obtained by TEE in four-chamber view ~0°, intercommissural view ~60°, or outflow section at ~120°);

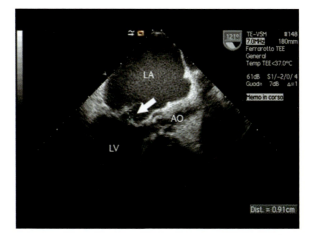

Fig. 2.57 Transesophageal echocardiogram at ~120°; flail gap <10 mm (*arrow*). *Ao*, aorta; *LA*, left atrium; *LV*, left ventricle

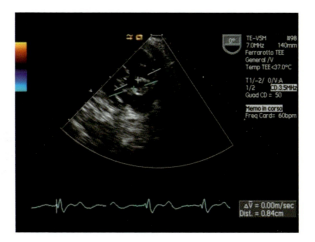

Fig. 2.58 Transesophageal echocardiogram at ~120°; flail width <10 mm

and *flail width*, the width of the floating segment measured along the coaptation line in short axis. The anatomical and morphological criteria for inclusion for MitraClip® implantation are a flail gap <10 mm (Fig. 2.57) and flail width <15 mm (Fig. 2.58).

2.2.4.3
Selection of Patients for Implantation

In addition to the anatomical eligibility criteria illustrated above, echocardiography also allows for search of the other parameters necessary to select an ideal

patient for percutaneous repair using MitraClip® [131, 139]. The exclusion criteria are:
- intracardial masses and/or thrombotic formations in the heart cavity (Figs. 2.59–2.61)
- prior mitral valve surgery (valvuloplasty or implantation of mechanical or biological device)
- patent foramen ovale (Fig. 2.62)
- prior implantation of an occlusive device in the atrium (Fig. 2.63)
- anatomical variants such as lipomatosis of the septum (Fig. 2.64), aneurysmal atrial septum, or hypoplasia or surgical closing of the left superior pulmonary vein; these should not be considered as absolute contraindications to the procedure, but the operator should be aware of them to decide the transseptal strategy or, as in the case of the pulmonary vein variants, to plan a different route for the catheters. Another condition, which can complicate the

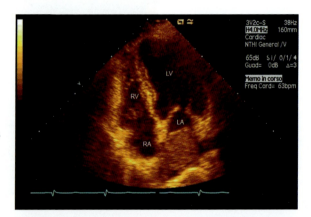

Fig. 2.59 Transthoracic echocardiogram; apical four-chamber view, presence of left atrial mass. *LA*, left atrium; *LV*, left ventricle; *RA*, right atrium; *RV*, right ventricle

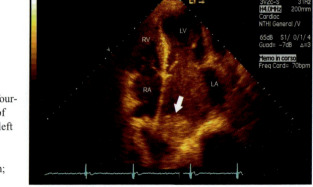

Fig. 2.60 Transthoracic echocardiogram. Apical four-chamber view, presence of thrombotic formation on left atrial roof (*white arrow*). *LA*, left atrium; *LV*, left ventricle; *RA*, right atrium; *RV*, right ventricle

2.2 Mitral Regurgitation

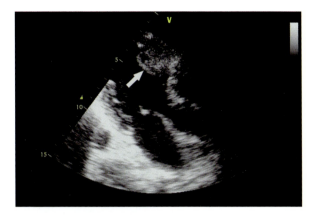

Fig. 2.61 Transthoracic echocardiogram. Apical three-chamber view, presence of thrombotic formation on anterior interventricular septum (*white arrow*)

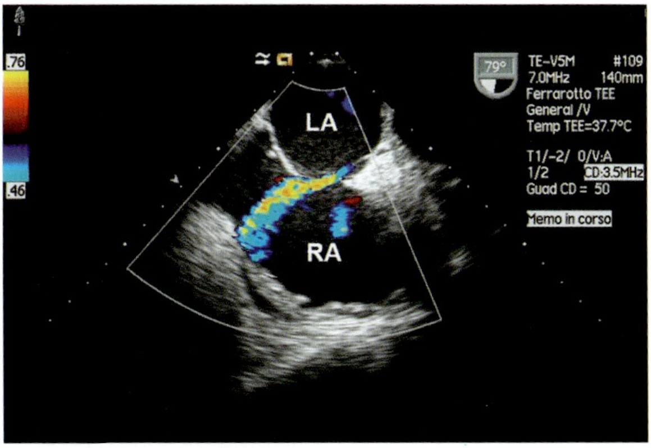

Fig. 2.62 Transesophageal echocardiogram at ~80°. Patent foramen ovale with left–right shunt at rest. *LA*, left atrium; *RA*, right atrium

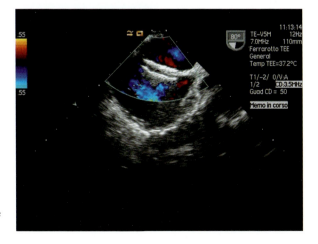

Fig. 2.63 Transesophageal echocardiogram at ~80°. Presence of occlusive device in interatrial septum

performance of the trans-septal strategy and needs to be signaled to the operator, is ectasia of the ascending aorta, aortic bulb, or sinuses of Valsalva. TEE should be used to assess the course of the ascending aorta (Fig. 2.65)
- hypertrophic cardiomyopathy and/or anterior systolic motion of a mitral leaflet (Fig. 2.66).

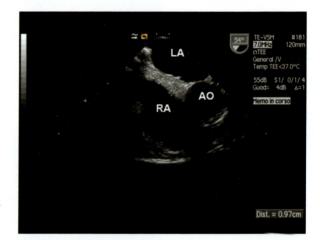

Fig. 2.64 Transesophageal echocardiogram at ~50°. Major thickening of interatrial septum. *Ao*, aorta; *LA*, left atrium; *RA*, right atrium

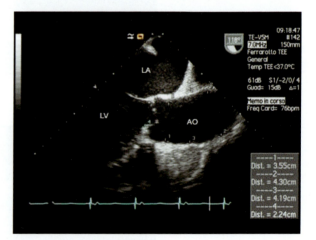

Fig. 2.65 Transesophageal echocardiogram at ~120°. Measurement of aortic annulus, bulb, sinuses of Valsalva, and ascending aorta. *Ao*, aorta; *LA*, left atrium; *LV*, left ventricle

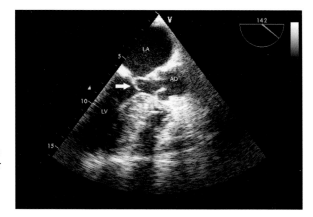

Fig. 2.66 Transesophageal echocardiogram at ~140°. View of anterior systolic motion of the anterior leaflet (*arrow*) in patient with major septal hypertrophy. *Ao*, aorta; *LA*, left atrium; *LV*, left ventricle

2.2.5 Percutaneous Therapy

Based on the results collected by the Euro Heart Survey [140], in order to treat the increasingly larger group of patients who are rejected for cardiac surgery due to the high surgical risk, the focus of research has shifted in recent years to the development of percutaneous techniques to treat MR, in order to restore valve function in a minimally invasive fashion, without any need for surgical incisions and extracorporeal circulation, and with a closed chest and beating heart.

The basic surgical concepts of annuloplasty and leaflet repair have been adapted for the development of catheter-based percutaneous approaches. These percutaneous approaches imitate aspects of the surgical procedures and are less invasive than the surgical alternatives. Transcatheter approaches for mitral repair have been implemented in clinical trials for the treatment of MR. Advances in both technique and development of novel devices have led to a variety of methods to treat MR using a percutaneous course.

Percutaneous techniques for transcatheter mitral valve repair include [141, 142] (Table 2.12):
- leaflets repair with edge-to-edge technique
- annulus remodeling using devices implanted in the coronary sinus device
- direct annuloplasty using a suture-based technique, or application of radio-frequency energy
- chamber remodeling using transventricular or transatrial devices.

Table 2.12 Overview of transcatheter mitral valve therapies

Device	Technology	Indication	Access	Trial	CAC[a]	Imaging
MitraClip®	Edge-to-edge repair	DMR or FMR	Trans-septal	EVEREST	(−)	E/F
MOBIUS Leaflet Repair System	Edge-to-edge repair	DMR or FMR	Trans-septal	Experimentation suspended	(−)	E/F
MONARC™ system	Coronary sinus device	FMR	RIJ vein (access to CS)	EVOLUTION	(+++)	F/E
CARILLON system	Coronary sinus device	FMR	RIJ vein (access to CS)	AMADEUS and TITAN	(+++)	F/E
PTMA device	Coronary sinus device	FMR	FMR (access to CS)	PTOLEMY	(+++)	F/E
Mitralign	Annuloplasty	DMR or FMR	FA (retrograde access to LV)	FIM	(−)	E/F
Quantum Cor™ radiofrequency technology	"Radiofrequency" annuloplasty	FMR	Under investigation (trans-septal)	Preclinical	(−)	Under investigation (ICE?)
AccuCinch™	"Suture" annuloplasty	FMR	RIJ vein (access to CS) and FA (retrograde access to LV)	Preclinical	(−)	E/F
Coapsys	Transventricular remodeling	FMR	Subxiphoid pericardial approach	VIVID	(++)	E/F
PS3 System™	Chamber and annulus remodeling	FMR	RIJ vein (access to CS) and trans-septal	Preclinical	(+)	F/E

[a]The number of + symbols indicates the potential for coronary artery occlusion with the device; + symbols indicate the greatest risk and a − symbol indicates no risk.

CAC, coronary artery compromise; *DMR*, degenerative mitral regurgitation; *FMR*, functional mitral regurgitation; *E*, echocardiography; *F*, fluoroscopy; *RIJ*, right internal jugular; *CS*, coronary sinus; *FA*, femoral artery; *LV*, left ventricle; *ICE*, intracardiac echocardiography

2.2.5.1 Leaflets Repair

The edge-to-edge repair has been used as a surgical technique in open-chest, arrested-heart surgery for the treatment of MR since the early 1990s [138,

143–145]. With this technique, a portion of the anterior leaflet is sutured to the corresponding portion of the posterior leaflet, creating a point of permanent coaptation ("approximation") of the two leaflets and resulting in a double-orifice [143–145]. More recently, several percutaneous methods to accomplish the double-orifice repair have been developed [131, 146, 147].

2.2.5.1.1
MitraClip®

The MitraClip® system (Fig. 2.67) consists on a catheter-based device designed to perform an edge-to-edge reconstruction of the insufficient mitral valve while the heart is beating, as an alternative to the conventional surgical approach. The MitraClip® system uses a tri-axial catheter system with an implantable clip.

The steerable guide catheter (SGC) is 24 Fr proximally and 22 Fr distally, and is delivered with an echogenic tapered dilator. A dial on the proximal end of the guide catheter allows deflection of the distal tip (Fig. 2.68).

The clip delivery system (CDS) has the MitraClip® attached to its distal end. This system uses two dials that permit medial-lateral and anteroposterior steering (Fig. 2.69).

The MitraClip® device (Fig 2.70) is a cobalt/chromium implant with two arms, covered with polyester fabric, pre-assembled to the tip of the disposable delivery catheter. On the inner portion of the clip are two "grippers" adjacent

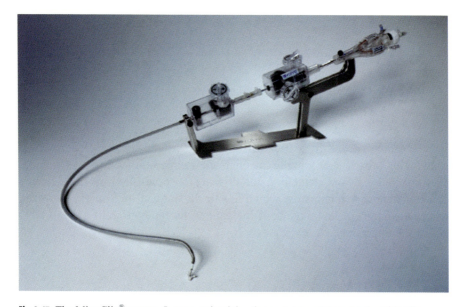

Fig. 2.67 The MitraClip® system. It uses a tri-axial catheter system with an implantable clip

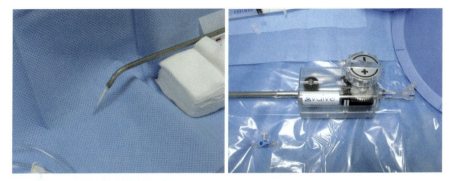

Fig. 2.68 The steerable guide catheter

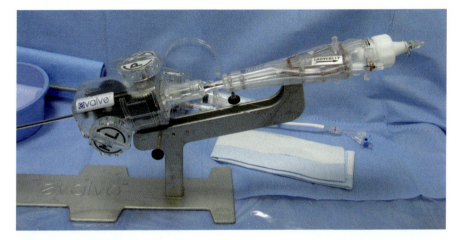

Fig. 2.69 The clip delivery system

to each arm to secure the leaflets as they are "captured" during closure of the arms. The clip has a locking mechanism to maintain closure. Opening, closing, locking, and detaching the clip are all controlled by the delivery catheter handle mechanisms, which are firmly lodged on a metal sterilized external support placed outside of the patient, on the bottom of a small table above the upper leg.

2.2 Mitral Regurgitation

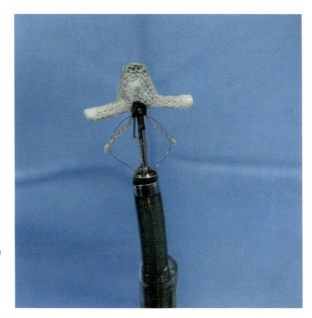

Fig. 2.70 The MitraClip® device. It consists of a cobalt/chromium device with two arms, each of which has two grippers, allowing for secure capture of the mitral leaflets

Procedure and Technical Aspects

Before initiating trans-septal catheterization, a pre-procedure TEE to confirm final eligibility is required. Before the procedure, all patients are administered a single dose of broad-spectrum antibiotic IV (intravenous) for prophylactic purposes. If a patient is on oral anticoagulant therapy, this must be put on hold for 3 days before the procedure to obtain an international normalized ratio (INR) ≤1.7, and replaced with heparin. If low molecular weight heparin (LMWH) is administered, it must be put on hold for 12 hours before the procedure, while unfractionated heparin (UFH) should be put on hold at least 4 hours before surgery. A loading dose of clopidogrel 300 mg is administered the day before the procedure.

The procedure is performed in the cardiac catheterization laboratory with echocardiography and fluoroscopic guidance while the patient is usually under general anesthesia. Emergency surgical back-up should be available for each procedure, because if complications arise during the procedure, it may be necessary to convert to an open surgical procedure. During the procedure, invasive arterial pressure is monitored through the radial or the femoral artery, and a central venous catheter is placed in the right internal jugular or subclavian vein. The right femoral vein is cannulated with a 7 Fr introducer sheath, and a baseline right heart catheterization is performed.

In order to evaluate the acute hemodynamic effects of the MitraClip® device, intracardiac pressure and flow measurements are performed at baseline and 10 minutes after device deployment (Box 2.3). Baseline activated clotting time

> **Box 2.3 Catheterization measurements obtained before clip implantation and ≥10 minutes post-clip deployment**
> - PCWP or left atrial pressure (a wave/v wave/mean pressure) with simultaneous left ventricular pressure
> - Pulmonary artery pressure (Systolic/Diastolic mean pressure)
> - Right atrial pressure
> - Left ventricular peak systolic and end-diastolic pressure
> - Systemic arterial pressure (S/D/mean)
> - Cardiac output

(ACT) has to be determined following venous access for the endovascular procedure. ACT and heparin administration should be recorded throughout the procedure and a final ACT level should be documented before leaving the catheterization laboratory

After the right catheterization is performed, the 7 Fr introducer is exchanged with an 8 Fr Mullins sheath over a 0.32 guidewire, and a trans-septal puncture is performed using a Brockenbrough needle under TEE guidance. This is a critical point of the procedure, because the puncture has to be located in the posterosuperior part of the interatrial septum in order to obtain enough room in the LA for a safe and optimal orientation of the steerable distal part of the CDS. Once the LA is entered with the 8 Fr sheath (Fig. 2.71), the left pulmonary vein is cannulated using a 6 Fr multipurpose catheter and a 260 cm Amplatz Super stiff guidewire is left in place (Fig. 2.71). Following trans-septal crossing, 100 IU/kg of UFH or alternative anticoagulation therapy is administered in accordance with standard hospital practice, maintaining an ACT of >250 s throughout the procedure. Then the 24 Fr guiding catheter is introduced into the LA and the dilator is carefully and slowly retrieved to avoid vacuum air bubbles. The delivery system is then advanced in the LA, and the distal steerable part is manipulated in the atrium for obtaining a perpendicular and central position with respect to the mitral valve leaflets' coaptation line (Fig. 2.71). Under echocardiography and fluoroscopic guidance, the clip is steered until axially aligned and centered over the origin of the regurgitant jet. The correct trajectory of the clip and the perpendicularity of the two arms with respect to the mitral leaflet coaptation line are checked using TEE standard views, described next.

Once the system has been aligned, the clip with opened arms is advanced into the left ventricle (Fig. 2.71), and under TEE guidance the arms grasp the leaflets. When a double orifice has been created and the echocardiography confirms regurgitation reduction and optimal and stable grasp of both leaflets, the clip arms are closed (Fig. 2.71), locked and detached, and the guiding

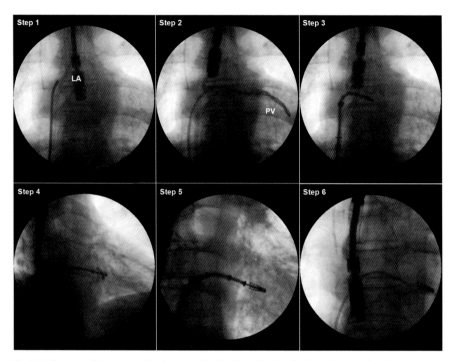

Fig. 2.71 Once the left atrium (*LA*) is entered with the 8 Fr sheath (Step 1), the left pulmonary vein (*PV*) is cannulated and a stiff guidewire is left in place (Step 2). Then the 24 Fr steerable guide catheter is introduced in the left atrium and the dilator is carefully and slowly retrieved to avoid vacuum air bubbles. The catheter delivery system is then advanced in the left atrium and the distal steerable part is manipulated in the atrium for obtaining a perpendicular and central position with respect to the mitral valve leaflet's coaptation line (Step 3). Once the system has been aligned, the clip with opened arms is advanced into the left ventricle (Step 4), and, under transesophageal guidance, the arms grasp the leaflets. When a double orifice has been created and the echocardiography confirms regurgitation reduction and optimal and stable grasp of both leaflets, the clip arms are closed (Step 5), locked, and detached, and the steerable guide catheter and clip delivery system are withdrawn (Step 6)

catheter and delivery system are withdrawn (Fig. 2.71). If the position is judged suboptimal by TEE evaluation, the clip can be reopened and repositioned; if the clip must be withdrawn into the LA, the arms may be inverted in the ventricle, providing a smooth profile for retraction to prevent entangling the *chordae tendineae* (Fig. 2.72). When necessary, for example in the case of degenerative MR or ruptured *chordae tendineae* with wide prolapse, a second clip can be implanted, paying attention to positioning it very closely to the first implanted clip (Fig. 2.73). While the implantation of a second clip is predictable when a flail is present, the need for a second clip in other scenarios is evaluated on a

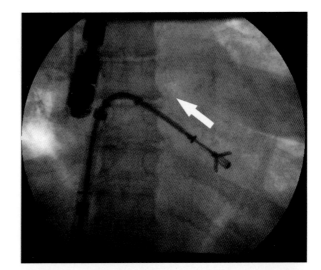

Fig. 2.72 Re-opening and repositioning of a clip judged by transesophageal echocardiography to be suboptimally deployed. The *arrow* shows the direction of clip retraction into the LA

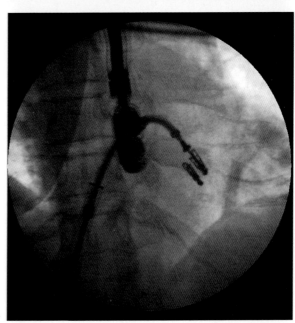

Fig. 2.73 In selected cases, a second clip can be implanted, paying attention to positioning it very close to the first implanted one

case-by-case basis. Right cardiac catheterization is finally performed to record the post-procedural pressure and the final results (Fig. 2.74). The guiding catheter is removed, ACT control is performed, heparin reversal with protamine sulfate is started, and venous femoral access is closed using a "figure-of-eight" superficial stitch (Fig. 2.75) [144].

2.2 Mitral Regurgitation

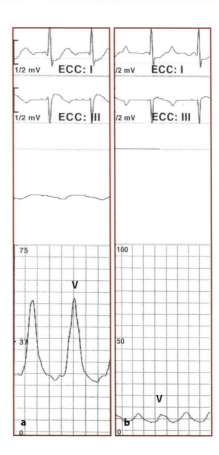

Fig. 2.74 Pulmonary wedge pressure recorded in basal condition shows a high V wave (**a**) secondary to severe mitral regurgitation. After clip implantation, the V wave is reduced (**b**). The parallel A wave reduction indicates diminished end-diastolic pressure. These variations in aggregate result in diminished mean wedge pressure after clip implantation

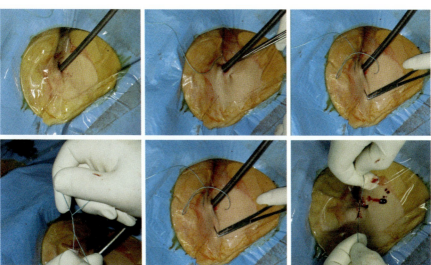

Fig. 2.75 Venous femoral access closing with a "figure-of-eight" superficial stitch

Post-procedural pharmacologic management includes aspirin 100 mg lifelong, and clopidogrel 75 mg for three months in patients without atrial fibrillation. Patients with atrial fibrillation are prescribed aspirin 100 mg and oral vitamin K antagonists.

Intraoperative Echocardiography Monitoring During MitraClip® Implantation

TEE during the procedure provides guidance to the operator and makes it possible to obtain information on the morphofunctional characteristics of the mitral valve, and to assess the degree of regurgitation and biventricular function (Fig 2.76), as well as the immediate result, and to exclude any complications.

Four views are mainly used during the procedure, and these are defined *"key views"*:

- *mid-esophageal view* (~0–90°), for the study (Fig. 2.77) of the inter-atrial septum (IAS) and to follow the catheters during the trans-septal approach and LA movements
- *two-chamber intercommissural view* (~60°), showing the anterolateral and posteromedial commissure and part of the mitral valve scallops (P3–A2–P1). This view allows for the mid-lateral (ML) orientation of the system
- *low-axis mid-esophageal view* (~120–150°), also defined as left ventricular outflow tract (LVOT) view. This view shows the P2–A2 scallops in addition to the aortic bulb and part of the ascending aorta. This view allows for the anteroposterior orientation of the system
- *transgastric short-axis view* (~0–30°), which shows the mitral valve in short axis. This view is essential to guide the clip perpendicularly to the coaptation line. (Fig. 2.78).

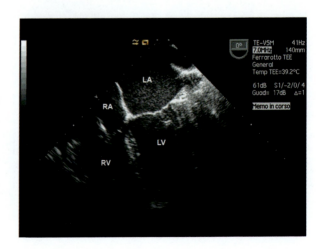

Fig. 2.76 Transesophageal echocardiogram at 0°. Apical four-chamber view. *LA*, left atrium; *LV*, left ventricle; *RA*, right atrium; *RV*, right ventricle

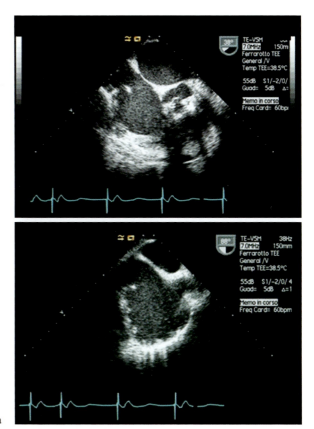

Fig. 2.77 Transthoracic echocardiogram at 0–90°. View for interatrial septum, aorta, and superior vena cava

The procedure can hence be illustrated in five basic steps:
1. performance of trans-septal puncture
2. axial orientation of the system
3. grasping of leaflets
4. post-grasping assessment
5. clip release.

Step 1 – performance of trans-septal puncture: in this procedure, the trans-septal puncture is a key moment and the puncture site is *"precise"* so fluoroscopic guidance and/or touch alone cannot be relied upon, as is the case, for instance, in mitral percutaneous valvuloplasty. A puncture of the septum in the posterior and superior position is required at about 4 cm above the mitral annular plane (Fig. 2.79). This distance is also important in degenerative diseases with a prolapsing leaflet. The catheter is visualized in all the views, in order to accurately find the point where the catheter is wedged inside the septum (Fig. 2.80), causing what is known as the "tenting effect", and to follow the

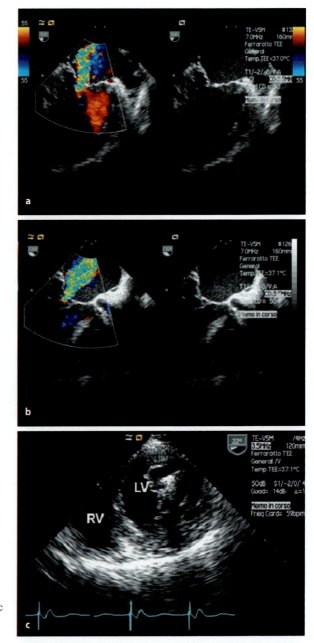

Fig. 2.78 Transesophageal echocardiogram at 0–180°. Intercommissural view (**a**), long axis (**b**) and transgastric short axis (**c**). *RV*, right ventricle; *LV*, left ventricle

needle until it passes the septum and enters the LA. A small quantity of saline solution is injected to confirm placement. After trans-septal puncture, TEE guides the catheters into the LA and the placement of the guiding catheter in the pulmonary vein (Fig. 2.81).

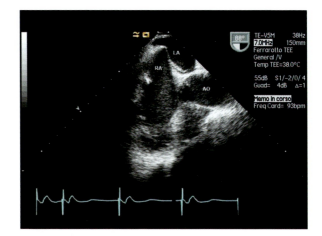

Fig. 2.79 Transesophageal echocardiogram at 90°. View with catheter wedged at ~4 cm from the valve. *Ao*, aorta; *LA*, left atrium; *RA*, right atrium

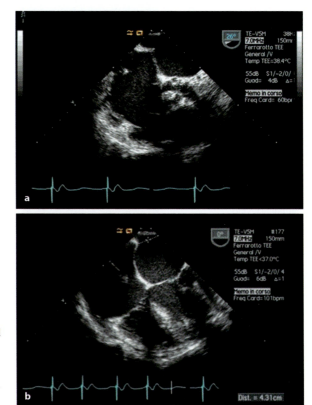

Fig. 2.80 Transesophageal echocardiogram. **a** Off axis view: relation of trans-septal needle compared to aorta. **b** 4-chamber view: distance between trans-septal puncture and mitral valvular plane

A radio-opaque and echogenic ring identifies the tip of the guiding catheter. The clip is advanced through this guidewire. The tip of the clip should be sought in the upper short-axis view, to avoid contact with the lateral and posterior walls of the LA (Fig. 2.82).

Step 2 – axial orientation of the system: once trans-septal puncture has been performed, the next step is the axial alignment of the clip perpendicularly to the mitral valve annular plane and parallel to the antegrade flow direction. The course of the system must be carefully followed by TEE to ensure proper passage into the LV and proper clip placement. The clip is oriented with small motions. Two useful views are those already described above:
- *LVOT long-axis view*, allowing anteroposterior clip orientation (Fig. 2.83)
- *intercommissural view*, allowing medial-lateral clip orientation (Fig. 2.84).

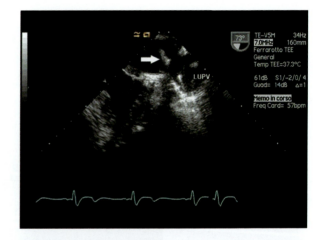

Fig. 2.81 Transesophageal echocardiogram at ~70°. Catheter in left superior pulmonary vein (*white arrow*). *LUPV*, left upper pulmonary vein

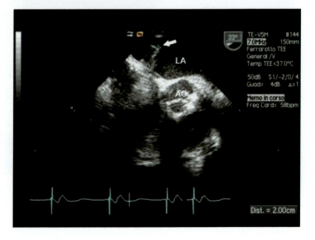

Fig. 2.82 Transesophageal echocardiogram at ~33°. Off-axis view: catheter measurement through the septum. *Ao*, aorta; *LA*, left atrium; *arrow*, catheter

2.2 Mitral Regurgitation

TEE makes it possible to closely follow the descent of the clip in the LV through the mitral valve (Fig. 2.85). Clip alignment perpendicular to the coaptation line is performed in transgastric short-axis view. This view is also used for further movements in either the anteroposterior or lateromedial direction (Fig. 2.86).

Step 3 – grasping of leaflets: once the device is satisfactorily oriented, both leaflets should be anchored, usually in long-axis LVOT view (120°) to better visualize the two leaflets. Special attention must be paid to proper insertion of the leaflets inside the clip to prevent embolism or device detachment. If grasping is inadequate, the clip can be released and repositioned. TEE is used not only to guide anchorage, but also to check grasping in the various views (Fig. 2.87).

Step 4 – post-grasping assessment: after checking the anchoring of both leaflets, residual MR and the transmitral diastolic gradient should be assessed

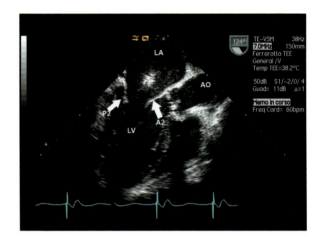

Fig. 2.83 Transesophageal echocardiogram at ~130°. LVOT long-axis view. *Ao*, aorta; *LA*, left atrium; *LV*, left ventricle

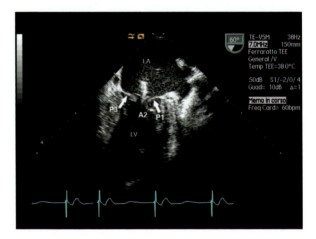

Fig. 2.84 Transesophageal echocardiogram at ~60°. Intercommissural two-chamber view, system orientation. *LA*, left atrium; *LV*, left ventricle

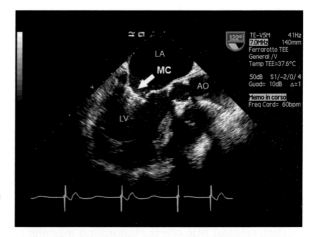

Fig. 2.85 Transesophageal echocardiogram at ~120°. LVOT long-axis view, insertion of MitraClip® (*MC*) in left ventricle (*LV*). *LA*, left atrium; *Ao*, aorta

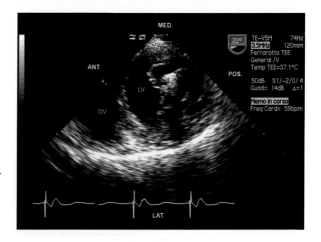

Fig. 2.86 Transesophageal echocardiogram at ~20°. Transgastric short-axis view. *ANT*, anterior; *LAT*, lateral; *LV*, left ventricle; *MED*, medial; *POS*, posterior; *RV*, right ventricle

with the aid of color Doppler before releasing the clip. Double-orifice insertion should be checked in both the intercommissural and short-axis views (Fig. 2.88). If the result is not satisfactory, the leaflets are released and the clip is repositioned. An adequate grasp of both mitral leaflets does not ensure an acceptable reduction in the degree of MR. It can also be due to suboptimal placement of the clip compared to the jet's origin, or to capture of the *chordae* or margin of the leaflets by the clip's arms, and it requires the placement of a second clip. Therefore, careful assessment of residual MR is carried out before releasing the clip. With the clip in situ, the regurgitant jet can become highly eccentric. It is absolutely mandatory that the Nyquist limits and color gain are identical to the initial assessments if there is no residual, as these factors may affect jet size.

Step 5 – clip release: after adequate reduction in the degree of regurgitation, the clip is released and the system and guidewire are withdrawn (Fig. 2.89).

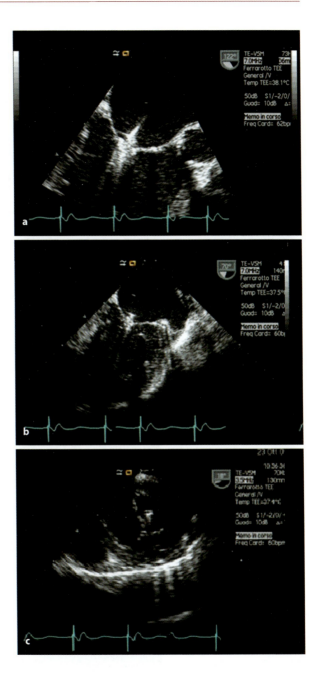

Fig. 2.87 Transesophageal echocardiogram. LVOT long-axis view (**a**), intercommissural (**b**) and transgastric short axis (**c**)

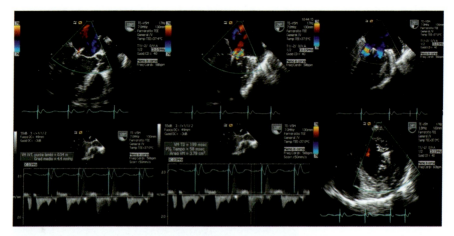

Fig. 2.88 Transesophageal echocardiogram. Assessment of residual MR, flow area, mitral gradient, and double orifice during diastole

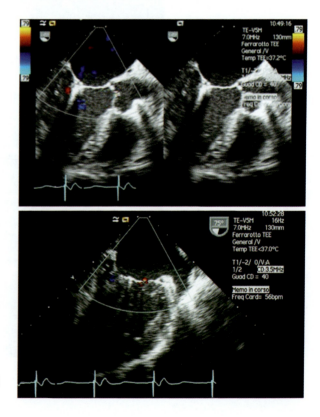

Fig. 2.89 Clip release and evaluation of residual mitral regurgitation

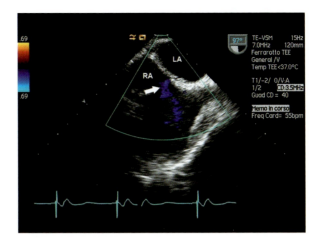

Fig. 2.90 Transesophaeal echocardiogram at ~90°. Assessment of any residual shunt (*arrow*). *LA*, left atrium; *RA*, right atrium

The data obtained from echocardiography are compared with the hemodynamic and angiographic data.

TEE also assesses whether there are any complications, focusing mainly on the detection of pericardial effusion and residual interatrial shunt after trans-septal puncture (Fig. 2.90).

Complications
The potential acute complications of this procedure are:
- *access site complications*, mainly related to the use of large-sized introducers (24 Fr)
- *complications related to trans-septal puncture* (pericardial effusion/cardiac tamponade). The puncture must be performed in the posterosuperior region of the interatrial septum, as already described; therefore, in situations marked by abnormal anatomy (e.g. large right atrium, kyphoscoliosis, bowed septum, aortic aneurysm), there is a greater risk associated with the trans-septal puncture
- *cerebrovascular events (stroke or TIA)*, following thromboembolism or gas embolism during the passage of catheters into the LA after trans-septal puncture
- *trauma to the mitral valve*, with risk of insult to the leaflets and *chordae tendineae*, during insertion of the delivery catheter in the LV and during device alignment and grasping maneuvers
- *clip detachment*, either partial or total, with embolization
- *worsening of MR*, due to improper device placement.

Results

Data on the safety and durability of the MitraClip® system were successfully reported in the initial EVEREST (Endovascular Valve Edge-to-edge Repair Study) Trial [131, 148]. A total of 107 patients were treated. In that cohort, 62% of patients were older than 65 years, 62% of patients were male, mean EF was 62%, and functional etiology accounted for 21% of patients. Acute procedural success was obtained in 74% of patients, and 64% were discharged with MR ≤1+. Ten (9%) had a major adverse events, including one non-procedural death (Table 2.13). Kaplan–Meier freedom from death was 95.9%, 94.0%, and 90.1%, and Kaplan–Meier freedom from surgery was 88.5%, 83.2%, and 76.3% at 1, 2, and 3 years, respectively. The composite primary efficacy endpoint (freedom from MR >2+, freedom from cardiac surgery for valve dysfunction, and freedom from death at 12 months) was 66%; at 24 and 36 months it was 65% and 63%, respectively. The 23 patients with functional MR had similar acute results and durability [148]. No clip embolization occurred at any time point. Partial clip detachment, defined as detachment of a single leaflet from the clip, occurred in 10 patients (9%). It occurred in three patients during the procedure, in one patient before hospital discharge, and in five patients between discharge and 30 days. In just one patient, a partial clip detachment was observed after 30 days. Mitral stenosis was not a problem [146]. Even when a clip was placed and surgery was required, subsequent surgical repair was possible after clip placement [149].

EVEREST II, a pivotal trial, will randomize patients with degenerative or functional MR ≥2+ to MitraClip® versus mitral valve surgery (2:1) [148, 150].

The study results have recently been disclosed [150a]. The primary safety endpoint was the occurrence of major adverse cardiac events at 30 days, including death, major stroke, re-operation of the mitral valve, urgent/emergent cardiovascular surgery, MI, renal failure, deep wound infection, ventilation >48 hours, new-onset permanent atrial fibrillation, septicemia, gastrointestinal complication requiring surgery and all transfusions >2 units. The primary effi-

Table 2.13 EVEREST Major adverse events at 30 days

Major adverse events	Number of patients
Death (related to clip)	0
Death (unrelated to clip)	1
Myocardial infarction	0
Stroke	1
Renal failure	0
Non-elective cardiac surgery (trans-septal complication)	2
Re-operation for failed surgery	1
Septicemia	0
Trasfusion ≥2 units of blood	5
Total major adverse events (patients)	10

cacy endpoint was clinical success rate defined as freedom from the combined outcome of death, mitral valve surgery or re-operation for valve dysfunction, and MR > 2+ at 12 months. A total of 184 patients were allocated to the device group and 95 were allocated to the control group. The primary safety endpoint met the superiority hypothesis (device group 9.6% versus control group 57.0%, p for superiority < 0.0001), while the primary efficacy endpoint met the non-inferiority hypothesis (device group 72.4% versus control group 87.8%, p for noninferiority < 0.0001).

Preliminary data of the High Risk Registry, collected from 78 patients enrolled in EVEREST II to assess the ability of the MitraClip® system to improve the clinical status of high-risk patients undergoing percutaneous repair for MR ≥3+ (59% affected by FMR, 41% by degenerative MR), show a 96% implant success rate; 2.6% partial clip detachment versus 9.3% incidence among patients of the preliminary cohort (n = 107); and a 30-day mortality of 7.7%. Major adverse events are shown in Table 2.14. At 30 days, 82% and 79% of patients with FMR and DMR respectively, had MR ≤2+; at 12 months 79% of patients with FMR and 75% of patients with DMR had MR ≤2+. Kaplan–Meier freedom from death was 76.4% at 12 months [151].

Preliminary studies yet to be published on reverse left ventricular remodeling in 49 out of 79 patients with MR ≤2+ at discharge and at 12 months show a significant reduction in left ventricular telediastolic and telesystolic volumes, LV mass and sphericity indices, and an improvement in the LVEF. In addition, no dilation of the septal-lateral annular dimension has been observed (Table 2.15) [152, 153].

In a study from Franzen et al., mitral valve repair using the MitraClip® system was shown to be feasible in 51 consecutive patients at high surgical risk with symptomatic functional [n = 35 (69%)] or organic MR [n = 16 (31%)] [153a]. Mean logistic EuroSCORE was 29 ± 22%; Society of Thoracic Surgeons (STS) score was 15 ± 11. MitraClip® implantation was successful in 49 patients (96%). Most patients [n = 34/49 (69%)] were treated with a single clip, whereas 14 patients (29%) received two clips and one patient received three clips. Forty-four of the 49 successfully treated patients (90%) showed clinical improvement at

Table 2.14 Major adverse events in High Risk Registry patients

Major adverse events (MAE)	Number of patients (%)
Death	6
Myocardial infarction	0
Stroke	0
Renal failure	0
Permanent atrial fibrillation	1
Ventilation >48 hours	1
Trasfusion ≥2 units of blood	11
Total major adverse events (patients)	19

Table 2.15 Data of reverse left ventricular remodeling from the preliminary EVEREST cohort

Echo parameters (number of patients)	Baseline	12 months	P value
Mitral regurgitation grade (49)	3.1	1.4	<0.0001
LVEDVI, ml/m^2 (47)	89	74	<0.0001
LVESVI ml/m^2 (47)	36	31	0.0007
Sphericity index (47)	0.62	0.59	0.01
Left ventricle mass, g (43)	182	158	0.0001
Septal lateral systolic annular dimension, mm (26)	3.7	3.8	NS
Septal lateral diastolic annular dimension, mm (26)	3.3	3.3	NS
LVEF, % (47)	60	58	NS
Forward stroke volume, ml (43)	59	68	<0.0001

LVEDVI, left ventricular end-diastolic volume index; *LVESVI*, left ventricular end-systolic volume index; *LVEF*, left ventricular ejection fraction

discharge [NYHA functional class ≥III in 48 patients (98%) before and 16 patients (33%) after the procedure (P < 0.0001)]. There were no procedure-related major adverse events and no in-hospital mortalities.

Italian Experience

Thirty-one patients (age 71 years, male 81%) were treated with the MitraClip® system between August 2008 and July 2009 in Italy in two centers, namely Ferrarotto Hospital (FH) of Catania and San Raffaele Hospital (SRH) of Milan [152]. Eighteen patients (58%) presented with functional disease and 13 patients (42%) with organic degenerative disease (P2 prolapse/flail 26%; bi-leaflets prolapsed/flail 10%; A2 prolapse/flail 6%). Among patients with functional MR, 67% had a previous history of coronary artery disease. Logistic EuroSCORE and STS scores were 14.3 ± 11.9% and 10.3 ± 8.8%, respectively. Mean pulmonary and wedge pressures assessed by right catheterization were 25.2 ± 10.8 and 18.4 ± 9.1 mmHg, respectively. Twenty-one procedures were performed at one site (FH) and ten at the other site (SRH). General anesthesia was employed in all patients except one, who was treated under a deep conscious sedation because of contraindications to anesthetic drugs. One clip was successfully implanted in each of 19 patients (61%) and two clips in each of 12 patients (39%). In no case was clip implantation unsuccessful. The etiology of MR was degenerative in 10% of patients who required one clip and 58% of patients who required two clips. There was no procedural mortality. Major adverse events (MAEs), defined as the composite of death, MI, non-elective cardiac surgery for adverse events, renal failure, transfusion of >2 units of blood, ventilation for >48 hours, deep wound infection, septicemia, and new onset of atrial fibrillation, occurred in two patients at 30 days, resulting in a primary safety endpoint of 93.6%. One patient, a 76-year-old man with thrombocytopenia and renal failure, and who was on hemodialysis, died two weeks after the procedure, from gastrointestinal bleeding. Another patient experienced

2.2 Mitral Regurgitation

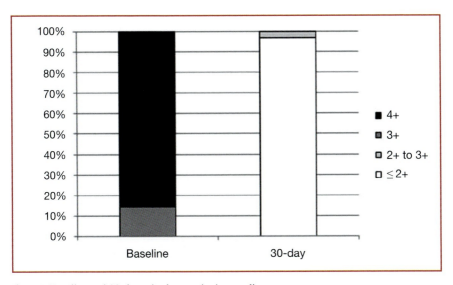

Fig. 2.91 Baseline and 30-day mitral regurgitation grading

intraprocedural cardiac tamponade, after trans-septal puncture, requiring surgical subxiphoid drainage and blood transfusion. Despite this complication, the clip was implanted successfully. No patient underwent emergency cardiac surgery for a failed clip implantation. No cases of clip detachment or embolization were observed. There were no other complications, including access site bleedings and transient ischemic attacks.

Acute device success was observed in 30 of 31 patients (Fig. 2.91). At 30 days, of the 28 patients with MR = 4+ before the procedure, 18 (58%) had MR graded as trivial to mild (0 to 1+), 9 (29%) had a MR graded as mild to moderate (1 to 2+), and 1 patient had MR graded as moderate to severe (2 to 3+). This latter patient was treated with two clips for degenerative MR. All three patients with MR = 3+ before the procedure had MR graded as trivial to mild (0 to 1+) at 30 days.

At baseline, NYHA functional class was I/II in 13% of patients and III/IV in 87% of patients. Thirty days after the procedure, all patients (100%) were in NYHA functional class I/II. Clinical symptoms were improved in all patients. In none of the patients was the dosage of diuretics increased after the procedure. Compared with baseline, diastolic left ventricular diameter, left ventricular volume, and annular septal–lateral dimension significantly diminished at 30 days. The mitral valve area by planimetry was 4.4 ±1.1 cm^2 at baseline and 2.8 ± 0.5 cm^2 at 30 days ($P < 0.001$). Systolic left atrial dimension and LVEF did not vary significantly.

2.2.5.1.2
Other Devices

The Edwards MOBIUS Leaflet Repair System (Edwards Lifesciences Inc.) uses a stitch, in 4-0 polypropylene, to create a double-orifice mitral valve (Fig. 2.92). The procedure is performed under intracardiac echocardiography and fluoroscopy [154] and a standard trans-septal approach is required to access the LA with a 10 Fr catheter. When the therapy catheter captures the free edges of the mitral valve, a 7 Fr fastener catheter deploys a nitinol suture clip and cuts the excess suture (Fig. 2.93). In the case of inadequate results, it is possible to remove the suture before deploying the clip. Feasibility studies in animals have provided encouraging results [155]. Acute procedural success of the first 15 patients treated with the MOBIUS system was present in 9 patients (60%). The degree of MR improved from a mean grade of 4+ to 2+ at discharge. At 30-day follow-up, the stitch was successfully in place with a significant reduction of MR in six patients (40%). However, because of poor intermediate durability results, further experimentation with the MOBIUS system has been suspended.

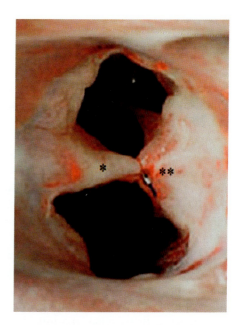

Fig. 2.92 Animal pathology specimen of the mitral valve with suture clip resulting in a double-orifice mitral valve. The * indicates the anterior mitral valve leaflet and ** the posterior leaflet

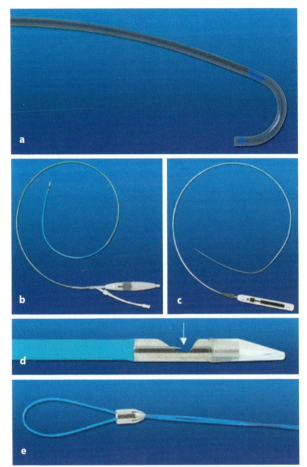

Fig. 2.93 a The 17 Fr guide catheter; **b** the 10 Fr therapy catheter; **c** the 7 Fr fastener catheter; **d** the end of therapy catheter with an orifice (*white arrow*) used to suction the mitral leaflet and deliver the suture; **e** nitinol suture-clip

2.2.5.2
Transcatheter Coronary Sinus Techniques

The stronghold of surgical therapy for MR has been ring reduction annuloplasty, either as a stand-alone treatment for MR or in conjunction with mitral leaflet repair [156]. Observation of the relationship of the coronary sinus to the mitral annulus has allowed development of transcatheter annuloplasty approaches [157]. Transcatheter coronary sinus techniques are performed through the right internal jugular vein, using reshaping devices implanted in the distal coronary sinus or great cardiac vein and in the coronary sinus ostium, to reduce the septal–lateral dimensions of the mitral annulus. The spatial relationship between the coronary sinus and mitral valve annulus plays a crucial role in these procedures [158]. A variety of devices delivered via a transjugular approach can be placed into the coronary sinus.

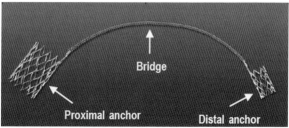

Fig. 2.94 The Edwards MONARC™ system: fully expanded distal and proximal anchoring self-expanding stents

2.2.5.2.1
MONARC™

The MONARC™ system (Edwards, Irvine, CA) is a catheter-deployed device consisting of nitinol (nickel–titanium alloy), and is inserted in the coronary sinus via the venous system (Fig. 2.94). The device is deployed in the coronary sinus vein, from the sinus ostium at the right atrium to the anterior interventricular vein (AIV). The device consists of two self-expanding stents that act as anchors at the AIV and at the entrance of the coronary sinus vein, and a connecting spring-like bridge with bioabsorbable suturing acting as a temporary spacer within the coil. The coil is designed to shorten the implanted device length as the bioabsorbable parts dissolve (gradually within 6 weeks), which results in shortening of the posterior portion of the mitral valve annulus that is in close proximity, thereby improving mitral valve coaptation in patients with functional MR. The rest of the mitral annulus is anatomically limited by the aortic and the tricuspid valves, and is therefore considered as a fixed portion, thereby allowing reduction of the total annular dimension by exerting compression from the direction of the coronary sinus [159, 160].

The Procedure
The procedures with the Edwards MONARC™ system are currently (2009–2010) performed within the EVOLUTION (EValuation Of the Edwards Lifesciences percUTaneous mItral annulOplasty system for the treatment of mitral regurgitatioN) II multicenter study [160–162]. Patients with symptomatic functional MR of 3–4/4 severity can be accepted for implantation after the relative anatomy of the coronary sinus and the circumflex/ramus/diagonal arteries are defined by coronary angiography and/or computed tomography (CT) scan and after the risk of significant coronary artery compression by the device is defined and considered non-existent. The procedure is performed in the cardiac catheterization laboratory without general anesthesia and without echocardiography monitoring. Access to the right internal jugular vein (12 Fr sheath) and a femoral artery (6 Fr sheath) is obtained. Coronary angiography is first performed and then a 12 Fr specially curved guiding sheath with its dilator is

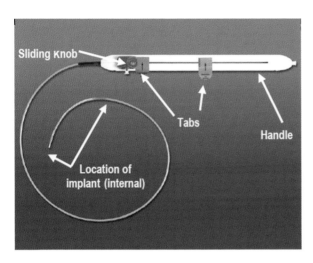

Fig. 2.95 Device characteristics. Delivery catheter used for placement and release of the stents via the hand-controlled retraction of a sliding knob. Access is provided via a specially curved jugular venous sheath. The current generation device includes a blunt curve on the free distal edge of the proximal anchor stent. Biodegradable components of the bridge allow its shortening within weeks of the implantation procedure

advanced in the right atrium and the dilator is removed. The coronary sinus ostium is located and engaged with manipulation of the guide catheter and with verification with contrast injections through its side port, and a guidewire is advanced inside the coronary sinus (usually the Magic Torque^{TM} or the hydrophilic ZIPwire^{TM}, Boston Scientific). The guide catheter is then advanced over the guidewire inside the coronary sinus, and simultaneous left coronary and coronary sinus angiography is performed in the LAO (left anterior oblique) and RAO (right anterior oblique) projections to delineate the courses of the AIV and the ramus, diagonal, and left anterior descending arteries. A higher-definition angiogram of the venous circulation is obtained if a Swan–Ganz catheter is advanced in the coronary sinus and its balloon is inflated before the contrast injection; this way most of the dye is successfully directed away from the blood flow direction, which allows delineation of the anterior interventricular vein. Typically, this allows a good-quality frame that can be used a "roadmap", and the wire can be directed carefully and successfully in the anterior interventricular venous system. Then a calibration guide catheter (Aurous Centimeter Sizing catheter, Cook Medical) is advanced over the wire, with its distal tip reaching the intended landing location for the distal stent of the device in the triangle of Brocq and Mouchet at the proximal part of the AIV. Angiography of the coronary sinus through the calibration guide catheter allows for measurement of the length of the coronary sinus and selection of the device length (100–160 mm) and stent diameters. Then the selected device (9 Fr) is flushed and advanced over the guidewire to the intended location, and the distal stent is released by slowly pulling the handle of the device, which withdraws its cover sheath (Figs. 2.94 and 2.95). After the distal stent is deployed, the device is pulled back with its proximal stent almost entirely outside of the coronary

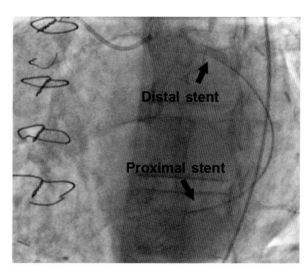

Fig. 2.96 The Edwards MONARC™ device implanted. The distal stent is typically in some proximity to diagonal branches; it should stay away from the left anterior descending artery, and the bridge should not cross a major non-bypassed obtuse marginal branch, due to the possibility of progressive compression of these arteries as a result of bridge shortening and the related tension of the coronary sinus on adjacent structures

sinus in the right atrium, and then it is rapidly released. The constant pull force before the release of the proximal stent takes all the slack out of the system so that the bridge coil confronts the inner surface of the coronary sinus arc that is in proximity to the mitral valve annulus. At the deployment of the proximal stent, the device springs this stent back in to anchor at the entrance of the coronary sinus. Finally, the position of the fully deployed device (Fig. 2.96) is checked with coronary sinus angiography through the guide catheter.

Results
The earlier EVOLUTION I trial was a prospective, multicenter feasibility study with the primary objective to evaluate the acute safety of the MONARC™ system in treating functional MR in heart failure patients, and a secondary objective to evaluate the reduction in MR by at least one grade at 90 days. Seventy-two patients with functional MR grade 2 to 4/4 and appropriate coronary sinus dimensions were enrolled, and the device was implanted in 59 of them. The cumulative event (death, cardiac tamponade, device migration and/or embolization, coronary sinus thrombosis, or pulmonary embolism) rates at 1, 6, 12, and 24 months were 9%, 17%, 19% and 28% respectively. Table 2.16 summarizes the prespecified safety analysis individual event rates at 90 days. The MR responders (reduction of MR by at least one grade) were 41% at 1 year and 47% at 2 years. However, the MR responders among those who had grade 3 to 4/4 at baseline (n = 5) was 100% at 1 year and 80% at 2 years. Furthermore, significant improvements in the NYHA functional status and in many echocardiographic indices of the MR (such as MR grade, mitral valve diameter, LV end-diastolic and end-systolic volumes) were observed, mainly in the subset with baseline MR of at least 3+. Therefore, further research with this device

Table 2.16 Event rates at 90 days after MONARC™ system implant

Clinical event	n (%)
Cardiac tamponade	2 (2.8)
Device migration	1 (1.4)
Device embolization	0 (0.0)
Coronary sinus thrombosis	0 (0.0)
Pulmonary embolism	1 (1.4)
Myocardial infarction	2 (2.8)
Death	5 (6.9)

focuses solely on patients with MR of 3–4+ and the surveillance criteria to avoid crossing (and risk of subsequent compression) of a significant arterial breach of the lateral wall have been heightened.

The EVOLUTION II trial is based on the above two contingencies and is currently ongoing with the primary safety endpoint the individual rate of death, MI (Q wave or non-Q wave having total creatine kinase [CK] >2× normal with any CK-MB > normal, or elevated troponin above the institution's upper level) and cardiac tamponade at 30 days, and the primary efficacy endpoint the percentage of subjects with an at least one-grade reduction in the severity of MR evaluated at 6 months as compared to baseline via TTE examination by an independent echocardiography core laboratory (Columbia University Medical Center, New York, USA). Enrolment in the trial includes angiographic and/or tomographic evaluation of the anatomic relationship between the lateral wall (diagonal, ramus, or obtuse marginal) and coronary braches, and evaluation of the MR severity and mechanism by independent analysis at the core laboratories before patient enrolment. Hence, a very careful patient screening is undertaken and no procedure can be performed on an ad hoc basis immediately after the first angiography hospitalization [160–162].

2.2.5.2.2
CARILLON

The CARILLON device (Cardiac Dimensions, Kirkland, Washington DC, USA) is a device placed in the coronary sinus via a jugular venous approach (Fig. 2.97) [157, 163]. It consists of a nitinol wire-shaping ribbon between proximal and distal figure-of-eight shaped anchors (Fig. 2.98) that are placed with one in the distal coronary sinus and one near the coronary sinus ostium. The distal anchor is released from the guide catheter and the catheter is pulled upward, resulting in tension on the coronary sinus with resultant shortening of the circumference of the coronary sinus.

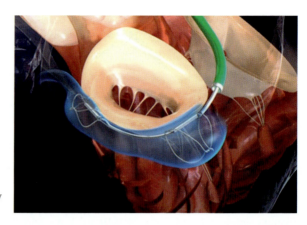

Fig. 2.97 The CARILLON device placed in the coronary sinus

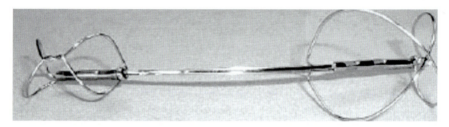

Fig. 2.98 The CARILLON Mitral Contour System consists of a proximal and distal helical anchor connected by a curved nitinol bridge

Patients with dilated cardiomyopathy, moderate to severe functional MR, EF <40%, and a six-minute walk distance between 150 and 450 m were enrolled in the CARILLON Mitral Annuloplasty Device European Union Study (AMADEUS). Of the 48 patients enrolled in the trial, 30 received the CARILLON device. Eighteen patients did not receive a device because of access issues, insufficient acute MR reduction, or coronary artery compromise. The major adverse event rate was 13% at 30 days. At 6 months, the degree of MR reduction among five different quantitative echocardiography measures ranged from 22% to 32%. Exercise tolerance, evaluated with the six-minute walking test, improved significantly at 6 months [164].

2.2.5.2.3
PTMA Device

A third technology that uses the coronary sinus route is the percutaneous transvenous mitral annuloplasty (PTMA) device (Viacor, Wilmington, MA, USA)

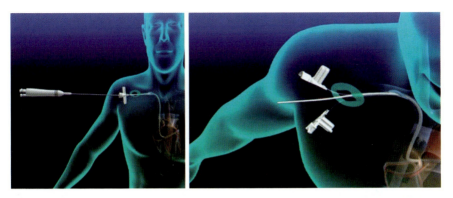

Fig. 2.99 Percutaneous subclavian access to insert the percutaneous transvenous mitral annuloplasty (PTMA) device

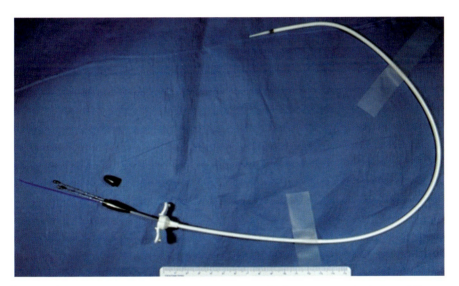

Fig. 2.100 The percutaneous mitral annuloplasty device (PTMA) consists of a 7 Fr multilumen delivery catheter that is placed in the coronary sinus. Up to three rods of varying stiffness, length, and tapers can be inserted into the parallel lumens of the delivery catheter to vary the tension of the delivery catheter

[165–167]. The device uses a novel mechanism. It is inserted via percutaneous subclavian access following similar methods of pacemaker placement (Fig. 2.99). It is composed of a 7 Fr trilumen delivery catheter that is placed in the coronary sinus (Fig. 2.100). The rods deform the shape of the midportion of the coronary sinus, which diminishes the septal to lateral dimension of the mitral annulus and reduces the severity of MR. The rod stiffness can be changed until some diminution and MR is achieved. While the major tension is placed in the center of the posterior leaflet, it is still possible for circumflex coronary compression to occur with this device. There is a small initial experience with this device from the PTOLEMY-1 trial (Percutaneous Mitral Annuloplasty). The study enrolled 27 patients and reported the ability of this device to reduce MR. Nine patients were excluded before implantation because of unsuitable coronary sinus anatomy. Of the 19 patients who underwent implantation, 13 had a reduction in MR severity, and in six the device was ineffective. Four patients subsequently required removal of the device: one patient at day 7 for device fracture, and three patients referred to surgery because of device migration and/or diminished efficacy. Five patients (18.5%) had long-term implants with reductions in MR severity [168]. The safety and efficacy of the PTMA device will be investigated in the PTOLEMY-2 trial that is currently under way, and will treat up to 60 patients.

2.2.5.3
Annuloplasty Techniques

Surgical suture annuloplasty, performed to reduce the size of the annulus while maintaining physiological annular and leaflet motion, is commonly recommended to complete mitral valve repair operations because its use has been associated with improved long-term durability [109, 145, 169].

Evidence suggests that a 20% relative reduction of the septal–lateral dimensions of the mitral annulus can significantly reduce the severity of regurgitation [170]. Transcatheter direct annuloplasty duplicates the surgical technique.

2.2.5.3.1
Mitralign

With the Mitralign system (Mitralign Inc., Tewksbury, MA, USA), percutaneous annuloplasty is accomplished by retrograde catheterization of the LV from the aorta. A catheter is located behind the posterior leaflet adjacent to the annulus, and three anchors are placed, leading to annular cinching. (Fig. 2.101) This approach is based on the concept of surgical suture annuloplasty [171, 172]. Anchors are placed directly through the mitral annulus and then tethered together. The anchors are tethered and put under tension to decrease the septal lateral dimensions of the mitral annulus. A triple-lumen catheter (Trident) (Fig. 2.102) and a new double-lumen catheter (Bident) (Fig. 2.103) are available; the latter makes the procedure simpler, as the device is easier to handle [173]. Percutaneous direct annuloplasty with this approach has been realized successfully in animal models. Mitralign is the first to report encouraging results in human studies, although long-term follow-up is still awaited.

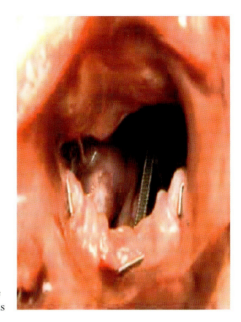

Fig. 2.101 Mitralign system. Three anchors in the posterior leaflet tensioned to decrease the septal lateral dimensions of the mitral annulus

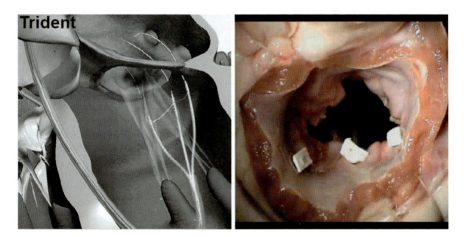

Fig. 2.102 Triple-lumen catheter (*Trident*) Mitralign system

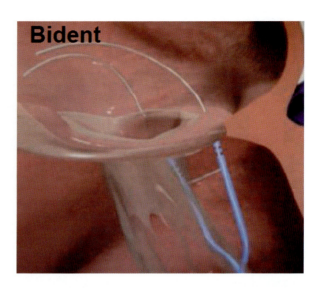

Fig. 2.103 Double-lumen catheter (*Bident*) Mitralign system

2.2.5.3.2
QuantumCor™

The QuantumCor™ device (QuantumCor, Bothell, WA) uses radiofrequency energy at subablative temperatures to produce contraction of the mitral valve annulus resulting in fibrosis, and theoretically reduces MR [174]. The initial prototype of the device involves a catheter with an endloop diameter of 40 mm that has 7 electrodes along with 14 thermocouples measuring 3 mm in length with 2 mm spacing (Fig. 2.104). This procedure has only been tested in animals, and no damage to the valve leaflets, coronary sinus, or coronary arteries has been detected. At 6-months' follow-up, chronic lesions created by radiofrequency did not compromise the structural integrity of the atrium or mitral leaflets, and the extramural coronary arteries, including the circumflex artery, were not involved in the thermal lesions and were microscopically normal [175]. This technology is in a very early stage of development and preclinical studies are currently in progress [176].

2.2.5.3.3
AccuCinch™

The AccuCinch™ device (Guided Delivery Systems, Inc., Santa Clara, CA, USA) utilizes a catheter with a proprietary design, allowing a retrograde approach to the subannular space of the mitral valve. The device concept is to place anchors connected by a cable from the first to the third scallop of the

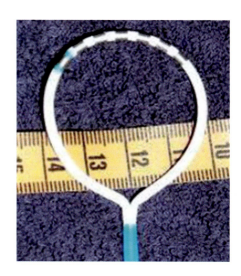

Fig. 2.104 The QuantumCor™ radiofrequency energy device

posterior mitral leaflet, apply traction on the cable to decrease the inter-anchor distance, and thus reduce mitral annular size. To date, only temporary implants have been performed in surgical patients [177]. The first human studies were initiated in Germany and Canada.

2.2.5.4
Chamber and Annular Remodeling

It is known that the SL mitral annular diameter is increased in functional MR [178, 179]. Recently, novel percutaneous techniques to create SL annular cinching, remodeling the left ventricular chamber and reducing the functional MR, have been developed.

2.2.5.4.1
Coapsys

The Coapsys device (Myocor Inc., Minneapolis, MN, USA) is composed of a pair of epicardial pads which are anchored on the LV surface, with a tensioning cable passed through the LV cavity to pull the pads together, thereby reducing the SL dimension of the mitral annulus and diminishing the LV chamber diameter (Fig. 2.105). This procedure is performed using both "open-chest" and "closed-chest" approaches. To date, greater experience is represented by the surgical approach. Over 150 patients have been treated with this surgical device,

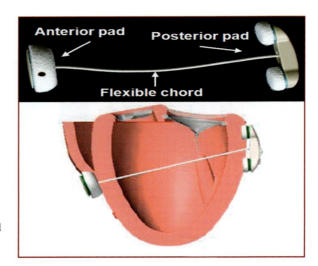

Fig. 2.105 The Coapsys device composed of two epicardial pads (anterior and posterior) connected by a flexible chord

and reductions in MR have been sustained for up to 12 months. The Coapsys device is a percutaneous adaptation of the surgical device. A transpericardial percutaneous approach has been developed and used successfully in animal models [180, 181]. Human implants have been realized in two patients, but the sponsoring company has unfortunately gone out of business.

2.2.5.4.2
PS3 System™

The percutaneous septal sinus shortening system (PS3 System™; Ample Medical, Inc., Foster City, CA, USA) is a transcatheter device that realizes chamber remodeling using anchors in the coronary sinus and fossa ovalis. It consists of a percutaneously placed interatrial septal anchor, coronary sinus anchor, and a connecting bridge element (Fig. 2.106). By tensioning the suture, the LV chamber decreases its dimensions, resulting in reduction of functional MR. The PS3 System™ has been shown in preclinical studies to acutely and chronically reduce functional MR in an ovine tachycardia model [182].

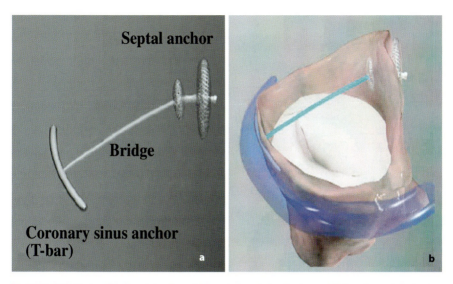

Fig. 2.106 PS3 System™. Consists of an atrial septal occluder device and T-bar element that act as anchors in the interatrial septum and coronary sinus, respectively (**a**). A bridging element traversing the left atrium connects the two anchors (**b**)

2.2.5.5
A Glimpse into the Future

A number of other transcatheter mitral valve therapies are currently in developmental stages: transcatheter mitral valve replacement, percutaneous neochordal implantation, and hybrid surgical-transcatheter strategies (e.g. a surgically implanted prosthetic annular ring that can, in case of future need, be adjusted mechanically in the catheterization laboratory percutaneously).

2.2.5.5.1
Transcatheter Mitral Valve Replacement

Various companies are currently working to develop percutaneous or minimally invasive devices for mitral valve replacement. Those most widely used in preclinical trial phases are stent-based bioprostheses inserted via a trans-septal or transapical approach [183].

Endovalve (Endovalve, Inc., CA, USA) is a mitral valve replacement device currently being developed for minimally invasive insertion. The device consists of a "foldable (non-stent)" structure in nitinol, which is inserted in the native valve apparatus thanks to anatomically appropriate grippers (Figure 2.107).

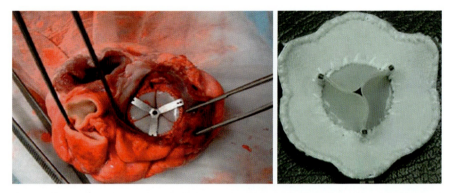

Fig. 2.107 Endovalve. The prosthesis includes a ring and bioprosthetic leaflets with a foldable tripod frame

The prosthesis includes a ring and bioprosthetic leaflets with a foldable tripod frame. It has integrated gripper features for fixation and attachment in the beating heart. The system is introduced via right minithoracotomy directly into the LA with a special delivery system and removable wires allowing for contraction, repositioning, and release. A sewn fabric skirt provides perivalvular sealing. In vivo sheep implants have demonstrated fixation, normal valve function, and lack of both left ventricular outflow tract obstruction and MR. A subsequent truly percutaneous delivery catheter using the same valve design is planned for later development [184].

2.2.5.5.2
Percutaneous Neochordal Implantation

This technique, which is currently under development, uses the standard surgical technique for the treatment of mitral valve prolapse. Maisano and colleagues have published their initial experience, utilizing a transapical beating heart approach, in six pigs [185]. Under intracardiac echo monitoring, after the apex was punctured, a 0.035 inch J tip guidewire was introduced in the LV and an ultra-stiff 14 Fr sheath (guide catheter) inserted through the apex. A suction-and-suture device was introduced into the LV. The mitral valve was crossed under echo guidance. Using suction, either the anterior or posterior leaflet was captured, and a loop of 4-0 polypropylene was thrown at the edge of the leaflet. The loop, with a pledget, was exteriorized through the introducer. The introducer was removed and the purse-string tied. Under echo guidance, the neochordae suture was pulled and tied over a pledget to evoke leaflet tethering. Data from this preclinical study show that this minimally invasive technique for mitral valve repair is feasible, although a prolapse model is needed to further demonstrate feasibility under pathologic conditions [185].

References

1. Wood P. An appreciation of mitral stenosis-I. BMJ 1954;4870:1051–1063.
2. Essop MR, Nkomo VT. Rheumatic and nonrheumatic valvular heart disease: epidemiology, management, and prevention in Africa. Circulation 2005;112:3584–3591.
3. Fae KC, Oshiro SE, Toubert A et al. How an autoimmune reaction triggered by molecular mimicry between streptococcal M protein and cardiac tissue proteins leads to heart lesions in rheumatic heart disease. J Autoimmun 2005;24:101–109.
4. Burge DJ, DeHoratious RJ. Acute rheumatic fever. Cardiovasc Clin 1993;23:3–23.
5. Guilherme L, Cury P, Demarchi LM et al. Rheumatic heart disease: proinflammatory cytokines play a role in the progression and maintenance of valvular lesions. Am J Pathol 2004;165:1583-1591.
6. Davutoglu V, Celik A, Aksoy M. Contribution of selected serum inflammatory mediators to the progression of chronic rheumatic valve disease, subsequent valve calcification and NYHA functional class. J Heart Valve Dis 2005;14:251–256.
7. Roberts WC. Morphologic aspects of cardiac valve dysfunction. Am Heart J 1992; 123:1610–1632.
8. Spencer FC. A plea for early, open mitral commissurotomy. Am Heart J 1978;95:668–670.
9. Carabello BA. Timing of surgery in mitral and aortic stenosis. Cardiol Clin 1991;9:229–238.
10. Hygenholtz PG, Ryan TJ, Stein SW et al. The spectrum of pure mitral stenosis. Am J Cardiol 1962;10:773-784.
11. Arani DT, Carleton RA. The deleterious role of tachycardia in mitral stenosis. Circulation 1967;36:511-516.
12. Schofield PM. Invasive investigation of the mitral valve. In: Wells FC, Shapiro LM (eds) Mitral valve disease. Oxford: Butterworth-Heineman, 1996.
13. Kennedy JW, Yarnall SR, Murray JA et al. Quantitative angiocardiography: relationships of left atrial and ventricular pressure and volume in mitral valve disease. Circulation 1970;41:817–824.
14. Choi BW, Bacharach SL, Barcour DJ et al. Left ventricular systolic dysfunction: Diastolic filling characteristics and exercise cardiac reserve in mitral stenosis. Am J Cardiol 1995;75:526–529.
15. Braunwald E, Turi ZG. Pathophysiology of mitral valve disease. In: Wells FC, Shapiro LM (eds) Mitral valve dsease. Oxford: Butterworth-Heineman, 1996.
16. Thompson ME, Shaver JA, Leon DF. Effect of tachycardia on atrial transport in mitral stenosis. Am Heart J 1977;94:297–306.
17. Stott DK, Marpole DGF, Bristow JD et al. The role of left atrial transport in aortic and mitral stenosis. Circulation 1970;41:1031–1041.
18. Diker E, Aydogdu S, Ozdemir M et al. Prevalence and predictors of atrial fibrillation in rheumatic valvular heart disease. Am J Cardiol 1996;77:96–98.
19. American College of Cardiology; American Heart Association Task Force on Practice Guidelines (Writing Committee to revise the 1998 guidelines for the management of patients with valvular heart disease); Society of Cardiovascular Anesthesiologists, Bonow RO, Carabello BA, Chatterjee K et al. ACC/AHA 2006 guidelines for the management of patients with valvular heart disease: a report of the American College of Cardiology/American Heart Association Task Force on Practice Guidelines (writing Committee to Revise the 1998 guidelines for the management of patients with valvular heart disease) developed in collaboration with the Society of Cardiovascular Anesthesiologists endorsed by the Society for Cardiovascular Angiography and Interventions and the Society of Thoracic Surgeons. J Am Coll Cardiol. 2006;48:1–148.

20. Vahanian A, Baumgartner H, Bax J et al. Task Force on the management of valvular heart disease of the European Society of Cardiology; ESC Committee for Practice Guidelines. Guidelines on the management of valvular heart disease: the task force on the management of valvular heart disease of the European Society of Cardiology. Eur Heart J 2007;28:230–268.
21. Braunwald E. Valvular heart disease. In: Braunwald E (ed) Heart disease. Philadelphia: WB Saunders, 1984; pp 1063–1135.
22. Nichol PM, Gilbert BW, Kisslo JA. Two-dimensional echocardiographic assessment of mitral stenosis. Circulation 1977;55:120–128.
23. Baumgartner H, Hung J, Bermejo J et al. Echocardiographic assessment of valve stenosis: EAE/ASE Recommendations for clinical practice. J Am Soc Echocardiogr 2009;22:1–23.
24. Messika-Zeitoun D, Brochet E, Holmin C et al. Three-dimensional evaluation of the mitral valve area and commissural opening before and after percutaneous mitral commissurotomy in patients with mitral stenosis. Eur Heart J 2007;28:72–79.
25. Wilkins GT, Weyman AE, Abascal VM et al. Percutaneous balloon dilatation of the mitral valve: an analysis of echocardiographic variables related to outcome and the mechanism of dilatation. Br Heart J 1988;60:299–308.
26. Iung B, Cormier B, Ducimetiere P et al. Functional results 5 years after successful percutaneous mitral commissurotomy in a series of 528 patients and analysis of predictive factors. J Am Coll Cardiol 1996;27:407–414.
27. Rahimtoola SH, Durairaj A, Mehra A, Nuno I. Current evaluation and management of patients with mitral stenosis. Circulation 2002;106;1183–1188.
28. Iung B, Cormier B, Ducimetiere P et al. Immediate results of percutaneous mitral commissurotomy. Circulation 1996;94:2124–2130.
29. Reid CL, McKay CR, Chandraratna PA et al. Mechanisms of increase in mitral valve area and influence of anatomic features in double-balloon, catheter balloon valvuloplasty in adults with rheumatic mitral stenosis: a Doppler and two-dimensional echocardiographic study. Circulation 1987;76:628–636.
30. Nishimura RA, Rihal CS, Tajik AJ, Holmes DR Jr. Accurate measurement of the transmitral gradient in patients with mitral stenosis: a simultaneous catheterization and Doppler echocardiographic study. J Am Coll Cardiol 1994;24:152–158.
31. Thomas JD, Newell JB, Choong CY, Weyman AE. Physical and physiological determinants of transmitral velocity: numerical analysis. Am J Physiol Heart Circ Physiol 1991;260:H1718–31.
32. Faletra F, Pezzano A Jr, Fusco R et al. Measurement of mitral valve area in mitral stenosis: four echocardiographic methods compared with direct measurement of anatomic orifices. J Am Coll Cardiol 1996;28:1190–1197.
33. Thomas JD, Weyman AE. Doppler mitral pressure half-time: a clinical tool in search of theoretical justification. J Am Coll Cardiol 1987;10:923–929.
34. Schwammenthal E, Vered Z, Agranat O et al. Impact of atrioventricular compliance on pulmonary artery pressure in mitral stenosis: an exercise echocardiographic study. Circulation 2000;102:2378–2384.
35. Thomas JD, Wilkins GT, Choong CY et al. Inaccuracy of mitral pressure half-time immediately after percutaneous mitral valvotomy. Dependence on transmitral gradient and left atrial and ventricular compliance. Circulation 1988;78:980–993.
36. Nakatani S, Masuyama T, Kodama K et al. Value and limitations of Doppler echocardiography in the quantification of stenotic mitral valve area: comparison of the pressure half-time and the continuity equation methods. Circulation 1988;77:78–85.
37. Messika-Zeitoun D, Fung Yiu S, Cormier B et al. Sequential assessment of mitral valve area during diastole using colour M-mode flow convergence analysis: new insights into mitral stenosis physiology. Eur Heart J 2003;24:1244–1253.

38. Currie PJ, Seward JB, Chan KL et al. Continuous wave Doppler determination of right ventricular pressure: a simultaneous Dopplercatheterization study in 127 patients. J Am Coll Cardiol 1985;6:750–756.
39. Braunwald E, Moscovitz HL, Mram SS et al. The hemodynamics of the left side of the heart as studied by simultaneous left atrial, left ventricular and aortic pressures; particular reference to mitral stenosis. Circulation 1955;12:69–81.
40. Gorlin R, Gorlin SG. Hydraulic formula for calculation of the area of the stenotic mitral valve, other cardiac valves, and central circulatory shunts. Am Heart J 1951;41:1–29.
41. Hugenholtz PG, Ryan TJ, Stein SW, Belmann WH. The spectrum of pure mitral stenosis: hemodynamic studies in relation to clinical disability. Am J Cardiol 1962;10:773–784.
42. Rowe JC, Bland EF, Sprague HB, White PD. The course of mitral stenosis without surgery: ten- and twenty-year perspectives. Ann Intern Med 1960;52:741–749.
43. Olesen KH. The natural history of 271 patients with mitral stenosis under medical treatment. Br Heart J 1962;24:349–357.
44. Selzer A, Cohn KE. Natural history of mitral stenosis: a review. Circulation 1972;45:878–890.
45. Munoz S, Gallardo J, Diaz-Gorrin JR, Medina O. Influence of surgery on the natural history of rheumatic mitral and aortic valve disease. Am J Cardiol 1975;35:234–242.
46. Ward C, Hancock BW. Extreme pulmonary hypertension caused by mitral valve disease: natural history and results of surgery. Br Heart J 1975;37:74–78.
47. Bonow RO, Carabello BA, Chatterjee K et al, American College of Cardiology/American Heart Association Task Force on Practice Guidelines. 2008 focused update incorporated into the ACC/AHA 2006 guidelines for the management of patients with valvular heart disease: a report of the American College of Cardiology/American Heart Association Task Force on Practice Guidelines (writing committee to revise the 1998 guidelines for the management of patients with valvular heart disease). Endorsed by the Society of Cardiovascular Anesthesiologists, Society for Cardiovascular Angiography and Interventions, and Society of Thoracic Surgeons. Circulation 2008;118:e523–e661.
48. Himelman RB, Stulbarg M, Kircher B et al. Noninvasive evaluation of pulmonary artery pressure during exercise by saline-enhanced Doppler echocardiography in chronic pulmonary disease. Circulation 1989;79:863–871.
49. Tamai J, Nagata S, Akaike M et al. Improvement in mitral flow dynamics during exercise after percutaneous transvenous mitral commissurotomy: noninvasive evaluation using continuous wave Doppler technique. Circulation 1990;81:46–51.
50. Leavitt JI, Coats MH, Falk RH. Effects of exercise on transmitral gradient and pulmonary artery pressure in patients with mitral stenosis or a prosthetic mitral valve: a Doppler echocardiographic study. J Am Coll Cardiol 1991;17:1520–1526.
51. Cheriex EC, Pieters FA, Janssen JH et al. Value of exercise Doppler-echocardiography in patients with mitral stenosis. Int J Cardiol 1994;45:219–226.
52. Tamburino C, Russo G, Di Paola G et al. La valvuloplastica percutanea nella stenosi mitralica. Cardiologia 1993;38:7–17.
53. Iung B, Garbarz E, Michaud P et al. Percutaneous mitral commissurotomy for restenosis after surgical commissurotomy: late efficacy and implications for patient selection. J Am Coll Cardiol, 2000;35:1295–1302.
54. Lip G, Wasfi MM, Hamil M et al. Percutaneous ballon valvuloplasty of stenosed mitral bioprosthesis. Int J Cardiol 1997;59:97–100.
55. Orbe LC, Sobrino N, Matè I et al. Effectiveness of balloon percutaneuos valvuloplasty for stenotic bioprosthetic valves in different positions. Am J Cardiol 1991;68:1719–1721.
56. Calvo OL, Sobrino N, Gamallo C et al. Balloon percutaneous valvuloplasty for stenotic bioprosthetic valves in the mitral position. Am J Cardiol 1987;60:736–737.

57. Spellberg RD, Mayeda GS, Flores JH. Balloon valvuloplasty of a stenosed mitral bioprosthesis. Am Heart J 1991;122:1785–1787.
58. Lin PJ, Chang JP, Chang CH. Balloon valvuloplasty is controindicated in stenotic mitral bioprosthesis. Am Heart J 1994;127:724–726.
59. Gupta A, Lokhandwala YY, Satoskar PR, Salvi VS. Balloon mitral valvotomy in pregnancy: maternal and fetal outcomes. J Am Coll Surg 1998;187:409–415.
60. Fawzy ME, Kinsara AJ, Stefadouros M et al. Long-term outcome of mitral balloon valvotomy in pregnant women. J Heart Valve Dis 2001;10:153–157.
61. Hameed A, Karaalp IS, Tummala PP et al. The effect of valvular heart disease on maternal and fetal outcome of pregnancy. J Am Coll Cardiol 2001;37:893–899.
62. de Souza JA, Martinez EE Jr, Ambrose JA et al. Percutaneous balloon mitral valvuloplasty in comparison with open mitral valve commissurotomy for mitral stenosis during pregnancy. J Am Coll Cardiol 2001;37:900–903.
63. Cohen DJ, Kuntz RE, Gordon SP et al. Predictors of long-term outcome after percutaneous balloon mitral valvuloplasty. N Engl J Med 1992;327:1329–1335.
64. Kamalesh M, Burger AJ, Shubrooks SJ. The use of transesophageal echocardiography to avoid left atrial thrombus during percutaneous mitral valvuloplasty. Cathet Cardiovasc Diagn 1993;28:320–322.
65. Tsai LM, Hung JS, Chen JH et al. Resolution of left atrial appendage thrombus in mitral stenosis after warfarin therapy. Am Heart J 1991;121:1232–1234.
66. Fatkin D, Roy P, Morgan JJ, Feneley MP. Percutaneous balloon mitral valvotomy with the Inoue single-balloon catheter: commissural morphology as a determinant of outcome. J Am Coll Cardiol 1993;21:390–397.
67. Reid CL, McKay CR, Chandraratna PA et al. Mechanisms of increase in mitral valve area and influence of anatomic features in double-balloon, catheter balloon valvuloplasty in adults with rheumatic mitral stenosis: a Doppler and two-dimensional echocardiographic study. Circulation 1987;76:628–636.
68. Palacios IF. Farewell to surgical mitral commissurotomy for many patients. Circulation 1998;97:223–226.
69. Palacios I, Block PC, Brandi S. Percutaneous ballon valvulotomy for patients with severe stenosis. Circulation 1987;75:778–784.
70. Davidson MJ, Baim DS. Percutaneous catheter-based mitral valve repair. Cohn LH (ed) Cardiac surgery in the adult. New York: McGraw-Hill, 2008; pp 1101–1108.
71. Marsocci G, Neri M, Natale N. Cardiopatie valvolari. Il Pensiero Scientifico Editore, Rome, 2004.
72. Inoue K. Percutaneous transvenous mitral commissurotomy using the Inoue balloon. Eur Heart J 1991;12:99–108.
73. Vahanian A, Acar J. Mitral valvuloplasty: the French experience. In: Topol EJ Textbook of interventional cardiology., Philadelphia: WB Saunders, 1994; pp 1206–1225.
74. Block PC, Palacios IF. Aortic and mitral balloon valvuloplasty: the United States experience. In: Topol EJ (ed) Textbook of interventional cardiology. Philadelphia: WB Saunders, 1994; pp 1189–1205.
75. Inoue K, Hungs JS. Percutaneous transvenous mitral commissurotomy (PTMC): the Far East experience. In: Topol EJ (Ed) Textbook of interventional cardiology. Philadelphia: WB Saunders, 1994; pp 1226–1242.
76. Tamburino C, Russo G, Calvi V et al. La valvuloplastica mitralica: risultati immediati e followup a 2 anni. Cardiologia 1993;38:367–375.
77. Ross J Jr. Catheterization of the left heart through the interatrial septum: a new technique and its experimental evaluation. Surg Forum 1959;9:297–301.
78. Zaki AM, Kasem HH, Bakhoum S et al. Comparison of early results of percutaneous metallic mitral commissurotome with Inoue balloon technique in patients with high mitral echocardiographic scores. Catheter Cardiovasc Interv 2002;57:312–317.

79. Inoue K, Owaki T, Nakamura T et al. Clinical application of transvenous mitral commissurotomy by a new balloon catheter. J Thorac Cardiovasc Surg. 1984;87:394–402.
80. Baim DS. Grossman's cardiac catheterization, angiography and intervention (7th edn). Philadelphia: Lippincott Williams and Wilkins, 2006.
81. Dean LS, Mickel M, Bonan R et al. Four-years follow up of patients undergoing percutaneous balloon mitral commissurotomy. A report from the National Heart, Lung, and Blood Institute Balloon Valvuloplasty Registry. J Am Coll Cardiol 1996;28:1452.
82. Palacios IF, Tuzcu ME, Weyman AE et al. Clinical follow-up of patients undergoing percutaneous mitral balloon valvulotomy. Circulation 1995;91:671–676.
83. Pan M, Medina A, Lezo JJ et al. Factors determining late success after mitral balloon valvulotomy. Am J Cardiol 1993;71:1181–1186.
84. Arora R, Kalra GS, Murty GS et al. Percutaneous transatrial mitral commissurotomy: immediate and intermediate results. J Am Coll Cardiol 1994;23:1327–1332.
85. Palacios IF, Block PC, Wilkins GT, Weyman AE. Follow-up of patients undergoing percutaneous mitral balloon valvotomy. Analysis of factors determining restenosis. Circulation 1989;79:573–579.
86. Thomas MR, Monaghan MJ, Michalis LK, Jewitt DE. Echocardiographic restenosis after successful balloon dilatation of the mitral valve with the Inoue balloon: experience of a United Kingdom centre. Br Heart J 1993;69:418–423.
87. Iung B, Garbarz E, Michaud P et al. Immediate and midterm results of repeat percutaneous mitral commissurotomy for restenosis following earlier percutaneous mitral commissurotomy. Eur Heart J 2000;21:1683–1689.
88. Vahanian A, Palacios IF. Percutaneous approaches to valvular disease. Circulation 2004;109:1572–1579.
89. Fenster MS, Feldman MD. Mitral regurgitation: an overview. Curr Probl Cardiol 1995;20:193–280.
90. Luther RR, Meyers SN. Acute mitral insufficiency secondary to ruptured *chordae tendineae*. Arch Intern Med 1974;134:568.
91. Hansen DE, Sarris GE, Niczyporuk MA et al. Physiologic role of the mitral apparatus in left ventricular regional mechanics, contraction synergy, and global systolic performance. J Thorac Cardiovasc Surg 1989;97:521–533.
92. Yun KL, Niczyporuk MA, Sarris GE et al. Importance of mitral subvalvular apparatus in terms of cardiac energetics and systolic mechanics in the ejecting canine heart. J Clin Invest 1991;87:247–254.
93. Yiu SF, Enriquez-Sarano M, Tribouilloy C et al. Determinants of the degree of functional mitral regurgitation in patients with systolic left ventricular dysfunction. Circulation 2000;102:1400–1406.
94. Grigioni F, Enriquez-Sarano M, Zehr KJ et al. Ischemic mitral regurgitation: long-term outcome and prognostic implications with quantitative Doppler assessment. Circulation 2001;103:1759–1764.
95. Enriquez-Sarano M, Avierinos JF, Messika-Zeitoun D et al. Quantitative determinants of the outcome of asymptomatic mitral regurgitation. N Engl J Med 2005;352:875–883.
96. Waller BF, Howard J, Fess S. Pathology of mitral valve stenosis and pure mitral regurgitation, part II. Clin Cardiol 1994;17:395–402.
97. Grossman W. Profiles in valvular heart disease. In: Baim DS, Grossman W (eds) Cardiac catheterization, angiography and intervention. Philadelphia: Lippincott Williams and Wilkins, 2006.
98. Ross J Jr. Adaptations of the left ventricle to chronic volume overload. Circ Res 1974;34–35.
99. Yun KL, Rayhill SC, Niczyporuk MA et al. Left ventricular mechanics and energetics in the dilated canine heart: acute versus chronic mitral regurgitation. J Thorac Cardiovasc Surg 1992;104:26–39.

100. Carabello BA, Nakano K, Corin W et al. Left ventricular function in experimental volume overload hypertrophy. Am J Physiol Heart Circ Physiol 1989;256:H974–H981.
101. Urabe Y, Mann DL, Kent RL et al. Cellular and ventricular contractile dysfunction in experimental canine mitral regurgitation. Circ Res 1992;70:131–147.
102. Starling MR, Kirsh MM, Montgomery DG et al. Impaired left ventricular contractile function in patients with long-term mitral regurgitation and normal ejection fraction. J Am Coll Cardiol 1993;22:239–250.
103. Nakano K, Swindle MM, Spinale F et al. Depressed contractile function due to canine mitral regurgitation improves after correction of the volume overload. J Clin Invest 1991;87:2077–2086.
104. Carabello BA, Crawford FA Jr. Valvular heart disease. N Engl J Med 1997;337:32–41.
105. Carabello BA, Nolan SP, McGuire LB. Assessment of preoperative left ventricular function in patients with mitral regurgitation: value of the end-systolic wall stress-end-systolic volume ratio. Circulation 1981;64:1212–1217.
106. Carabello BA, Williams H, Gash AK et al. Hemodynamic predictors of outcome in patients undergoing valve replacement. Circulation 1986;74:1309–1316.
107. Grossman W, Braunwald E, Mann T et al. Contractile state of the left ventricle in man as evaluated from end-systolic pressure-volume relations. Circulation 1977;56:845–852.
108. Borow KM, Green LH, Mann T et al. End-systolic volume as a predictor of postoperative left ventricular performance in volume overload from valvular regurgitation. Am J Med 1980;68:655–663.
109. Carpentier A. Cardiac valve surgery: the French correction. J Thorac Cardiovasc Surg 1983;86:323–337.
110 Carpentier A, Chauvaud S, Fabiani J et al. Reconstructive surgery of mitral valve incompetence: ten-year appraisal. J Thorac Cardiovasc Surg 1980;79:338–348.
111. Wells FC. Conservation and surgical repair of the mitral valve. In: Wells FC, Shapiro LM (eds) Mitral valve disease. Oxford: Butterworth-Heineman, 1996.
112. Dagum P, Timek TA, Green GR et al. Coordinate-free analysis of mitral valve dynamics in normal and ischemic hearts. Circulation 2000;102:62–69.
113. Ngaage DL, Schaff HV. Mitral valve surgery in non-ischemic cardiomyopathy. J Cardiovasc Surg 2004;45:477–486.
114. Rahimtoola SH, Dell'Italia LJ. Mitral valve disease. In: Fuster V, Alexander RW, O'Rourke RA et al Hurst's The Heart)11th edn). New York: McGraw-Hill, 2004; pp1669–1695.
115. Zoghbi W.A, Eriquez-Sarano M, Foster E et al. Recommendations for evaluation of the severity of native valvular regurgitation with two-dimensional and Doppler echocardiography. J Am Soc Echocardiogr 2003;16:777–802.
116. Bargiggia GS, Tronconi L, Sahn DJ et al. A new method for quantitation of mitral regurgitation based on color flow Doppler imaging of flow convergence proximal to regurgitant orifice. Circulation 1991;84:1481–1489.
117. Simpson IA, Shiota T, Gharib M, Sahn DJ. Current status of flow convergence for clinical applications: is it a leaning tower of "PISA"? J Am Coll Cardiol 1996;27:504–509.
118. Baumgartner H, Schima H, Kuhn P. Value and limitations of proximal jet dimensions for the quantitation of valvular regurgitation: an in vitro study using Doppler flow imaging. J Am Soc Echocardiogr 1991;4:57–66.
119. Sahn DJ. Instrumentation and physical factors related to visualization of stenotic and regurgitant jets by Doppler color flow mapping. J Am Coll Cardiol 1988;12:1354–1365.
120. Pu M, Griffin BP, Vandervoort PM et al. The value of assessing pulmonary venous flow velocity for predicting severity of mitral regurgitation: a quantitative assessment integrating left ventricular function. J Am Soc Echocardiogr 1999;12:736–743.
121. Thomas L, Foster E, Schiller NB. Peak mitral inflow velocity predicts mitral regurgitation severity. J AmColl Cardiol 1998;31:174–179.

122. Braunwald E, Awe W. The syndrome of severe mitral regurgitation with normal left atrial pressure. Circulation 1963;27:29–35.
123. Tricon BH, Felker GM, Shaw LK et al. Relation of frequency and severity of mitral regurgitation to survival among patients with left ventricular systolic disfuncion and heart failure. Am J Cardiol 2003;91:538–543.
124. Tribouilloy CM, Enriquez-Sarano M, Schaff HV et al. Impact of preoperative symptoms on survival aftersurgical correction of organic mitral regurgitation: rationale for optimizing surgical implications. Circulation 1999;99:400–405.
125. Enriquez-Sarano M, Freeman WK, Tribouilloy et al. Functional anatomy of mitral regurgitation: accuracy and outcome implications of TEE. J Am Coll Cardiol 1999;34:1129–1136.
126. Thamilarasan M, Griffin B. Choosing the most appropriate valve operation and prosthesis. Cleveland Clin J Med 2002;69:668–703.
127. Lee EM, Shapiro LM, Wells FC. Superiority of mitral valve repair in surgery for degenerative mitral regurgitation. Eur Heart J 1997;18:655–663.
128. Enriquez-Sarano M, Schaff HV, Orszulak TA et al. Valve repair improves the outcome of surgery for mitral regurgitation. A multivariate analysis. Circulation 1995;91:1022–1028.
129. Pu M, Thomas JD, Gillinov MA, Griffin BP et al. Importance of ischaemic and viable myocardium for patients with chronic ischaemic mitral regurgitation and left ventricular dysfunction. Am J Cardiol 2003;92:862–864.
130. Roques F, Nashef SA, Michel P et al. EuroSCORE study group. Risk factor for early mortality after valve surgery in Europe in the 1990s: lessons from the EuroSCORE pilot program. J Heart Valve Dis 2001;10:572–577.
131. Feldman T, Wasserman HS, Herrmann HC et al. Percutaneous mitral valve repair using the edge-to-edge technique six-month results of the EVEREST phase 1 clinical trial. J Am Coll Card 2006;46:2134–2140.
132. Silvestry FE, Rodriguez LL, Herrmann HC et al. Echocardiographic guidance and assessment of percutaneous repair for mitral regurgitation with the Evalve MitraClip: lessons learned from EVEREST I. J Am Soc Echocardiog 2007;20:1131–1140.
133. Rohatgi S, Wasserman HS, Block PC et al. Mitral stenosis is not produced by percutaneous edge-to-edge repair of mitral regurgitation. Circulation 2005;112:520.
134. Herrmann HC, Kar S, Siegal R et al. Effect of percutaneous mitral repair with the MitraClip device on mitral valve area and gradient. EuroIntervention 2009;4:437–442.
135. De Bonis M, Lapenna E, La Canna G et al. Mitral valve repair for functional mitral regurgitation in end-stage dilated cardiomyopathy. Circulation 2005;112(Suppl I):1402–1408.
136. Calafiore AM, Contini M, Iacò AL et al. Mitral valve repair for degenerative mitral regurgitation. J Cardiovasc Med 2008;8:114–118.
137. Foster E, Wasserman HS, Gray W et al. Quantitative assessment of severity of mitral regurgitation by serial echocardiography in a multicenter clinical trial of percutaneous mitral valve repair. Am J Cardiol 2007;100:1577–1583.
138. Maisano F, Schreuder JJ, Oppizzi M et al. The double-orifice technique as a standardized approach, to treat mitral regurgitation due to severe myxomatous disease: surgical technique. Eur J Cardiothorac Surg 2000;17:201–205.
139. Herrmann HC, Wasserman HS, Whitlow P et al. Percutaneous edge-to-edge mitral valve repair using the Evalve MitraClip™ device: initial one-year results of the EVEREST phase 1 trial. Circulation 2005;112(Suppl):520.
140. Mirabel M, Iung B, Baron G et al. What are the characteristics of patients with severe, symptomatic, mitral regurgitation who are denied surgery? Eur Heart J 2007;28:1358–1365.
141. Piazza N, Asgar A, Ibrahim R, Bonan R. Transcatheter mitral and pulmonary valve therapy. J Am Coll Cardiol 2009;53:1837–1851.
142. Feldman T, Leon MB. Prospects for percutaneous valve therapies. Circulation 2007;116;2866–2877.

143. Lorusso R, Borghetti V, Totaro P, et al. The double-orifice technique for mitral valve reconstruction: predictors of outcome. Eur J Cardiothorac Surg 2001;20:583–589.
144. Bagai J, Zhao D. Subcutaneous "figure-of-eight" stitch to achieve hemostasis after removal of large-caliber femoral venous sheaths. Cardiac Interventions Today I 2008; July/August:22–23.
145. Alfieri O, Maisano F, DeBonis M et al. The edge-to-edge technique in mitral valve repair: a simple solution for complex problems. J Thorac Cardiovasc Surg 2001;122:674–681.
146. Herrmann HC, Rohatgi S, Wasserman et al. Mitral valve hemodynamic effects of percutaneous edge-to-edge repair with the MitraClip™ device for mitral regurgitation. Catheter Cardiovasc Interv 2006;68:821–828.
147. Condado JA, Acquatella H, Rodriguez L et al. Percutaneous edge-to-edge mitral valve repair: 2 year follow-up in the first human case. Catheter Cardiovasc Interv 2006;67:323–325.
148. Feldman T, Kar S, Rinaldi M et al. for the EVEREST investigators percutaneous mitral repair with the MitraClip system: safety and midterm durability in the Initial EVEREST (Endovascular Valve Edge-to-edge Repair Study) cohort. J Am Coll Cardiol 2009;54;686–694.
149. Dang NC, Aboodi MS, Sakaguchi T et al. Surgical revision after percutaneous mitral valve repair with a clip: initial multicenter experience. Ann Thorac Surg 2005;80:2338–2342.
150. Feldman T, Wasserman HS, Herrmann HC et al. Edge-to-edge mitral valve repair using the evalve MitraClip: one year results of the EVEREST phase I clinical trial. Am J Cardiol 2005;96(Suppl 7A):49H.
150a. Feldman T. Endovascular Valve Edge-to-Edge REpair Study (EVEREST II) Randomized Clinical Trial: Primary Safety and Efficacy Endpoints. Presented at American College of Cardiology Congress, March 14, 2010, Atlanta.
151. Patrick L, Whitlow. Presented at Transcatheter Cardiovascular Therapeutics (TCT) Congress, 21–25 September 2009, San Francisco.
152. Tamburino C, Ussia GP, Maisano F et al. Percutaneous mitral valve repair with the Mitraclip system: acute results from a real world setting. Eur Heart J 2010, epub ahead of print.
153. Scott Lim. Presented at Transcatheter Cardiovascular Therapeutics (TCT) Congress, 21–25 September 2009, San Francisco.
153a. Franzen O, Baldus S, Rudolph V, et al. Acute outcomes of MitraClip therapy for mitral regurgitation in high-surgical-risk patients: emphasis on adverse valve morphology and severe left ventricular dysfunction. Eur Heart J 2010, epub ahead of print.
154. Naqvi TZ, Zarbatany D, Molloy MD et al. Intracardiac echocardiography for percutaneous mitral valve repair in a swine model. J Am Soc Echocardiogr 2006;19:147–153.
155. Naqvi TZ, Buchbinder M, Zarbatany D et al. Beating-heart percutaneous mitral valve repair using a transcatheter endovascular suturing device in an animal model. Catheter Cardiovasc Interv 2007;69:525–531.
156. Grossi EA, Goldberg JD, La Pietra A et al. Ischemic mitral valve reconstruction and replacement: comparison of long-term survival and complications. J Thorac Cardiovasc Surg 2001;122:1107–1124.
157. Maniu CV, Patel JB, Reuter DG et al. Acute and chronic reduction of functional mitral regurgitation in experimental heart failure by percutaneous mitral annuloplasty. J Am Coll Cardiol 2004;44(8):1652–1661.
158. Piazza N, Bonan R. Transcatheter mitral valve repair for functional mitral regurgitation: coronary sinus approach. J Interv Cardiol 2007;20:495–508.
159. Webb JG, Harnek J, Munt BIet al. Percutaneous transvenous mitral annuloplasty; initial human experience with device implantation in the coronary sinus. Circulation 2006;113:851–855.

160. Webb JG. MONARC Percutaneous transvenous mitral annuloplasty. Presented at Transcatheter Vale Therapies (TVT) Summit; 2009; Seattle.
161. Frerker C, Schäfer U, Schewel D et al. Percutaneous approaches for mitral valve interventions, a real alternative technique for standard cardiac surgery? Herz 2009;34:444–450.
162. Harnek J. 2-year interim results of the percutaneous MONARC™ system for the treatment of functional mitral regurgitation. Presented at Transcatheter Cardiovascular Therapeutics (TCT) Congress, 21–25 September 2009, San Francisco.
163. Kaye DM, Byrne M, Alferness C, Power J. Feasibility and short-term efficacy of percutaneous mitral annular reduction for the therapy of heart failure-induced mitral regurgitation. Circulation. 2003;108:1795–1797.
164. Schofer J, Siminiak T, Haude M et al. Percutaneous mitral annuloplasty for functional mitral regurgitation: results of the CARILLON Mitral Annuloplasty Device European Union Study. Circulation 2009;120:326–333.
165. Liddicoat JR, MacNeill BD, Gillinov AM et al. Percutaneous mitral valve repair: a feasibility study in an ovine model of acute ischemic mitral regurgitation. Catheter Cardiovasc Interv 2003;60:410–416.
166. Daimon M, Shiota T, Gillinov AM et al. Percutaneous mitral valve repair for chronic ischemic mitral regurgitation: a real-time threedimensional echocardiographic study in an ovine model. Circulation 2005;111:2183–2189.
167. Dubreuil O, Basmadjian A, Ducharme A et al. Percutaneous mitral valve annuloplasty for ischemic mitral regurgitation: first in man experience with a temporary implant. Catheter Cardiovasc Interv 2007;69:1053–1061.
168. Ellis S. Percutaneous mitral annuloplasty: Viacor PTOLEMY I update. Presented at Transcatheter Cardiovascular Therapeutics (TCT) Congress, 2008, Washington DC.
169. Gillinov AM, Cosgrove DM, Blackstone EH et al. Durability of mitral valve repair for degenerative disease. J Thorac Cardiovasc Surg. 1998;116:734–743.
170. Tibayan FA Rodriguez F, Liang D et al. Paneth suture annuloplasty abolishes acute ischemic mitral regurgitation but preserves annular and leaflet dynamics. Circulation 2003;108:128–133.
171. Burr LH, Krayenbuhl C, Sutton MS. The mitral plication suture: a new technique of mitral valve repair. J Thorac Cardiovasc Surg 1977;73:589–595.
172. Nagy ZL, Peterffy A. Mitral annuloplasty with a suture technique. Eur J Cardiothoracic Surg 2000;18:739–741.
173. Buellesfeld L. Presented at Transcatheter Cardiovascular Therapeutics (TCT) Congress, 21–25 September 2009, San Francisco.
174. Heuser RR, Witzel T, Dickens D, Takeda PA. Percutaneous treatment for mitral regurgitation: the QuantumCor system. J Interv Cardiol 2008;21:178–182.
175. Goel R, Witzel T, Dickens D et al. The quantumcor device for treating mitral regurgitation: an animal study. Catheter Cardiovasc Interv. 2009;74:43–48.
176. Heuser RR. Presented at Transcatheter Cardiovascular Therapeutics (TCT) Congress, 21–25 September 2009, San Francisco.
177. Starksen N, Guided delivery system. Presented at Transcatheter Cardiovascular Therapeutics (TCT) Congress, 2008.
178. Kono T, Sabbah HN, Rosman H et al. Left ventricular shape is the primary determinant of functional mitral regurgitation in heart failure. J Am Coll Cardiol. 1992;20:1594–1598.
179. Sabbah HN, Rosman H, Kono T et al. On the mechanism of functional mitral regurgitation. Am J Cardiol. 1993;72:1074–1076.
180. Pedersen WR, Block PC, Feldman TE. The Coapsys Repair System for the percutaneous treatment of functional mitral insufficiency. Eurointervention 2006;1:A44–48.
181. Pedersen WR, Block P, Leon M et al. Coapsys mitral valve repair system: percutaneous implantation in an animal model. Catheter Cardiovasc Interv 2008;72:125–131.

182. Rogers JH, Macoviak JA, Rahdert DA et al. Percutaneous septal sinus shortening: a novel procedure for the treatment of functional mitral regurgitation. Circulation 2006; 113;2329–2334.
183. Lozonschi L, Quaden R, Edwards NM et al. Transapical mitral valved stent implantation. Ann Thorac Surg 2008;86:745–748.
184. Herrmann HC. Transcatheter mitral valve implantation. The advantages of MIS-tMVI may make it the ideal choice for high-risk patients. Cardiac Interventions Today August/September 2009.
185. Maisano F, Michev I, Rowe S et al. Transapical endovascular implantation of neochordae using a suction and suture device. Eur J Cardiothorac Surg. 2009;36:118–122.

Aortic Valve Disease

3

3.1
Aortic Stenosis

3.1.1
The Pathophysiology of Aortic Stenosis

Aortic stenosis (AS) is an obstruction to blood ejection from the left ventricle (LV) due to a fixed or dynamic stenosis located in the valve either over (supravalvular) or below it (subvalvular) [1].

Supra- and subvalvular stenoses have a congenital genesis. AS is the most frequent form, and it accounts for the majority of congenital forms and all of the acquired forms. In most cases the etiopathogenesis of acquired AS is ascribable to a fibrocalcific degenerative process of the valve [2]. The characteristic morphological appearance of the non-rheumatic calcific AS consists of the presence of calcification in the cusps, preventing valve opening during outflow. The cusps have a calcific, fibrous and thickened appearance (Fig. 3.1). In some cases there can be a pathoanatomical condition marked by severe calcification of the walls of the ascending aorta, namely "porcelain aorta", which is a high-risk picture for surgical aortic valve replacement. Calcification starts in the fibrous part of the valve, and the stratified microscopic structure is usually preserved. In degenerative AS, unlike in the rheumatic variety, there is no commissural fusion.

Congenital bicuspid aortic valve disease occurs in 1–2% of the population (Fig. 3.2). In most cases the cusps have different dimensions and a median raphe is often present due to their incomplete splitting. At birth, bicuspid aortic valves are not usually stenotic, but they are predisposed to gradually become stenotic owing to sclerosis and calcifications of mechanical origin. The raphe is the site where calcifications develop most frequently.

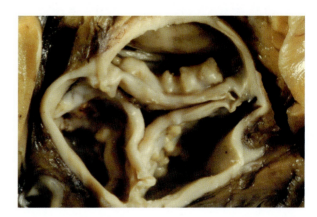

Fig. 3.1 Calcific aortic stenosis

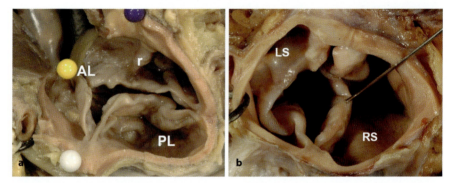

Fig. 3.2 Bicuspid aortic valve. Anteroposterior (**a**) and right–left (**b**) patterns. *AL*, anterior leaflet; *LS*, left sinus; *PL*, posterior leaflet; *r*, raphe; *RS*, right sinus

The aortic valve area (AVA) in adults amounts to about 3.0 cm² and varies within a range of 2.5 to 5 cm² depending on body surface area. In males, a transvalvular gradient can be measured when the AVA is reduced by at least 50% compared to normal [3, 4]. Valve stenosis exerts a resistance to ventricular outflow and, in order to maintain its outflow, the LV develops a higher systolic pressure. Pressure overload leads to concentric hypertrophy of the ventricular walls, namely the heart's main compensation mechanism to cope with LV outflow obstruction. As a result of hypertrophy, left ventricular diastolic compliance tends to reduce, while telediastolic pressure rises without necessarily giving rise to ventricular decompensation [5]. In this case, left atrial contraction plays an important role in ensuring adequate filling pressure in the LV. In these patients, the loss of synchronous and vigorous pump function, as in the case of atrial fibrillation or atrioventricular dissociation, can cause rapid clinical deterioration [6]. With a further rise in afterload, the LV adopts additional compensatory mechanisms such as increase in preload and myocardial contractility. Both of these expedients maintain normal left ventricular systolic pump function [1]. When the preload reserve limit is reached (afterload mismatch) [7], or myocardial contractility is reduced, left ventricular systolic pump function becomes abnormal. Clinically manifest heart failure is usually the result of this alteration in pump function. There is hence a rise in pulmonary artery pressure in the right ventricle and atrium. The increase in myocardial muscle mass due to left ventricular hypertrophy leads to increase of myocardial oxygen demand. There can also be interference with the coronary flow, as the pressure on the artery exceeds the coronary perfusion pressure, and this often leads to ischemia, especially at a subendocardial level and during tachycardia either with or without hemodynamically significant stenosis [8–10].

3.1.2
Diagnosis

3.1.2.1
Non-invasive Diagnosis

A diagnosis of AS is reached through thorough clinical and instrumental assessment of patients. The symptomatic forms are characterized by angina, dyspnea, and syncope, but the diagnostic suspicion can be corroborated by the presence of typical physical signs such as harsh diamond-shaped systolic murmur, often matched by a more intense fremitus along the right upper sternal margin and irradiated to the neck, *parvus et tardus* pulse, and fourth sound. In asymptomatic forms, physical findings can be the only evidence of aortic valve disease.

With regard to instrumental examinations, standard electrocardiogram (ECG) can highlight signs of left ventricular hypertrophy (Fig. 3.3). However, even in the more severe forms of AS, ECG may not show any alteration.

Chest x-ray commonly shows a normal cardiac picture with dilation of the proximal ascending aorta (post-stenotic) and valve calcification in the lateral views. The increase in cardiac area and signs of pulmonary edema can be seen in the case of heart failure.

The staple examination for non-invasive diagnosis of AS is *transthoracic echocardiogram* (TTE) with color-Doppler.

This method consists of:
- assessing the presence, etiology, and severity of valve stenosis
- identifying associated valve diseases and assessing the degree of heart function impairment
- assessing valve apparatus anatomy.

TEE echocardiogram gives very accurate morphological and functional information on the aortic valve, identifying the number of cusps, the thickening

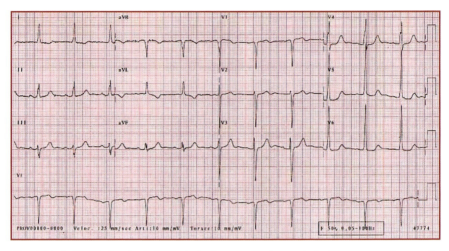

Fig. 3.3 Typical ECG showing left ventricular hypertrophy in a patient with severe aortic stenosis

pattern, and motility [11]. It allows for the detection of some anatomical features of the valve apparatus, which can guide diagnosis, such as, for instance, the presence of bicuspid aortic valve disease, which can be better visualized in parasternal short-axis view and during systole; marked calcifications in degenerative forms, which are predictors of rapidly progressing valve disease; or commissural fusion, typically present in rheumatic forms. Moreover, although the degree of stenosis should be assessed using Doppler, leaflet motility can help estimate the severity of valve disease. It is unlikely that severe stenosis is present if the cusps open well or if a cusp opens well and the other two are stiff, while a calcified and immobile aortic valve is the sign of a severe stenosis (Fig. 3.4).

Doppler assessment allows estimation of the severity of AS by considering the following parameters [12]:
- peak velocity of the antegrade aortic systolic jet
- transvalvular gradient
- valve area by means of the continuity equation.

The antegrade systolic jet velocity through a narrow aortic valve is measured by continuous wave (CW) Doppler [13] (Fig. 3.5). The ultrasound beam should be aligned as best as possible with the jet direction and, in order to obtain a satisfactory Doppler velocity scan, various acoustic windows can be used: apical, suprasternal, right parasternal, and, on rare occasions, subcostal. AS jet velocity is defined as the highest velocity signal obtained from any acoustic window after thorough assessment. It is important not to mistake a Doppler systolic signal due to AS with a signal secondary to mitral regurgitation (MR). The two signals have the same direction compared to the transducer's position, but the two Doppler scans can be distinguished based on the different

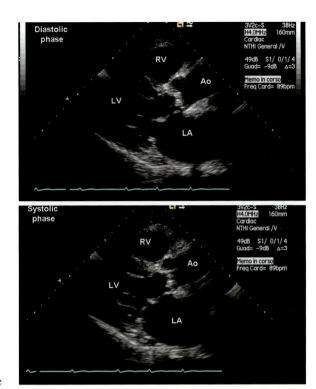

Fig. 3.4 Transthoracic echocardiogram, long-axis view, showing a calcified and stenotic aortic valve. During systolic phase the reduced opening of aortic leaflets is clear. *Ao*, aorta; *LA*, left atrium; *LV*, left ventricle; *RV*, right ventricle

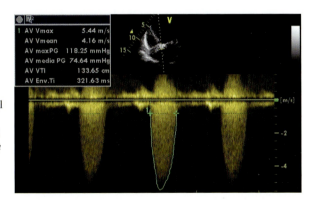

Fig. 3.5 Continuous wave Doppler recordings at the level of a stenotic aortic orifice in five-chamber apical view. Peak velocity (*AV* V_{max}) is more than 5 m/s and the mean gradient (*AV media PG*), obtained tracking the velocity wave, is about 75 mmHg

morphology: the aortic signal starts later on and ends earlier compared to a MR signal, and it seldom reaches the high velocities recorded in the mitral regurgitant jet.

The shape of the Doppler velocity curve allows assessment of the severity of AS, as the maximum peak is later and the curve has a rounded shape in the more severe obstructions; in addition, it can be useful in distinguishing fixed obstructions from dynamic obstructions, as the latter have a late peak, often with a concave curve at the beginning of the systole. Based on the jet velocity, an AS is defined as severe when the jet peak velocity at CW Doppler is greater than 4.0 m/s (Table 3.1); by applying the modified Bernoulli equation ($\Delta P = 4V^2_{max}$), where P is pressure and V is velocity, a velocity of 4.0 m/s corresponds to a maximum transvalvular gradient of 64 mmHg.

Another important parameter to determine the severity of AS is the mean transaortic gradient, calculated by means of the Doppler velocity curve as the mean value of the instantaneous gradients during the ejection period [13] (Fig. 3.5). Of course, an underestimated aortic Doppler velocity gives a proportionally greater underestimation of the gradients, considering the relationship that exists between velocity and pressure gradient. Underestimated Doppler gradients are usually the result of inadequate signal recording or inaccurate alignment of the ultrasound beam, while overestimation can be secondary to a high cardiac output, and associated subvalvular stenosis. Stenosis is defined as severe when the mean pressure gradient is over 40 mmHg according to US guidelines, or over 50 mmHg according to European guidelines [14, 15] (Table 3.1).

Another parameter that is useful to quantify the extent of stenosis is the aortic valve area (AVA). This is calculated using echocardiography by resorting to the continuity equation, which is based on the flow conservation principle by which the flow through the stenotic cross-section is the same as that passing through the left ventricular outflow tract (LVOT) [16]. Since the flow quantity is given by the product of the cross-sectional area (A) and the velocity (V), it follows that the cross-sectional area at the left ventricular outflow tract (A_{lvot}) multiplied by the flow velocity at this level (V_{lvot}) is equal to the stenotic valve cross-sectional area (A_{av}) multiplied by the velocity at the stenotic aortic valve (V_{av}). The calculation of the AVA (A_{av}) by means of the continuity equation

$$A_{av} = [A_{lvot} \times V_{lvot}]/V_{av}$$

requires three measurements: jet velocity in the AS by means of CW Doppler (V_{av}), the diameter of the LVOT to calculate the LVOT cross-sectional area (A_{lvot}), and LVOT velocity at pulsed wave Doppler (V_{lvot}). LVOT diameter

Table 3.1 Criteria for the definition of aortic valve stenosis severity

Criteria	Mild	Moderate	Severe
Aortic jet velocity (m/s)	2.6–2.9	3.0–4.0	>4.0
Mean gradient (mmHg)	<20[a]	20–40[a]	>40[a]
	(<30)[b]	(30–50)[b]	(>50)[b]
Aortic valve area (cm^2)	>1.5	1.0–1.5	<1
Indexed aortic valve area (cm^2/m^2)	>0.85	0.60–0.85	<0.6
Velocity ratio	>0.50	0.25–0.50	<0.25

[a]American Heart Association (AHA)/American College of Cardiology (ACC) guidelines
[b]European Society of Cardiology (ESC) guidelines

should be calculated on two-dimensional (2D) images using the distance between the inner margin of the septal endocardium and the inner margin of the anterior mitral leaflet during systole in parasternal long-axis view (Fig. 3.6). The velocity at the LVOT should be recorded using the apical approach by means of pulsed wave (PW) Doppler, by positioning the sample volume in apical five-chamber view, right below the aortic valve plane (Fig. 3.7). The mean velocity at the stenotic orifice is determined by CW Doppler (Fig. 3.5). Stenosis is severe when it has an AVA below 1 cm^2, or less than 0.6 cm^2/m^2 if indexed based on the body surface area (Table 3.1) [14, 15]. However, it has been proven that AS should be considered severe when the valve area reaches the critical value of 0.8 cm^2, since at this value valve resistance becomes very high and the onset of symptoms occurs [17].

The main source of errors in calculating the continuity equation lies in the measurement of the LVOT diameter. Therefore, when it is not possible to obtain an adequate image at TTE, transesophageal echocardiogram (TEE) is recommended [12]. It must be borne in mind that the continuity equation measures the

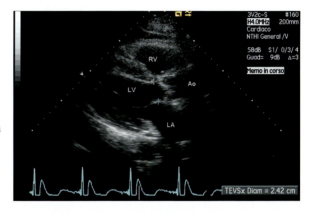

Fig. 3.6 Measurement of the diameter of the left ventricle outflow tract in parasternal long-axis view, carried out in mid-systole, at 0.5–1.0 cm from the aortic orifice. *Ao*, aorta; *LA*, left atrium; *LV*, left ventricle; *RV*, right ventricle

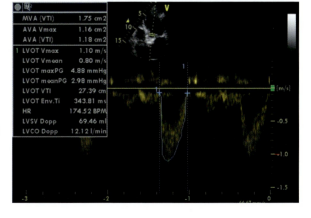

Fig. 3.7 Pulsed wave Doppler recording of the left ventricle outflow tract (LVOT), obtained in five-chambers apical view, with sample volume placed about 0.5 cm below the aortic valve

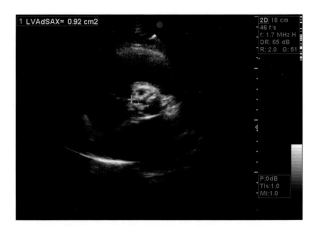

Fig. 3.8 Planimetry of the aortic orifice, transthoracic echocardiogram, short-axis view

effective area, i.e. the flow area, and not the anatomical area. However, direct planimetry is not used, since, especially in case of an extremely calcified aortic valve, orifice identification is difficult (Fig. 3.8). It must also be borne in mind that the valve area calculated with the continuity equation is affected by flow changes, with minimal effects in the case of AS and normal left ventricular function, but more evident in the case of low ejection fraction [18].

There is a simplified continuity equation using peak velocities instead of mean velocities, considering that the systolic ejection time and morphology of the velocity curves in the LVOT and at the stenotic aortic valve are very similar [19]. Based on the same concept, the velocity ratio has been introduced. It consists of the relationship between the velocity in the LVOT, measured by PW Doppler, and the velocity at the aortic valve, measured by CW Doppler. The purpose of this method is to reduce error due to the calculated LVOT diameter. In the absence of stenosis, the velocity ratio is about 1; in the case of severe stenosis it is 0.25 or less and corresponds to a valve area less than 25% of normal.

In the global assessment of a patient, it is necessary to check for associated valve and/or heart diseases, for both therapeutic and prognostic purposes. MR should be carefully assessed both with regard to the severity, as it affects the prognosis, and with regard to the pathophysiological mechanisms of MR (functional, ischemic, post-rheumatic, degenerative). However, it must be borne in mind that MR can often be overestimated due to high left ventricular pressures secondary to AS.

Aortic regurgitation (AR) is present in about 80% of patients with AS, but in most cases it is either mild or moderate [12] (Figs. 3.9 and 3.10). Severe aortic or mitral regurgitation can impair an accurate assessment of AS, since severe AR, by causing a high transaortic flow, can lead to overestimation of the mean gradient, while severe MR, by reducing the transaortic flow, can lead to underestimation of valve stenosis.

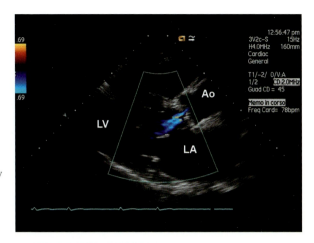

Fig. 3.9 Transthoracic echocardiogram, long-axis view: examples of color flow recordings of a calcified aortic valve with mild regurgitation. *Ao*, aorta; *LA*, left atrium; *LV*, left ventricle

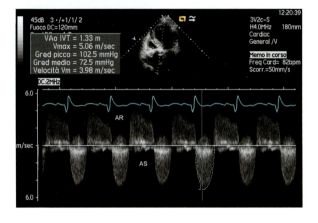

Fig. 3.10 CW Doppler recording, apical five-chamber view, in patient with stenosis and aortic regurgitation. The high-velocity systolic jet of the aortic stenosis (*AS*) and the regurgitant diastolic jet (*AR*) are easily identifiable

The morphological and functional assessment of the left and right chambers (diameters, wall thickness, volumes, ventricular contractile function) provides information on AS severity, left ventricular hypertrophy, and systolic and diastolic function, with obvious prognostic and therapeutic implications (Figs. 3.11 and 3.12). Similar considerations apply to estimation of the pulmonary pressure, and the resulting overload affecting the right ventricle (Fig. 3.13).

The presence of severe AS with severe left ventricular dysfunction, a condition defined as "low-flow, low-gradient AS" as it is characterized by reduced AVA, and low jet velocity and mean transvalvular pressure gradient, is a clinical entity that should be carefully assessed, as it is a form with a severe prognosis, which, however, may lead, at times, to diagnostic errors. Assessment of AS is hence more difficult in the case of concomitant severe left ventricular dysfunction. In a similar situation, the reduced AVA with a low pressure gradient can

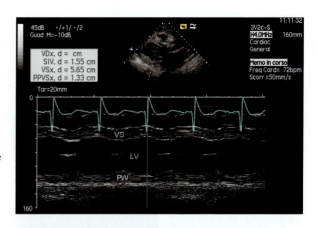

Fig. 3.11 M-mode echocardiogram in a patient with severe aortic stenosis who has developed moderate left ventricular hypertrophy. *LV*, left ventricle; *PW*, posterior wall; *VS*, ventricular septum

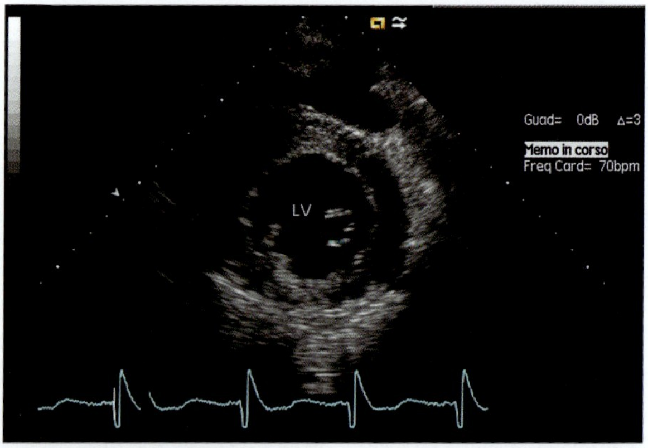

Fig. 3.12 2D echocardiogram, short-axis view, showing concentric left ventricular hypertrophy in a patient with aortic stenosis. *LV*, left ventricle

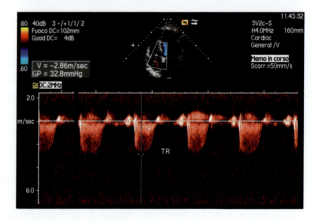

Fig. 3.13 CW Doppler recording showing the tricuspid regurgitant jet velocity. *TR*, tricuspid regurgitation

depend either on severe stenosis proper, in which the stenotic lesion itself is the cause of the impaired left ventricular systolic function due to the increase in the afterload, or on a primary left ventricular dysfunction, which does not generate sufficient contractile strength to overcome the inertia to open the valve (pseudo-severe AS). In these cases, a stress test with dobutamine should be performed to distinguish a morphologically severe AS from a reduced orifice area secondary to low cardiac output. If there actually is AS, infusion of dobutamine at gradually increasing doses (starting from 2.5–5 µg/kg/min with 5 µg/kg/min increases every 3–5 min until a maximum dose of 10–20 µg/kg/min is reached), by increasing cardiac output, also increases the pressure gradient, leaving the AVA unaltered; on the other hand, in the case of aortic pseudostenosis, the increase in cardiac output increases the valve area with a minimal change in gradient [20, 21]. The stress test with dobutamine is also useful in assessing the LV's contractile reserve for prognostic purposes; in cases in which there is no increase in ejection fraction or cardiac output, i.e. if there is a lack of contractile reserve, the prognosis is bad and the risk of operative mortality is high [22, 23].

The test on effort is contraindicated in symptomatic patients with AS. In asymptomatic patients, it can be performed under close monitoring and it has great prognostic value. Reduced tolerance to effort and the onset of symptoms or abnormal pressures, such as an increase in arterial pressure of less than 20 mmHg, are associated with an unfavorable outcome, so these patients should be considered as symptomatic [24].

Cardiac magnetic resonance imaging (MRI) and multislice computed tomography (MSCT) scan can be useful to assess the ascending aorta or, in the case of MSCT scan, to quantify the degree of aortic valve calcification. Their use is currently rather limited due to the high costs limiting their spread.

3.1.2.2
Invasive Diagnosis

The main role of cardiac catheterization in AS patients consists of determining whether there is concurrent coronary artery disease in patients to be treated surgically or percutaneously for valve disease. Careful hemodynamic study to determine the severity of stenosis is indicated when echocardiography data leave doubts or are of non-optimal quality, when there is a discrepancy between clinical information and echocardiography findings, and when AS is associated with low cardiac output or altered LV function [15, 25]. In the latter case, the hemodynamic assessment of AS severity at rest and during maneuvers to increase the flow through the aortic valve (e.g. by infusing dobutamine) can provide crucial information for the difficult assessment of the indications to treatment; indeed, severe AS patients show an increase in transvalvular gradient without changes in the AVA during dobutamine infusion, while those without AS show an increase in the calculated valve area [23].

In general, valve obstructions produce a pressure gradient through a stenosis or narrowing of a duct or chamber. The pressure gradient is affected by physiological variables, like blood flow velocity, resistance to flow, pressure, and compliance of the proximal chamber, and by anatomical variables, like the shape and width of the valve orifice. In clinical practice, the most useful measurements are the assessments of the peak transvalvular gradient (Fig. 3.14) and AVA. The method to calculate AVA uses the Gorlin formula [26] or the simplified Hakke method [27], which differs from the Gorlin method by 18 ± 13% in patients with bradycardia (<65 beats/min [bpm]) or tachycardia (>100 bpm) [28]. Moreover, in low-output conditions, the Gorlin equation overestimates the severity of valve stenosis. In these cases (cardiac output <2.5 l/min), the Gorlin formula should be modified [26].

However, despite their proven effectiveness, AVA measurements have both practical and theoretical limits. The area is a planar measurement, which does not consider mitral inflow with its funnel shape, or aortic outflow with a tubular shape. AVA calculation is based on a laminar flow of a non-compressible fluid. Turbulence is hence not considered. As a result, valve areas <0.7 cm^2 are almost always associated with clinical symptoms, and areas >1.1 cm^2 are not usually associated with symptoms, but the intermediate areas are in a gray zone. Another hemodynamic parameter that has proven its clinical utility is the calculation of valve resistance, although it is a complementary index that cannot be used instead of valve area assessment [26]. Based on these considerations, according to guidelines, hemodynamic assessment of AS is not necessary on a routine basis [15].

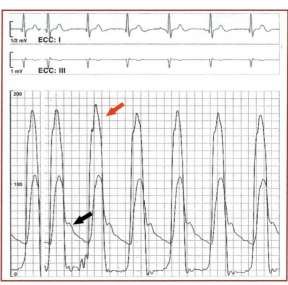

Fig. 3.14 Pressure waves recorded at left cardiac catheterization. The *black arrow* indicates the aortic pressure wave, the *red arrow* indicates the left ventricle pressure wave. The transvalvular gradient is calculated by measuring the difference between the peak pressures in the left ventricle and aorta (peak-to-peak gradient)

3.1.3
Timing of Interventions

Senile degenerative AS is a pathology whose clinical history is marked by an asymptomatic period of latency with a variable duration, during which the risk of sudden death is lower than 1% [29–33], followed by the onset of the typical symptoms characterizing an unfavorable prognosis [34] (Fig 3.15). The predictors of AS progression and a severe prognosis in asymptomatic patient are [15]:
- advanced age and the presence of risk factors of atherosclerotic disease
- echocardiography parameters indicative of AS severity (marked valve calcification, increase in aortic ejection peak velocity >0.3 m/s in a year, low ejection fraction)
- onset of typical symptoms during effort test.

The elements of interest with major implications on the indication and timing of treatment of this valve disease are:
- continual increase in AS prevalence in the age group over 65 years of age
- associated comorbidities in elderly patients, which affect surgical risk
- development in techniques and materials used to treat AS, such that high-risk patients can be treated with minimally invasive techniques.

The rise in the general population's mean age is leading to the need today to treat patients with severe AS, who are over 80 years of age and have pathologies affecting other systems and organs, in whom cardiac surgery is excluded and medical treatment alone has proven to be ineffective.

Elderly age, while not a surgical risk factor per se, is associated with a greater frequency of comorbidities, which contribute as a whole to increasing surgical risk and making the choice of the most appropriate treatment of a single patient more complicated. However, open-heart cardiac surgery to replace the native diseased valve with a mechanical or biological device is currently the therapeutic gold standard for severe AS [15].

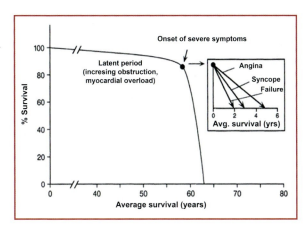

Figure 3.15 Survival curve describing the natural history of aortic stenosis. This is characterized by a variable asymptomatic period, where the risk of sudden death is lower than 1%, followed by the onset of characteristic symptoms: dyspnea, angina pectoris, and syncope. In these cases the prognosis is severe, with a mean two-year survival rate that varies from 0% to 50%

For the indication to intervention, two groups of patients need to be distinguished: symptomatic patients and asymptomatic ones.

3.1.3.1
Symptomatic Patients

Valve replacement is indicated in symptomatic patients with severe stenosis. As stated above, the typical symptoms are dyspnea, angina pectoris, and syncope, although many patients develop more subtle symptoms marked by fatigue and dyspnea after effort; in this regard, an accurate assessment of the development of symptoms over the course of time is essential to define this class of patients. The risk of sudden death is high once the symptoms are manifest even to a mild degree [18, 24, 34]. When symptoms appear, aortic valve area is <1 cm^2 and velocity at Doppler is >4 m/s; in this case, the indication for surgical replacement is loud and clear [15]. Nonetheless, some patients are symptomatic even with a valve area between 1 and 1.5 cm^2 or with a velocity at Doppler of 3–4 m/s. In these cases, other diagnostic instruments (coronarography, chest x-ray, etc) are recommended to exclude other causes for the symptoms; with clear symptoms not due to any other reason, valve replacement can be considered in these cases, if the valve has major calcifications, even though stenosis is moderate [22].

3.1.3.2
Asymptomatic Patients

In asymptomatic patients, surgical risk must be carefully assessed compared to the risk of any event in the case of non-intervention. Aortic valve repair is not a valid option. Therefore, device duration and the correlated risks must be considered as well. If symptoms are not clear, an effort test can be useful to determine any clinical or hemodynamic changes under effort.

As noted above, patients with reduced tolerance to effort, with a drop in pressure during exercise (>20 mmHg), or onset of symptoms should be considered symptomatic and hence referred for invasive treatment [15]. In any case, the effort test in severe AS patients must be carried out with the utmost caution. Even with a severe obstruction, the risk of sudden death is low (<1%) in asymptomatic patients [22]. In theory, early surgery could prevent the onset of systolic and diastolic ventricular dysfunction, but sound data supporting this hypothesis are still lacking. Therefore, to date, the most correct management of asymptomatic patients consists of a "wait-and-see" approach, and intervention should be put off until the onset of symptoms.

However, there are various exceptions in which surgery is recommended despite the lack of symptoms [15]:
- in asymptomatic patients with severe AS who need to undergo other cardiac surgery procedures (aortocoronary bypass, ascending aorta surgery, etc)
- in asymptomatic patients with moderate AS who need to undergo other cardiac surgery procedures (aortocoronary bypass, ascending aorta surgery, etc)
- in patients with left ventricular function impairment (ejection fraction <50%)
- in patients with evidence of a rapid evolution in the degree of obstruction (0,3 m/s a year)
- in patients with thickened interventricular septum (≥15mm), not of hypertensive origin.

The complete picture of the indications for surgery in AS patients, according to European guidelines [15], is provided in Table 3.2.

In general, surgical replacement allows for a marked improvement in clinical

Table 3.2 Indications for valve replacement in aortic stenosis, adapted from 2007 European guidelines for the treatment of valve diseases

Indication	Recommendation
Patients with severe aortic stenosis and any symptoms	IB
Patients with severe aortic stenosis undergoing coronary artery bypass graft, surgery of the ascending aorta, or another valve	IC
Asymptomatic patients with severe aortic stenosis and systolic left ventricular dysfunction (LVEF <50%) unless due to other cause	IC
Asymptomatic patients with severe aortic stenosis and abnormal exercise test showing symptoms on exercise	IC
Asymptomatic patients with severe aortic stenosis and abnormal exercise test showing fall in blood pressure below baseline	IIaC
Patients with moderate aortic stenosis undergoing coronary artery bypass graft, surgery of the ascending aorta, or another valve	IIaC
Asymptomatic patients with severe aortic stenosis and moderate-to-severe valve calcifications and a rate of peak velocity progression ≥0.3 m/s per year	IIaC
Aortic stenosis with low gradient (<40 mmHg) and left ventricular dysfunction with contractile reserve	IIaC
Asymptomatic patients with severe aortic stenosis and abnormal exercise test showing complex ventricular arrhythmias	IIbC
Asymptomatic patients with severe aortic stenosis and excessive left ventricular hypertrophy (≥15 mm) unless this is due to hypertension	IIbC
Aortic stenosis with low gradient (<40 mmHg) and left ventricular dysfunction without contractile reserve	IIbC

LVEF, left ventricular ejection fraction

symptoms and in long-term survival in most patients, with an intraoperative mortality of 3–5% for patients below 70 years of age undergoing aortic valve replacement alone for the first time; this percentage rises to 5–15% in patients aged over 70 years [35].

The risk of operative mortality is increased by the following factors:
- elderly age
- comorbidities
- female gender
- advanced New York Heart Association (NYHA) class
- ventricular dysfunction
- pulmonary hypertension
- atherosclerotic coronaropathy
- prior cardiac surgery.

The predictors of intraoperative mortality have been identified based on a long series of cardiac surgery patients, and have been correlated with cardiac diseases, patient age, comorbidity, and type of surgical procedure [36].

In this regard, there are two main models utilized to evaluate surgical risk: The Society of Thoracic Surgery Predicted Risk of Mortality (STS-PROM) [37] and the European System for Cardiac Operative Risk Evaluation (EuroSCORE) [38]. These systems are based on the assessment of cardiac and extra-cardiac factors. Although these represent the sole objective methods to estimate short-term mortality after surgical aortic valve replacement, they have several limitations, although the STS-PROM seems to reproduce more closely the operative and 30-day mortality for the highest-risk patients having aortic valve replacement [37]. First of all they are not specifically designed for AS and tend to overestimate or sometimes underestimate the real risk [37, 38]. Also, they are not widely applicable, as it is now well accepted that the risk is also related to the particular surgical team; moreover, there are a series of clinical conditions, such as previous mediastinal irradiation, the presence of porcelain aorta, anatomical abnormalities of the chest wall, a history of mediastinitis, liver cirrhosis, or patient's frailty, which have not been taken into account in these risk scores, but which very often are a contraindication or make surgery particularly risky. Despite these limitations and the need for further validation, the use of these systems has significantly reduced the subjectivity of surgical risk and risk–benefit assessments.

In clinical practice, although indications for aortic valve replacement are well defined by guidelines and clearly recommend surgery in symptomatic patients with severe AS, regardless of age, there is a tendency to consider patients over 70 years of age as inoperable *tout court* [15]. The EuroHeart Survey [39], a prospective study, published in 2001 and carried out on over 5000 patients affected by moderate-to-severe valve diseases enrolled in 92 centers in 25 European countries, showed that, while there is general agreement between the decision to intervene surgically and existing guidelines on the treatment of symptomatic patients, recourse to surgery in patients with serious symptoms is less frequent for several, often groundless, reasons.

In the EuroHeart Survey, at least one-third of the elderly patients with comorbidities and AS were not considered operable. The reason for non-intervention was:
- in 31% of patients with only severely diseased aortic valve, patient refusal to undergo surgery
- regression of symptoms with medical therapy (about 39%)
- end-stage disease in 18%
- symptoms ascribed to a concurrent coronary artery pathology (14%) with recent myocardial infarction in 7%.

Alongside the cardiac causes, the presence of at least one extra-cardiac condition was considered a contraindication to surgery in 55.3% of cases. The most frequent reasons reported were:
- advanced age (27.6%; sole reason in 1.3% of cases)
- chronic obstructive pulmonary disease (13.6%)
- kidney failure (6.1%)
- patient refusal (16%)
- low life expectancy (19.3%).

Clearly, the use of the EuroScore and STS score to quantify surgical risk is just one of the factors for assessment of the therapeutic approach; it must be corroborated by other essential elements like the patient's life expectancy and quality of life, as well as requests and expectations of patients and their families. It has been proven that, despite high surgical risk, patients over 80 years of age have a much better prognosis after surgery compared to medical therapy alone. Therefore, the development of a less invasive treatment to reduce the cardiovascular complications due to general anesthesia, thoracotomy and extra-corporeal circulation to a minimum, is essential for elderly patients affected by severe AS associated with comorbidities, which, without adequate treatment, would inevitably lead to death in a few months.

3.1.4
Patient Selection

As explained, aortic valve replacement is currently still the "gold-standard" treatment of AS [15]. It hence follows that percutaneous treatment, as underscored by the consensus of European cardiology, invasive cardiology, and cardiac surgery societies published in 2008, is a valid option only when there are conditions contraindicating surgery [40].

In this regard, setting up a multidisciplinary team comprising a cardiologist, cardiac surgeon, and anesthesiologist working together is essential for the proper selection of candidates for the percutaneous approach [41].

This is done in four steps:
- confirmation of AS severity
- assessment of symptoms
- analysis of surgical risk, life expectancy, and quality of life
- assessment of the procedure feasibility and any contraindications to percutaneous treatment.

The first three items were addressed in the sections on the timing of intervention and invasive and non-invasive diagnosis. In this section we will discuss the clinical and anatomical indications to percutaneous aortic valve implantation and its contraindications.

In order to determine the eligibility for transcatheter device implantation, coronary anatomy should be assessed. If there is critical coronary artery disease requiring a percutaneous, surgical, or mixed approach, the timing of treatment should be assessed case by case, based on the patient's clinical and anatomical conditions [40].

In general, percutaneous implantation is not indicated in patients with proximal coronary stenosis not treatable by angioplasty [40]. MSCT or standard angiography is especially useful to assess the relations between the coronary ostia and the valve leaflets [42] (Fig 3.16). Proper valve measurement is essential to reduce the incidence of malpositioning to a minimum, as this may lead to prosthetic dysfunction due to frame hypo-expansion or damage due to compression on adjacent cardiac structures (in the case of placement of oversized devices), or inadequate anchoring such that it may cause significant perivalvular regurgitation or device embolization (in the case of undersized devices) (Fig 3.17).

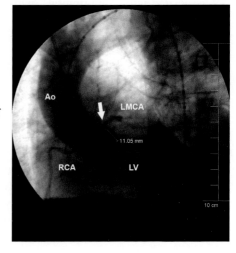

Fig. 3.16 Aortography in left anterior oblique projection: *white arrow* indicates the take-off of the left main coronary artery (*LMCA*); accurate measurement of the distance from the aortic valve annulus and origin of the coronary ostia is mandatory to prevent its impairment during balloon valvuloplasty or prosthesis deployment, caused by calcified aortic cusp put against the Valsalva sinus wall. *Ao*, aorta; *LV*, left ventricle; *RCA*, right coronary artery

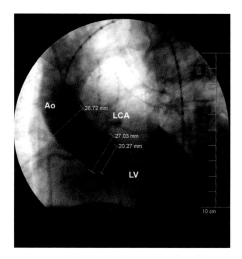

Fig. 3.17 Aortography in left anterior oblique projection: measurement of the main structures of the aortic root; from the bottom to the top of the figure: annulus, sinus of Valsalva weight, and sinotubular junction. *Ao*, aorta; *LCA*, left coronary artery; *LV*, left ventricle

However, the gold standard method for measuring the various anatomical structures has not yet been determined. Transthoracic and/or transesophageal echocardiography, for cases of non-optimal acoustic window, have proven to be effective methods especially for measuring the outflow tract of the LV and ascending aorta. MSCT, too, is an instrument of proven efficacy and utility in selecting patients for percutaneous aortic valve implantation. The three-dimensional (3D) reconstructions provided by this examination offer accurate information on the anatomy of the aortic root, aorta, coronary arteries, and peripheral vessels. Therefore, MSCT is a valid non-invasive imaging instrument to confirm the baseline pathology, select the patients to be treated, and choose the proper size of the device [42]. MSCT is especially useful in patients with high acoustic impedance in the chest and in those with contraindications to TEE. Scanning is generally carried out by asking the patient to hold his breath for 10–15 s; in the meantime, the computed tomography (CT) ECG device is synchronized with the patient's QRS, to perform scans during both systole and diastole. During this interval of time, non-iodinated contrast medium is administered, the quantity of which varies from 60 to 100 ml depending on the patient's build. Image post-processing starts with reconstruction of the coronal and single-oblique sagittal views (like a parasternal long-axis view) passing through the aortic valve. Then, centering of both views on the aortic valve allows for processing of the double-oblique transverse view (like a short-axis parasternal view) at the aortic valve; the latter view offers an in-depth anatomical and morphological analysis of the valve, which makes it possible to distinguish between bicuspid and tricuspid valves and to detect and quantify build-up of calcium [43] (Fig. 3.18). It is important to study the arrangement of the calcifications, as these formations may exert resistance to the expansion of the devices, leading to a non-circular shape and hence paraprosthetic leaks. By delimiting the cusps, the double-oblique transverse view with reconstruction during the systolic phase (about 35% of the R–R interval after the R wave) is useful to measure the valve area with an accuracy comparable to that of TEE [44, 45]. With regard to the assessment of the aorto-iliac-femoral axis, MSCT can provide important information, not only with 3D reconstruction of the vessels, which allows for easy identification of the twists, but also by illustrating calcifications, which may hinder the insertion of the catheters and cause tears in the arteries (Figs. 3.19 and 3.20).

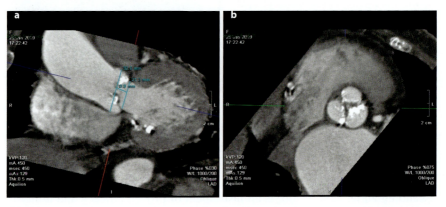

Fig. 3.18 64 MSCT image, coronal view (**a**), showing the aortic valve apparatus with measurement of the annulus, sinuses of Valsalva, and height of the sinuses of Valsalva, and, in transverse view (**b**), showing the tricuspid aortic valve with calcified cusps

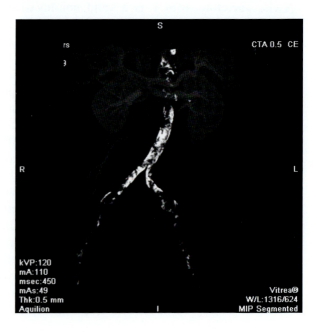

Fig. 3.19 Angio-CT, 3D reconstruction, showing aorto-iliac-femoral vascular tree: vessels are calcified without significant stenosis and tortuosity

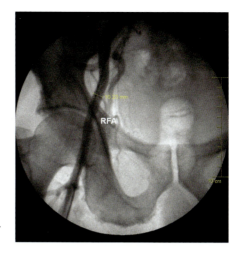

Fig. 3.20 Peripheral angiography in anteroposterior projection, shows the right femoral artery (*RFA*) >10 mm. This vascular access is suitable for 18 Fr (CoreValve®), 22- and 24 Fr (Edwards-SAPIEN™) catheters

During assessment for eligibility for transcatheter implantation of aortic valve devices, with self-expanding and balloon-expandable prostheses, a series of morphological and functional parameters should be measured. These parameters can be either general or specific to the device or approach used [2], and are discussed under the next headings.

3.1.4.1
Valve Annulus

A precise measurement of aortic annulus diameters is crucial in the choice of devices with the right size. Annulus diameter is measured during systole in parasternal long-axis view with zoom of the image, which clearly shows the LVOT, aortic valve, and root (Fig 3.21). At least three measurements and their

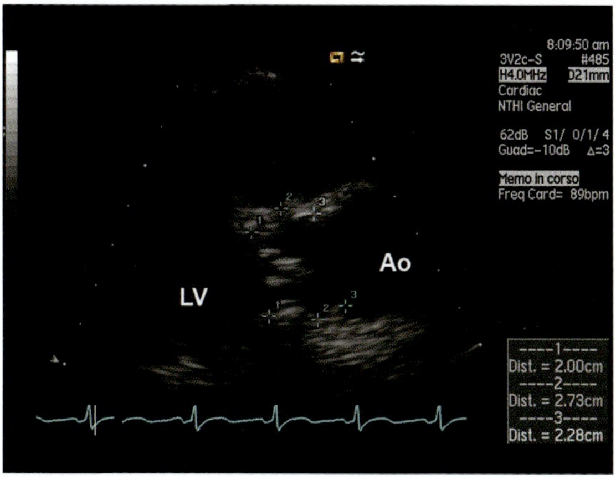

Fig. 3.21 Transthoracic echocardiogram, long-axis projection: standard measurement of the aortic root, 1 = aortic annulus; 2 = sinus of Valsalva; 3 = sinotubular junction). *Ao*, ascending aorta; *LV*, left ventricle

mean should be taken; in the case of a non-optimal acoustic window, TEE needs to be performed (Fig 3.22).

Sources of error include: failure to identify cusp avulsion due to prior valvuloplasty (a presence of significant AR following aortic valvuloplasty should give rise to suspicion) or the presence of substantial valve and cusp calcifications, which make the identification of annulus margins difficult. Only two device sizes (small and large) can currently be found commercially and they cover a range of valve annuli of 20–27 mm for self-expanding valves (CoreValve® ReValving System [CRS], Medtronic Inc., MN, USA) and 18–25 mm for balloon expandable valves (Edwards-SAPIEN™ [ES] Edwards Lifesciences, Irvine, California, USA) (Table 3.3). Precise annulus measurement is a critical factor for the procedure's efficacy, especially in borderline cases in which annulus diameters are halfway between the size of small and large valves (23–24 mm for CRS, 21–22 for ES). Generally speaking, it should be borne in mind that TTE tends to underestimate the actual aortic annulus.

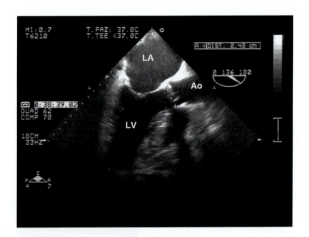

Fig. 3.22 Transesophageal echocardiogram with measurement of the aortic annulus. *Ao*, ascending aorta; *LA*, left atrium; *LV*, left ventricle

Table 3.3 Anatomical criteria for eligibility for current devices with CE mark

Diameters (mm)	CoreValve ReValving System®		Edwards-SAPIEN™ heart valve	
	CRS-26 mm	CRS-29 mm	ES-23 mm	ES-26 mm
Ascending aorta	≤40	≤45	NA	NA
SV width	≥27	≥31	NA	NA
SV height	>12 >	12	10–12	10–12
Annulus	20–23	24–27	18–21	22–25
Vascular access	>6		>9	

CRS, CoreValve ReValving System®; *ES*, Edwards-SAPIEN™; *SV*, sinus of Valsalva; *NA*, not available

3.1.4.2
Sinuses of Valsalva (Width and Height)

The width of the sinuses of Valsalva, measured in left parasternal long axis both as absolute diameter and related to the device type and diameter, is an important piece of information to avoid obstacles to coronary perfusion.

There are minimal diameters for device implantation (27 mm for small CRS, 29 mm for large CRS; Table 3.3) to leave enough space for proper perfusion of the coronary arteries (Fig 3.21). This is needed because the device's outer diameter may crush the thickened and calcified aortic valve cusps inside the sinuses, thus obstructing the coronary ostia. For this reason, the width of the sinuses of Valsalva should also be referred to the height of the sinuses. The minimum height required for CRS is 12–15 mm and 10–12 mm for the Edwards device (Table 3.3).

Transcatheter aortic valve implantation (TAVI) is indicated with:
- an aortic valve with sinuses of Valsalva that are wide and short enough or vice versa
- large annulus, narrow and tall sinuses of Valsalva
- large annulus, wide and short sinuses of Valsalva.

TAVI is not indicated with:
- an aortic valve with small annulus and narrow and short sinuses of Valsalva
- an aortic valve with large annulus and sinuses of Valsalva near the lower width and height limits.

3.1.4.3
Sinotubular Junction (STJ)

This measure is more useful for the CRS than the ES device (Fig 3.21). An STJ of less than 23–25 mm may not be suitable for large CRS implantation, as it may prevent proper expansion. Generally speaking, the diameter of the STJ is always equal to or smaller than that of the annulus, except for aorto-annular ectasia.

3.1.4.4
Left Ventricular Outflow Tract

Measurement of LVOT has gained importance with experience acquired from the first implants. A narrow LVOT with concurrent severe septal hypertrophy may be a contraindication to implantation, as the valve protrudes with its still terminal part into the LVOT. A severely hypertrophic septum makes the implantation of a CRS valve rather difficult, as it often requires a lower implantation position to ensure device stability; this means that the device protrudes more inside the ventricle. However, a low implantation position increases the risk of total atrioventricular block (AVB) and may be the cause of MR due to distortion of the mitral annulus near the mitral-aortic junction. An LVOT greater than 24 mm with valve annulus of 23–24 mm (borderline) and adequate sinuses of Valsalva may lead to choosing a large device rather a small one; vice versa, for a borderline annulus with small LVOT, it may better to lodge a small device.

3.1.4.5
Ascending Aorta

This measure is more important for the CRS than for the ES device. The distal portion of the device is softer and has a wider mesh compared to the central and proximal portions; it is 40–45 mm wide and its purpose is to align the valve with the central axis of the ascending aorta, thus ensuring further stability. If the diameter of the ascending aorta is >43 mm, there is a relative contraindication (Table 3.3). The specific contraindications to the transfemoral or transapical approach have not been defined yet and the indication should be based on the patient's conditions and the center's experience.

3.1.4.6
Iliac-femoral and Subclavian Artery

The study of peripheral accesses is a crucial step in patient selection: assessment of the feasibility, and especially the safety of a femoral approach, is generally the first step to be made when a patient is considered for TAVI; in this regard, various aspects must be borne in mind:
- assessment of the peripheral arterial vessels for risk of distal ischemia; patients with superficial femoral artery occlusion are at risk of acute ischemia if there are small emboli in the deep arteries
- assessment of the common femoral arteries as a puncture site and for potential risks of occlusion or extensive bleeding in the presence of severe calcifications or vessels with a small gauge
- assessment of the iliac arteries for risk of rupture or perforation in the presence of severe calcifications or diseased vessels
- assessment of the thoracic and abdominal aorta for risk of mobilizing emboli when the release device is advanced or in the case of device retraction due to malapposition or device migration
- assessment of the angle and calcification of the aortic arch and ascending aorta, for the risk of valve misplacement, stroke, and aortic dissection.

Study of the subclavian artery is useful when using the CRS device, as it may be

implanted using this approach in the case of inappropriate femoral accesses. There are criteria contraindicating this approach with regard to the risk of causing subclavian artery dissection in patient in whom the left internal mammary artery (LIMA) has already been used for prior cardiac bypass:
- artery diameter <6.5 mm from the origin of the subclavian artery at the LIMA ostium
- severe LIMA bending
- circumferential calcification or atherosclerosis of the subclavian artery at the origin of the LIMA (risk of dissection)
- atherosclerotic lesions requiring treatment by angioplasty.

Generally speaking, the following conditions are considered contraindications to the transfemoral approach:
- iliac arteries with severe calcification, bends, or a diameter of <6–9 mm depending on the device used or prior aortofemoral bypass (Table 3.3)
- aorta with narrow curves, aortic coaptation, or aneurysm of the abdominal aorta (Fig. 3.23) with mural thrombi
- calcium masses in the ascending aorta
- transverse ascending aorta (ES device).

The contraindications to the transapical approach are:
- prior left ventricular surgery with patch placement (Dor procedure)
- cutaneous disease due to prior radiation therapy of the chest
- calcified pericardium
- severe respiratory failure
- apex of the left ventricle not reachable.

The clinical exclusion criteria are:
- confirmed hypersensivity/allergy to one of the drugs used in the peri- or post-procedure period
- active sepsis or endocarditis
- atherosclerosis, calcification, or bending of the femoral and iliac arteries and aorta
- aortic aneurysm
- bleeding diathesis/coagulopathy
- myocardial infarction or recent cerebrovascular events (<1 month)
- severe mitral or tricuspid regurgitation (>3/4)
- uncontrolled atrial fibrillation with high ventricular response (>100 bpm), despite drug therapy
- atheromatous disease (plaques >70%) in the carotid or vertebral arteries, accompanied by symptoms.

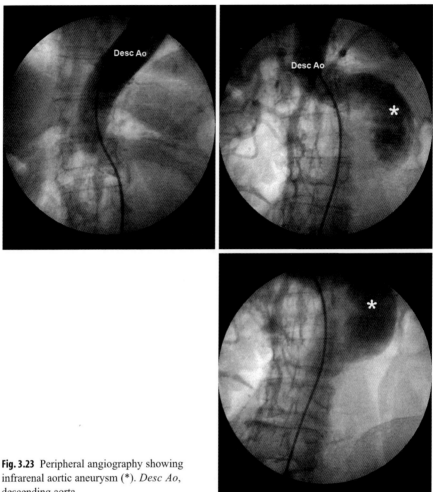

Fig. 3.23 Peripheral angiography showing infrarenal aortic aneurysm (*). *Desc Ao*, descending aorta

3.1.5
Percutaneous Therapy

For many years, percutaneous treatment of AS consisted of balloon aortic valvuloplasty, a method capable of temporarily improving symptoms without having an impact on survival [46–51] (Fig 3.24). The explanation for this lies in the principle on which the technique is based: dilating a calcified valve with a balloon temporarily increases the aortic valve area, thus creating microfractures in the fibrocalcific cusps and increasing the elasticity of the aortic valve apparatus. These changes do not, however, affect the disease's natural history, as calcification, accelerated flow, and turbulence in the valve, namely the main pathophysiological mechanisms in AS, continue to persist [49].

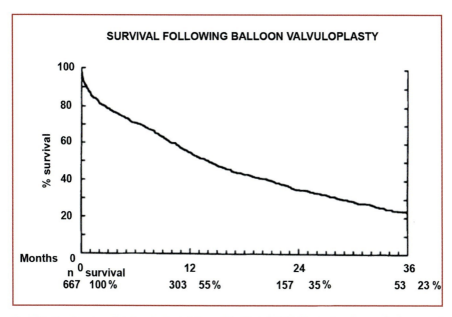

Fig. 3.24 Graph extrapolated and adapted from Otto C et al [49], illustrating the survival curve of a population of 667 patients affected by severe aortic stenosis receiving palliative valvulopathy. Survival was 55% at 1 year, 35% at 2 years, and 23% at 3 years. Most of the deaths were due to cardiac causes (70%)

Over the years and with improvement in techniques and materials, percutaneous aortic valvuloplasty has become a safer method, with a drastic reduction in peri-procedural complications, without any impact, however, on survival and progression of the valve disease. Therefore, in order to address the growing number of patients who are denied cardiac surgery due to high surgical risk [52], in recent years, research has focused on the development of percutaneously implantable devices, by experimenting with minimally invasive implantable systems that ensure valve function comparable to the devices used in cardiac surgery [53].

Various percutaneous devices are currently available. Of these, only the ES [54] and CRS prosthesis [55] have the CE mark, being at an advanced experimentation level with more than 10 000 patients treated with each device, for which several case histories have been published, demonstrating safety and short- and medium-term efficacy [56–73].

3.1.5.1
Edwards-SAPIEN™ Valve

3.1.5.1.1
Device Description

The Edwards-SAPIEN™ percutaneous heart valve consists of a tricuspid valve made of bovine pericardium and implanted on a stainless steel stent (Fig. 3.25). Initially, there was just a single size: 23 mm at maximum diameter, and 14.5 mm high. Currently, this percutaneous device comes in two diameters (23 × 14.5 mm and 26 × 16 mm) compatible with 22 and 24 Fr catheters respectively. The 23 mm device is suitable for an annulus between 18 and 21 mm; and the 26 mm device is suitable for an annulus between 22 and 25 mm.

The device has various components (Fig. 3.26):
- percutaneous aortic valve device
- delivery system composed of a flexible catheter (RetroFlex 3, Edwards Lifesciences, Irvine, California, USA) (Fig. 3.27)
- 24 Fr introducer
- RetroFlex dilator kit
- RetroFlex valvuloplasty balloon
- Atrion™ indeflators
- Crimper.

The valve is mounted on a flexible guiding catheter and implanted using a balloon (Z-MED II™, NuMed, Inc., Hopkinton, New York, USA), which fits on the inside using the crimper (Fig. 3.28), and is inflated, thus expanding the prosthesis and anchoring it on the degenerated native aortic valve.

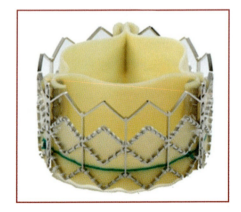

Fig. 3.25 Edwards-SAPIEN Transcatheter Heart Valve™ (courtesy of Edwards Lifesciences Inc.)

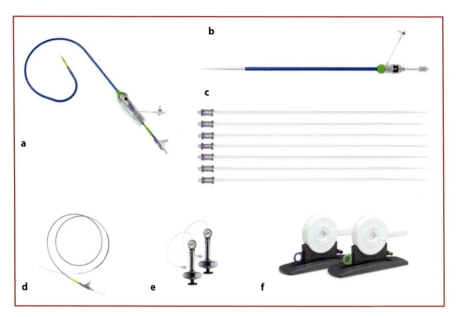

Fig. 3.26 Components of the Edwards-SAPIEN™ device: **a** RetroFlex 3 delivery system; **b** 24 Fr introducer; **c** RetroFlex dilators kit; **d** RetroFlex valvuloplasty balloon; **e** Atrion indeflators; **f** Crimper systems for the 23-mm (*green crimper*) and the 26-mm (*purple crimper*) Edwards SAPIEN valve (courtesy of Edwards Lifesciences Inc.)

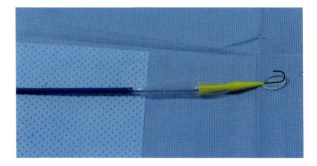

Fig. 3.27 Distal part of RetroFlex 3 catheter

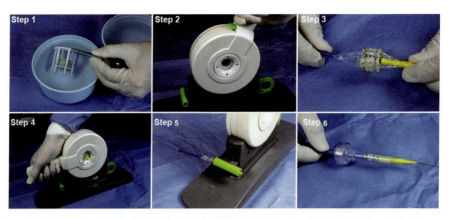

Fig. 3.28 Crimping systems of the Edwards-SAPIEN™ device. **Step 1**: take the valve basket from the package, place it in a tray with saline solution, and rinse the valve, moving the basket quickly up and down to make the leaflets move. **Step 2**: after releasing the device from the basket, crimp the valve alone to reduce the diameter by about 30%. **Step 3**: place the valve on the balloon, between the two markers on the inside and make sure to orient the device correctly (the green seam in the valve indicates the ventricular side). **Step 4**: progressively crimp the valve until you reach the bottom, and maintain it in position for 10 s; make sure that the position between the markers does not change (crimping must be performed several times until the desired profile is obtained). **Step 5**: using the crimper's gauge, previously washed, make sure that the valve is duly crimped and, in case of attrition, continue crimping. **Step 6**: approach the RetroFlex catheter to the valve and fit the loader on the catheter (the loader must completely cover the valve)

3.1.5.1.2
Procedure and Technical Aspects

Three approaches are used for implantation:
- antegrade approach (Fig. 3.29)
- retrograde approach (Fig. 3.30)
- transapical approach (Fig. 3.31).

The antegrade approach was the first to be used by Cribier in 2002 [54]; it is achieved by using catheters inserted in the femoral vein and advanced to the left atrium, left ventricle, and aortic root after crossing the inter-atrial septum [56, 57].

This procedure, like the other approaches, is performed in the catheterization laboratory with cardiac surgery back-up, under mild sedation and local anesthesia. A 5 Fr pigtail is inserted into the right femoral artery and advanced to the ascending aorta to allow continual monitoring of systemic pressure. Contralateral femoral artery access is thus obtained, and a 23 mm valvuloplasty balloon is inserted through it. The stenotic native valve is dilated using the standard technique, and the balloon is then withdrawn; after trans-septal puncture,

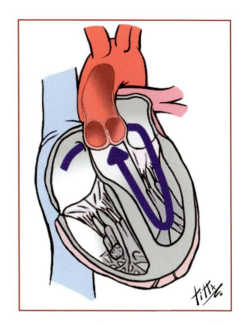

Fig. 3.29 Scheme of antegrade approach

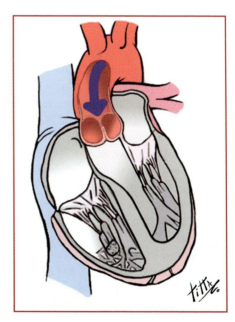

Fig. 3.30 Scheme of retrograde approach

the device is inserted through the right femoral vein and a straight 0.035" guidewire is advanced through a floating balloon catheter into the left atrium and is passed through the aortic annulus. Once the guidewire is placed in the ascending aorta, it is replaced with a long 260 cm stiff guidewire, which is

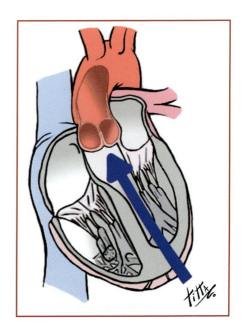

Fig. 3.31 Scheme of transapical approach

fastened and extracted from the introducer in the left femoral artery. This creates a single circuit, starting from the right femoral vein and reaching the left femoral artery.

The 24 Fr introducer is then inserted in the right femoral vein, and the inter-atrial septum is dilated using a 10 mm balloon. Thanks to the crimping system, the device is mounted on a 23/30 mm balloon (Z-MED, Numed Inc.) and the catheter is easily advanced through the right femoral vein, into the inferior vena cava, through, the inter-atrial septum, into the left ventricle, and finally placed on the aortic annulus. Using valve calcifications as markers, under fluoroscopic guidance and after administering contrast medium through the pigtail, the biological device is expanded and positioned, crushing the native valve during pacing at 180–220 bpm; the latter must start a few seconds before inflating the balloon and be stopped a few seconds after deflation; once this is done, the release catheter is retracted and a control aortography is performed to assess the efficacy and adequacy of the implant (Fig. 3.32); once the procedure is completed, all the catheters are retracted and arterial hemostasis is achieved using a percutaneous sealing system: Angio-Seal™ (St Jude Medical), ProGlide™ 5 Fr (Abbott Vascular Devices, Redwood City, California, USA), FemoSeal® (Radi Medical Systems AB, Uppsala, Sweden).

However, this antegrade approach has been abandoned, as it is technically demanding, carries additional risks due to trans-septal puncture, and is poorly tolerated by some patients, especially those with hemodynamic instability. In

3.1 Aortic Stenosis

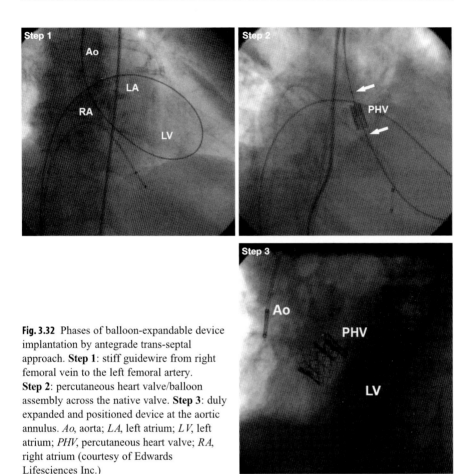

Fig. 3.32 Phases of balloon-expandable device implantation by antegrade trans-septal approach. **Step 1**: stiff guidewire from right femoral vein to the left femoral artery. **Step 2**: percutaneous heart valve/balloon assembly across the native valve. **Step 3**: duly expanded and positioned device at the aortic annulus. *Ao*, aorta; *LA*, left atrium; *LV*, left atrium; *PHV*, percutaneous heart valve; *RA*, right atrium (courtesy of Edwards Lifesciences Inc.)

the use of this approach, there have been reports of lesions to the anterior leaflet of the mitral valve caused by the catheters, which must be advanced first from the left atrium into the ventricle and then into the ascending aorta.

The same valve, with duly modified dimensions and components, is currently implanted with success using the retrograde approach with a more flexible and smaller catheter, inserted by the retrograde route from the femoral artery to the aortic root. Although this approach is more convenient compared to the antegrade one, and affords fewer intraprocedure complications, the diameter of 24 and 22 Fr catheters used requires an anatomy that is favorable to arterial access [58–60]. In this case as well, the procedure is performed in the catheterization laboratory, under mild sedation and fluoroscopic guidance.

A new generation of balloon-expandable devices (SAPIEN XT, Edwards Lifesciences) (Fig. 3.33) has been recently introduced. They are made of cobalt chromium and available in 4 sizes (20, 23, 26 and 29 mm), allowing for use

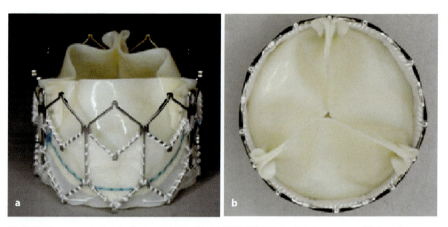

Fig. 3.33 New-generation balloon-expandable SAPIEN™ XT device (courtesy of Edwards Lifesciences Inc.)

with 20-Fr and 22-Fr catheters, and two more flexible delivery catheters (NovaFlex™, Edwards Lifesciences, Irvine, California, USA), both equipped with a more favorable profile [61,62]. The NovaFlex™ delivery system allows for a further reduction in catheter diameter to 18 Fr for 23 mm devices and 19 Fr for 26-mm devices; this allows use in patients with iliac and femoral artery diameters of 6 mm for 18 Fr and 6.5 mm for 19 Fr. The delivery catheter incorporates an outer deflectable catheter and an inner balloon catheter with a tapered crossing tip. The valve itself is crimped on the inner catheter proximal to the inflatable balloon. This reduces the maximal diameter of the delivery catheter and allows for a reduction in sheath size.

For the retrograde approach both the right and left femoral artery accesses and a venous access are obtained; the purpose of the latter access is to allow the placement of a temporary pacemaker. A 5 Fr pigtail is introduced through a femoral artery for angiography. In the contralateral femoral artery through which the delivery catheter is inserted, percutaneous sutures are preimplanted by means of a dedicated device for the hemostasis of arterial breaches cannulated with large-diameter catheters (Prostar™ XL 10 Fr, Abbott Vascular Devices, Redwood City, California, USA); on the other hand, surgical isolation of the femoral artery could be also obtained. After performing an aortography and orienting the fluoroscopic view to align all three sinuses and the aortic cusps on a same plane (Fig. 3.34), the native valve is crossed by the stiff guidewire (Teflon®-coated wire [e.g.: Medtronic PTFE guidewire, Medtronic Vascular, Danvers, Massachusetts, USA] or Amplatz Extra Stiff J Guidewire [William Cook Europe, Bjaeverskov, Denmark]). Numerous catheters can be used for crossing the aortic valve; 5 Fr or 6 Fr left coronary Amplatz catheters should be preferred: Amplatz left-2 (AL-2) is usually chosen in patients with an enlarged or a horizontal aortic root, whereas the Amplatz left-1 (AL-1) is preferred in cases with a small and vertical aortic root. Once the stiff guidewire is accurately positioned in the LV, aortic valvuloplasty is performed with stan-

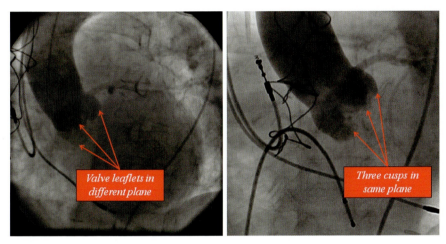

Fig. 3.34 Preimplantation aortography must be performed in a view allowing the three valve cusps to be aligned on the same plane. The image on the left obtained from a left cranial view (left anterior oblique) shows that the alignment is not optimal. The image on the right, obtained from an anteroposterior view, shows a view of the three cusps on the same plane

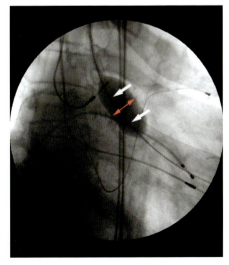

Fig. 3.35 Preimplantation aortic valvuloplasty with standard technique using Z-MED balloon (Numed Inc.). The *white arrows* indicate the radio-opaque markers of the balloon, the *red arrows* show the expansion of the balloon

dard technique using a balloon with a slightly smaller diameter (3 mm) compared to the device to be implanted (Z-MED, Numed Inc.) (Fig. 3.35).

After valvuloplasty, keeping the guidewire in the LV, the access site where the Prostar is placed or surgical isolation was obtained, is dilated gradually using dilators to allow for the placement of the introducer, which is advanced beyond the iliac artery to the aorta. The flexible catheter is then introduced and advanced to the ascending aorta. Thanks to its flexibility, the catheter, with the balloon and device mounted on its tip, is advanced and carefully guided through the aorta and annulus (Fig. 3.36): several angiograms are performed to find the optimal position and orientation for valve implantation and once obtained during pacing at 220 bpm (lasting a few seconds more than the inflation time), and, under fluoroscopic guidance, the balloon is inflated and the device is expanded, crushing the native aortic valve (Fig. 3.37). Once the device is placed, an aortogram is performed to detect any peri-prosthetic leaks (Fig. 3.38), and the pigtail is advanced in the LV to assess the residual gradient.

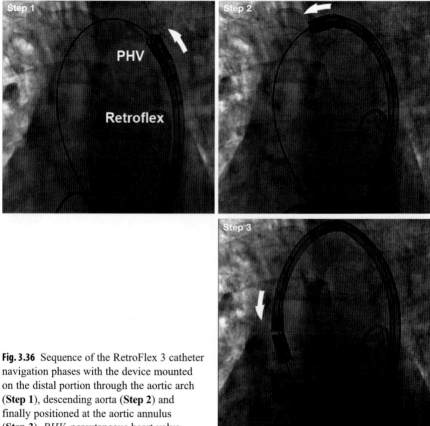

Fig. 3.36 Sequence of the RetroFlex 3 catheter navigation phases with the device mounted on the distal portion through the aortic arch (**Step 1**), descending aorta (**Step 2**) and finally positioned at the aortic annulus (**Step 3**). *PHV*, percutaneous heart valve

Post-dilations can be performed if the operator deems that the device has not been perfectly expanded. Once the procedure is completed, all the catheters are retracted and femoral hemostasis is performed using percutaneous or surgical sutures.

If the arterial accesses are not deemed appropriate (small gauge, major bending, stenosis), the transcatheter apical approach is used. In this case, device insertion requires the Ascendra Transapical Delivery System (Edwards Life-

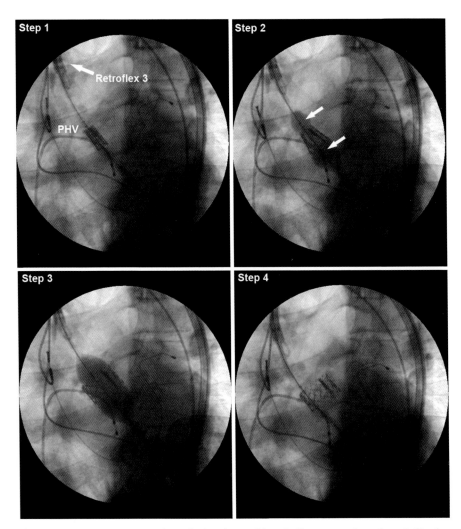

Fig. 3.37 Step 1, balloon-mounted prosthetic valve positioned adjacent to native valve calcification (*arrow*). **Step 2**: partial inflation of the deployment balloon; the *white arrows* indicate the radio-opaque markers of the balloon. **Step 3**: full inflation of the deployment balloon. **Step 4**: deflation of the balloon. *PHV*, percutaneous heart valve

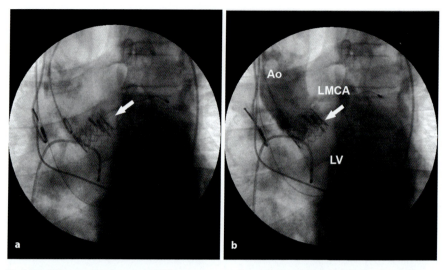

Fig. 3.38 a Fluoroscopic image and (**b**) aortogram performed after placing the device (*white arrow*) to highlight any intraprosthetic regurgitation, perivalvular leaks and no obstruction of the coronary artery ostia. *Ao*, aorta; *LMCA*, left main coronary artery; *LV*, left ventricle

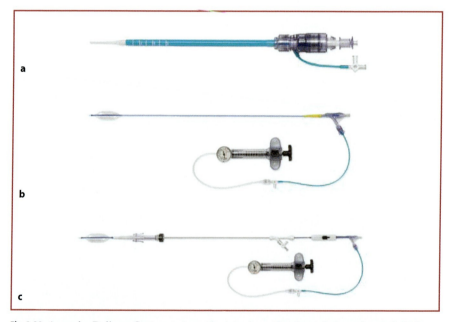

Fig. 3.39 Ascendra Delivery System. **a** Ascendra introducer sheath set; **b** Ascendra aortic balloon valvuloplasty catheter; **c** Ascendra balloon catheter (courtesy of Edwards Lifesciences Inc.)

science) (Fig. 3.39). The procedure is performed in the operating room with beating heart, total anesthesia, and orotracheal intubation, under fluoroscopic and TEE guidance, with close cooperation between the cardiac surgeon and interventional cardiologist.

A left anterolateral thoracotomy is performed first (Fig. 3.40) (a CT scan should be performed in advanced to determine the relationships between the ventricle's apex and the chest wall and to identify the precise location of the incision site) generally speaking, a lower incision, rather than a higher one, should be made, since the apex can be distracted downward with pericardial traction sutures. The pericardium is opened longitudinally and the positioning of stable sutures allows adequate apex exposure. The next step is to identify the site of the anterior interventricular branch of the left coronary artery. Two apical purse-string sutures (Prolene 2-0, large needle with five interrupted Teflon® pledgets; Ethicon Inc., Somerville, NJ, USA) are placed with sufficiently deep bites in the myocardium (approximately 3–5 mm, but not penetrating into the left ventricular cavity), close to the apex and lateral to the left anterior descending coronary artery (Fig. 3.41). The apex is punctured with a needle, and a soft guidewire is inserted and advanced through the native aortic valve in antegrade direction. A 14 Fr (30 cm long) soft-tip sheath is then placed across the aortic valve; a 260 cm × 0.035" J-tipped guidewire (Amplatz Super Stiff; Boston Scientific, Natick, MA, USA) is inserted and advanced through the aortic arch and descending aorta (Fig. 3.42). A 20 × 40 mm balloon (Z-MED, Numed Inc.) is placed in the ascending aorta and the 14 Fr catheter tip is withdrawn into the LV. In this case as well, valvuloplasty is carried out during pacing at 170–220 bpm (Fig. 3.43); during dilation, arterial pressure must be kept over 60 mmHg to avoid hemodynamic deterioration (valvuloplasty must not be performed if the pre-inflation pressure is <100 mmHg). Once the

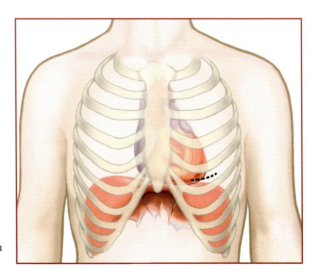

Fig. 3.40 Anterolateral mini-thoracotomy at the 5th or 6th intercostal space

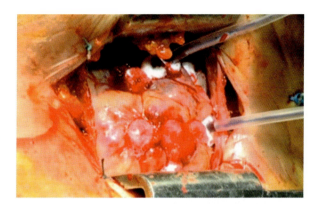

Fig. 3.41 Exposure of the left ventricle apex with Teflon®-reinforced purse-string sutures (Ethicon Inc., Somerville, NJ, USA)

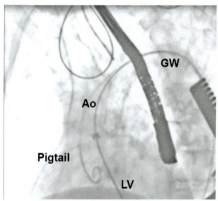

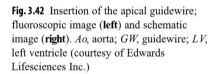

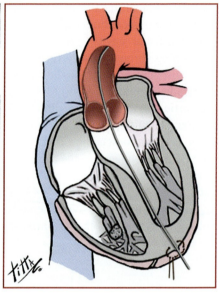

Fig. 3.42 Insertion of the apical guidewire; fluoroscopic image (**left**) and schematic image (**right**). *Ao*, aorta; *GW*, guidewire; *LV*, left ventricle (courtesy of Edwards Lifesciences Inc.)

balloon is withdrawn along with the 14 Fr catheter, leaving only the stiff guidewire in place, the 26 Fr sheath is positioned 4–5 cm under the aortic annulus; after advancing the catheter, air on the inside can be removed from the loader, and the black screw should be slightly closed.

The prosthetic valve is then inserted and positioned through the annulus, and the pusher is retrieved back into the delivery sheath; if the pusher is not pulled back several centimeters prior to valve deployment, subsequent balloon expansion will be impeded and the valve will be pushed obliquely forward. Device placement is performed under fluoroscopic and TEE guidance; during this phase, exact device orientation perpendicular to the annulus is of crucial importance for proper positioning (Fig. 3.44); once the device is perfectly aligned,

3.1 Aortic Stenosis

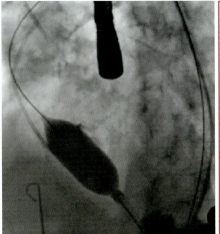
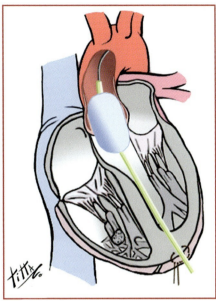

Fig. 3.43 Dilation of native aortic valve; fluoroscopic image (**left**) and schematic image (**right**); (Courtesy of Edwards Lifesciences Inc.)

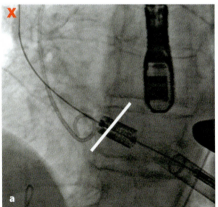
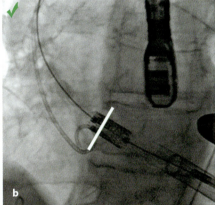

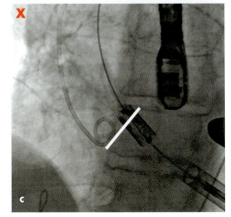

Fig. 3.44 Positioning of devices. **a** rightward oblique position due to slack of the wire; **b** proper perpendicular placement compared to the annulus axis; **c** leftward oblique position due to a tight wire (courtesy of Edwards Lifesciences Inc.)

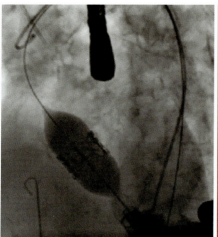

Fig. 3.45 Dilation of native aortic valve; fluoroscopic image (**left**) and schematic image (**right**); (courtesy of Edwards Lifesciences Inc.)

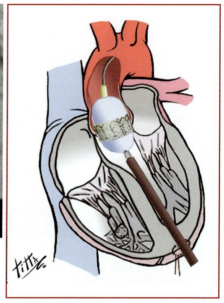

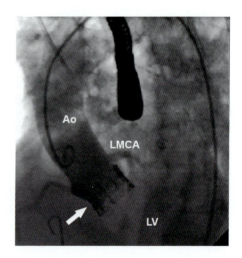

Fig. 3.46 Final angiographic assessment after transapical implantation of the aortic valve device (*arrow*). *Ao*, aorta; *LMCA*, left main coronary artery; *LV*, left ventricle (courtesy of Edwards Lifesciences Inc.)

pacing and inflation of the balloon inside the device are performed (Fig. 3.45). After deploying the device, pacing is stopped, the balloon is pulled back, and an aortogram is performed to make sure that there is no perivalvular regurgitation (Fig. 3.46).

Once implantation is completed, both the catheter and the stiff guidewire are pulled back simultaneously. The apex is closed through the previously placed two purse-string sutures. Other suture points (usually Teflon®-reinforced; Ethicon Inc.) may be needed for complete hemostasis. Sutures are also applied to close the pericardium, and a drain tube is placed [63–67].

The main advantage of this device compared to the self-expanding model described further later is that it can also be implanted in patients with major hypertrophy of the interventricular septum or ascending aorta aneurysm, conditions that are, per se, a contraindication to the implantation of the current self-expanding device. Complications of the procedure will be discussed in a dedicated section.

3.1.5.1.3
Essential Bibliography

The first case history published by Cribier in 2004 [56] proved the feasibility of TAVI using balloon-expandable devices; success was achieved in five out of six patients, with a decrease in transaortic gradient and an increase in valve area. In this initial experience, the antegrade approach was used and, as already stated, it was abandoned for the retrograde and transapical approach. These two approaches were investigated by a French team that studied 33 patients [57]; 27 were treated with success (75%) – 23 with the retrograde approach and 4 with the transapical technique. The aortic gradient dropped from 37 ± 13 mmHg to 9 ± 2 mmHg ($P < 0.0001$) and the valve area rose from 0.60 ± 0.11 cm^2 to 1.70 ± 0.10 cm^2 ($P < 0.0001$). The incidence of major adverse cardiac and cerebrovascular events (MACCEs) at 30 days and at 6 months was 26% (6 deaths) and 37% (10 deaths) respectively.

A series of implants by retrograde approach performed by Webb et al [58] showed an initial success rate of 78%, which rose to 96% after the first 25 cases, thus proving the importance of the learning curve [59]. Thirty-day mortality was 12% as opposed to the expected 28%. At follow-up there was no evidence of valve deterioration, embolization, or intraprosthetic failure. Perivalvular regurgitation was observed at 1 month in three cases, while in most patients there was a slight leak without any significant hemodynamic consequences. In the most recent case history published by Webb and colleagues [60] in 2009, the overall success rate was 94.1%; intraprocedure mortality was 1.2%, and 30-day mortality was 11.3%, lower in the transfemoral group compared to the transapical group (8.0% versus 18.2%; $P = 0.07$). Overall mortality dropped from 14.3% in the first half to 8.3% in the second half of the experience, from 12.3% to 3.6% ($P = 0.16$) in patients receiving the transfemoral approach, and from 25% to 11.1% ($P = 0.30$) in the transapical group. The functional class significantly improved at over one year of follow-up ($P < 0.001$), and survival at 1, 12, and 24 months was 88.7%, 73.8%, and 60.9%, respectively. In this case history as well, no device deterioration phenomena were detected.

For the transapical approach, the first data published by Lichtenstein et al

[63] related to seven patients: implantation was successfully performed in all cases and there were no intraprocedural deaths. An improvement of the aortic valve area was seen in all patients. Thirty-day mortality was less than expected (14% versus 35%) [16, 17]. Walther et al [65] reported a procedural success rate of 93.2% with an incidence of conversion to surgery of 6.8%. Thirty-day mortality was 13.6%, while the expected mortality was 26.8%; recourse to extracorporeal circulation was frequent (47%) at the beginning of the experience, with a progressive reduction in subsequent procedures.

A recently published US-based feasibility study has shown effective transapical device implantation in 90% of cases, matched by a persistent improvement in symptoms, valve area, mean gradient, and quality of life [66]. Survival was 81.1% at 1 month, 71.7% at 3 months, and 58.7% at 6 months. MACCEs were observed in 65% of cases and included: stroke (5%), urgent cardiac surgery (2.5%), and myocardial infarction (17.5%). Ye et al. [67] reported a case history of 26 patients with a follow-up at 12 months: of these, six patients died within 30 days (30-day mortality, 23%), and three died due to non-cardiovascular causes after 30 days (late mortality, 12%). Of the patients who survived at least 30 days, survival at 12 months was 85%. No late complications correlated with the device were observed.

3.1.5.2
CoreValve® ReValving System

3.1.5.2.1
Device Description

The CoreValve® aortic valve device (Fig. 3.47) consists of a tricuspid valve made of porcine pericardial tissue mounted and sutured inside a frame of self-expanding nitinol. The valve inner diameter measures 21 mm. The frame is laser modeled using a 50 mm nitinol tube. The lower part of the device has great radial strength, allowing for self-expansion and exclusion of the calcified native valve leaflets, which are crushed against the wall of the aortic root, at the same time preventing collapse of the device on itself. The central portion of the stent supports the valve; it has a narrow shape to avoid interfering with the coronary artery ostia. The upper part is widened so that the frame can be fastened to the ascending aorta to ensure the valve's longitudinal stability (Figs. 3.48 and 3.49).

Over the years, the device has undergone several modifications to increase efficiency and, at the same time, facilitate implantation. The first-generation device used bovine pericardial tissue and was implanted using 24 Fr catheters. The second generation of devices made of porcine pericardial tissue had a

3.1 Aortic Stenosis

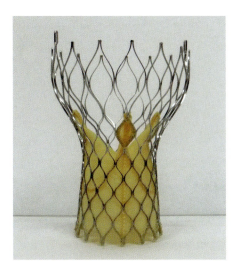

Fig. 3.47 18 Fr third-generation self-expanding CoreValve® device

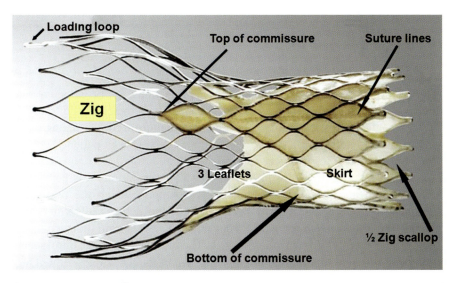

Fig. 3.48 The CoreValve® device is made by suturing valve leaflets made of a single layer of porcine pericardium in a trileaflet configuration using PTFE sutures. The leaflets are attached to a three-piece scalloped skirt on the inflow aspect of the valve. The pericardial tissue has been completely fixed in buffered glutaraldehyde solution using standard and well-established methods. A final sterilization step is carried out with glutaraldehyde and isopropyl alcohol as active ingredients. This sterilization process is identical to the process used by currently available surgical-type tissue heart valves

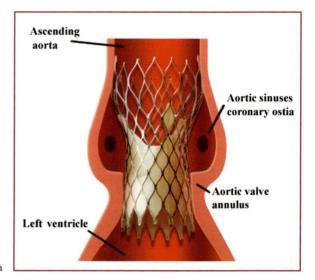

Fig. 3.49 Relations of the CoreValve® device with the aortic valve apparatus structures; from the bottom up, the device fitted to the valve annulus, sinuses of Valsalva, and ascending aorta

smaller profile so that they could be implanted using 21 Fr catheters and allowed access through a vascular bed with a smaller diameter. In addition, this device was marked by a wider upper segment for a more secure fastening to the wall of the ascending aorta to allow for implantation also in patients with an ascending aorta diameter of over 45 mm.

The implantation of the 24 Fr and 21 Fr valve generations was performed under general anesthesia with extracorporeal support, using the retrograde approach. Various changes have been made to the devices allowing for a gradual reduction in catheter gauge from the 24 Fr of the initial device to the 18 Fr of the current third-generation device. The introduction of the third-generation device has led to a significant improvement of the technique, without any differences in terms of safety and results. To date, two device sizes are available, 26 and 29 mm respectively. The 26 mm device is suitable for an annulus between 20 and 23 mm, while the 26 mm device is suitable for an annulus between 24 and 27 mm (Scheme 3.1).

The reduction in diameter from 24 Fr to 18 Fr has made the retrograde approach much easier and more feasible, solving most of the difficulties constituted by the vascular accesses and the passage from the aortic arch to the ascending aorta. The procedure has been streamlined, substantially reducing procedure time and eliminating surgical preparation of the access site and the need for cardiopulmonary bypass with extracorporeal membrane oxygenation (ECMO) or TandemHeart® (CardiacAssist Inc.).

3.1 Aortic Stenosis

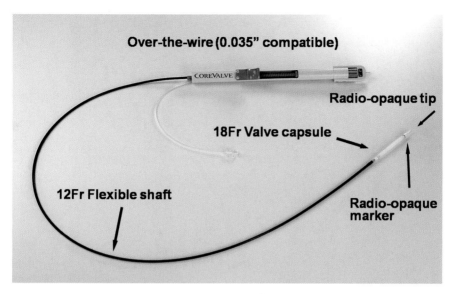

Fig. 3.50 18 Fr delivery catheter system. The CoreValve® delivery catheter system is an over-the-wire catheter, which can accommodate a guidewire up to 0.035" in diameter. The distal part of the catheter carries the prosthesis and delivers it to the deployment site. It incorporates the flexibility, trackability, and rigidity required to navigate to the aortic annulus and has an integral handle for precise control of delivery of the bioprosthesis (courtesy of Medtronic Inc. MN, USA)

The third-generation device now allows for a genuinely percutaneous approach for aortic valve replacement. The CoreValve® ReValving System 18 Fr device is composed of:
- a percutaneous aortic valve device
- a delivery catheter system (DCS) (Fig. 3.50) with over-the-wire guiding catheter consisting of:
    - a distal part with an 18 Fr diameter hosting the collapsed valve covered by a protective sheath (Fig. 3.51)
    - a central 12 Fr part
    - a terminal part with manual control to load the valve and release it (Fig. 3.52)
- the loading system used to compress and load the valve in the guiding catheter (Fig. 3.53).

Scheme 3.1 Indications for use according to the CE mark

Elements below reflect indications for use according to the CE mark								
Diagnostic Findings	Non-invasive			Angiography			Selection Criteria	
	Echo	CT/MRI	LV	Ao Root	CAG	Vascular	Recommended	Not Recommended
Atrial or Ventricular Thrombus	X						Not Present	Present
Sub Aortic Stenosis	X	X	X				Not Present	Present
LV Ejection Fraction	X		X				≥20%	<20% without contractile reserve
Mitral Regurgitation	X						≤Grade 2	>Grade 2 Organic Reason
Vascular Access Diameter		X				X	≥6 mm Diameter	<6 mm Diameter
Aortic and Vascular Disease		X				X	None to Moderate	Sever Vascular Disease
Indications for 26 mm CoreValve® Device								
Annulus Diameter	X	X					20-23 mm	<20 mm or >23 mm
Ascending Aorta Diameter		X		X			≤40 mm	>40 mm
Indications for 29 mm CoreValve® Device								
Annulus Diameter	X	X					24-27 mm	<24 mm or >27 mm
Ascending Aorta Diameter		X		X			≤43 mm	>43 mm

(cont. ↓)

Scheme 3.1 *(continued)*

General medical guidance for use of CoreValve®*

Diagnostic Findings	Non-invasive		Angiography				Selection Criteria	
	Echo	CT/MRI	LV	Ao Root	CAG	Vascular	Recommended	Moderate-High Risk
LV Hypertrophy	X	X					Normal to Moderate 0.6 - 1.6 cm	Severe > 1.7 cm
Coronary Artery Disease		X			X		None, Mid or Distal >70%	Proximal Lesions >70%
Aortic Arch Angulation		X				X	Large Radial Turn	Sharp Turn
Aortic Root Angulation		X				X	<30 degrees	30-45 degrees
Aortic and Vascular Disease		X				X	No or Light Vascular Dosease	Moderate Vascular Disease
Vascular Access Diameter		X				X	>6 mm	Calcified and elongated >7 mm
Anatomic Considerations for 26 mm CoreValve® Device								
Sinus of Valsalva Width	X	X		X			≥27 mm	<27 mm
Sinus of Valsalva Height	X	X		X			≥15mm	<15mm
Anatomic Considerations for 29 mm CoreValve® Device								
Sinus of Valsalva Width	X	X		X			≥29 mm	<29 mm
Sinus of Valsalva Height	X	X		X			≥15mm	<15mm

*General medical guidance reflects the experience to date with the product, but final judgment remains with the implanting physicians(s)
CT, Computed Tomography; *MRI*, Magnetic Resonance Imaging; *LV*, Left Ventricle; *Ao*, Aorta; *CAG*, Coronary Artery Graft

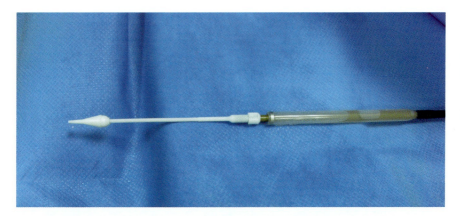

Fig. 3.51 Distal end of the DCS where the device is loaded. The CoreValve® device's frame is made of a heat-shrinking material and it can be shaped and hence loaded inside the DCS only when it is at a low temperature; for this reason, this maneuver is carried out in a basin full of ice and water

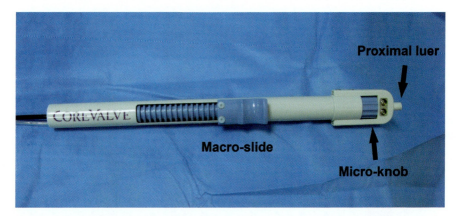

Fig. 3.52 CoreValve® delivery catheter handle. The handle features a micro-adjustment knob and macro-movement knob. The macro-slide and micro-knob are used to facilitate the loading of the bioprosthesis into the delivery catheter. After initial positioning of the delivery catheter across the aortic annulus, the micro-knob is used for slow progressive sheath retrieval and delivery of the bioprosthesis

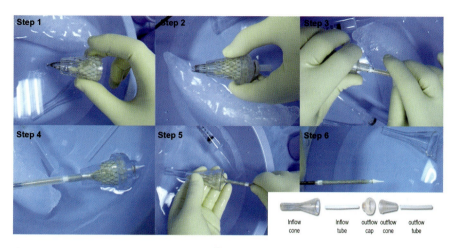

Fig. 3.53 Crimping systems of the CoreValve® device. **Step 1**: the outflow part of the cold bioprosthesis frame is gently squeezed and inserted into the outflow cone. **Step 2**: after securing the outflow cap onto the outflow cone, the inflow tube (non-tapered) is carefully inserted into the outflow cap and advanced until the frame loops begin to separate. **Step 3**: the distal tip of the catheter is inserted into the inflow tube, it is carefully manipulated, and the exposed frame loops are attached to the catheter tabs. **Step 4**: frame loops are covered by the catheter sheath by using the micro-knob, and the outflow tube is advanced past the radio-opaque marker band. **Step 5**: once the outflow cap and inflow tube are removed from the outflow cone, the bioprosthesis is advanced into the inflow cone until the outflow tube contacts the inside of the inflow cone. **Step 6**: the catheter sheath is slowly advanced over the bioprosthesis until the sheath comes within approximately 5 mm of the catheter tip. Bottom right, the image shows the device-loading system inside the DCS; it is specifically designed not to damage the device structure and it can be used only once

3.1.5.2.2
Procedure and Technical Aspects

The procedure is performed in the catheterization laboratory with cardiac surgery back-up. Besides fluoroscopic guidance, intraprocedural TEE guidance can also be used. In this case, general anesthesia is required; otherwise, deep sedation and analgesia are sufficient.

The vascular accesses are obtained percutaneously without surgical incision. The left femoral vein or right internal jugular vein are cannulated with a 5 or 6 Fr introducer, through which the electrocatheter of the temporary pacemaker is inserted and positioned at the apex of the right ventricle.

Once the artery through which the valve-release catheter is to be introduced is chosen, the contralateral femoral artery is cannulated with a 5 Fr catheter and the contrast medium is injected to visualize the femoral artery receiving the 18 Fr introducer (William Cook Europe, Bjaeverskov, Denmark) (Fig. 3.54); after visualizing the artery at fluoroscopy (Fig. 3.55), it is punctured with an

18 gauge needle using a high degree of inclination to reduce the distance between the skin and vessel to a minimum; a standard 0.035" guidewire is inserted through the needle and advanced to the common femoral artery. A 9 Fr introducer is inserted to further dilate the breach and it is then replaced with the Prostar™ XL 10 Fr device; the guidewire is pulled back and the device is advanced through the artery. Once two sutures are applied for effective and complete closing of the femoral breach at the end of the procedure by creating a tobacco pouch, the Prostar is removed, and the 9 Fr introducer is inserted again. Sodium heparin (100 IU/kg IV) is administered to maintain an activated clotting time (ACT) between 200 and 300 s.

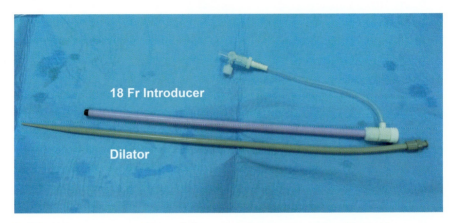

Fig. 3.54 18 Fr introducer and dilator (William Cook Europe, Bjaeverskov, Denmark)

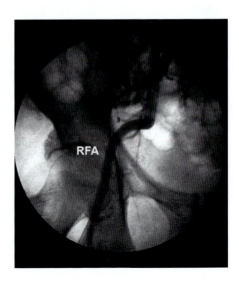

Fig. 3.55 Before the arterial puncture, an angiogram is performed on the femoral artery accommodating the 18 Fr introducer. *RFA*, right femoral artery

A 5 Fr gauged catheter is advanced to the ascending aorta, and the tip of the catheter is placed at the base of the non-coronary cusp of the native aortic valve (the tip of the pigtail is also important as the point of reference during device release). Small injections of contrast medium make it possible to determine the ideal angiographic view to visualize the aortic annulus. When it is reached, a larger quantity of contrast medium is injected to obtain an angiographic image of the valve apparatus and ascending aorta. As described in the section on the implantation of the Edwards-SAPIEN™ device, the ideal view is the one in which the three sinuses and three valve cusps are aligned on a same plane (Fig. 3.35). A left 5 or 6 Fr Amplatz catheter (AL-1 or AL-2) is inserted through the femoral artery contralateral to the one receiving the pigtail and advanced up to the ascending aorta, and the standard guidewire is changed with a stiff 0.035" guidewire (ASS, Super Stiff – Amplatz Cook, Inc., Bloomington, Indiana, USA), which makes it easier to pass across the stenotic valve. After crossing the valve, the Amplatz catheter is advanced inside the left ventricle, the guidewire is removed, and it is connected to the transducer (Fig. 3.56).

Having done this much, and using both catheters at the same time, the transvalvular gradient is recorded. The guidewire is inserted again and positioned at the apex of the left ventricle. Under direct fluoroscopic guidance, the 9 Fr introducer is replaced with an 18 Fr, and the valvuloplasty balloon is inserted through it and advanced to the aortic annulus (the most used balloon is the Nucleus, NuMed Inc., Canada; Fig. 3.57). Valvuloplasty is performed using a 50 ml syringe and, during inflation, a rapid pacing of the right ventricle is performed with pacing at 180/220 bpm for 5 s, in order to drastically reduce left ventricular systolic output (Fig. 3.58).

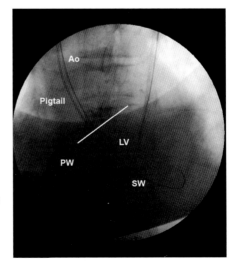

Fig. 3.56 Stiff guidewire after crossing the stenotic aortic valve and being placed inside the left ventricle. Proper stiff guidewire placement is essential for a safe procedure and to ensure adequate support during release of the self-expanding device. The *white line* shows the aortic valve plane. *Ao*, aorta; *GW*, guidewire; *LV*, left ventricle; *PW*, pacing wire

The balloon is then removed while maintaining the Super Stiff guidewire in the LV, the delivery system with the valve on the inside is advanced through the aorta (Fig. 3.59), and it is positioned on the native valve (Fig. 3.60); the best view for correct device release is the one in which the radio-opaque ring positioned in the distal portion of the DCS appears as a segment and not as a circle or ellipse (Fig. 3.61). The device can now be expanded in a stepwise manner, using the handle on the distal part of the release system and slowly pulling back the catheter. With the aid of repeated small injections of contrast medium, the catheter is pulled back by turning the release system's handle counterclockwise, thus allowing total expansion of the device (Fig. 3.62); During deployment it has to be considered that when one-third of the CoreValve® is expanded, neither the native nor the prosthetic valves work appropriately, resulting in temporary

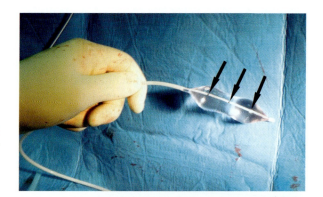

Fig. 3.57 Nucleus balloon™ (NuMed Inc., Canada). The *black arrows* indicate the radio-opaque markers of the balloon

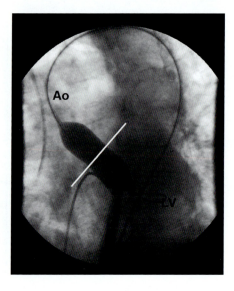

Fig. 3.58 Preimplantation valvuloplasty performed with ventricular pacing at 180–220 bpm. The *white line* shows the aortic valve plane. *Ao*, aorta; *LV*, left ventricle

systemic pressure fall; therefore, this phase has to be carried out as quickly as is possible. When the distal two-thirds of the frame are expanded, the prosthetic valve works normally. Once it is completely expanded, the DCS is pulled back and its proper positioning is assessed, namely about 6–8 mm below the aortic annulus (Fig. 3.63), by means of fluoroscopy and, when performed, by TEE.

Fluoroscopic control in at least two views is important to ascertain optimal frame expansion (Fig. 3.64). Then, left cardiac catheterization is performed with aortography, the transprosthetic gradient is measured, and the presence of intra- or peri-prosthetic regurgitation is assessed. Once the procedure is completed, the 18 Fr introducer is pulled back and effective hemostasis is performed with two sutures previously positioned with the 10 Fr Prostar (Fig. 3.65). Hemostasis of the controlateral femoral artery is achieved by using the percutaneous closing

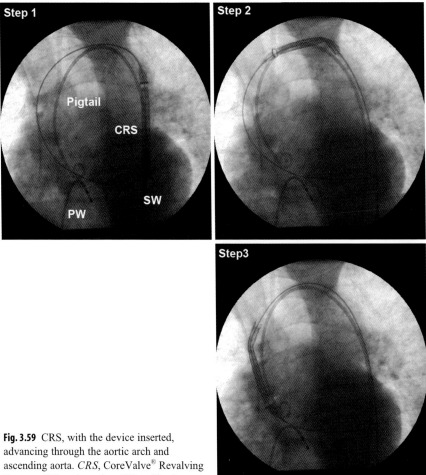

Fig. 3.59 CRS, with the device inserted, advancing through the aortic arch and ascending aorta. *CRS*, CoreValve® Revalving System; *PW*, pacing wire; *GW*, guidewire

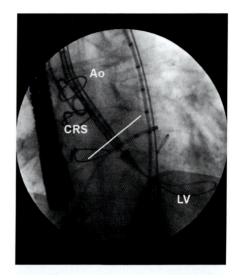

Fig. 3.60 CRS placed on the aortic annulus. The *white line* shows the aortic valve plane. *Ao*, aorta; *CRS*, CoreValve® Revalving System; *LV*, left ventricle

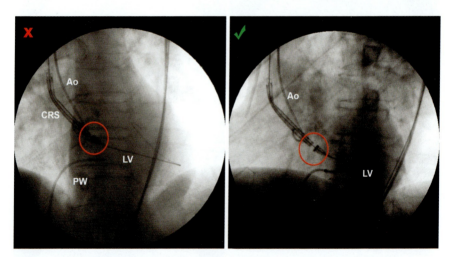

Fig. 3.61 Fluoroscopic view before device release is of major importance for its proper positioning. The image **on the left** shows a non-optimal view for release, as the radio-opaque ring in the distal portion of the DCS is shaped like an ellipsis; **on the right**, the same view is rotated cranially by 20° and the radio-opaque ring looks like a single segment. *Ao*, aorta; *CRS*: CoreValve® Revalving System; *LV*, left ventricle; *PW*, pacing wire

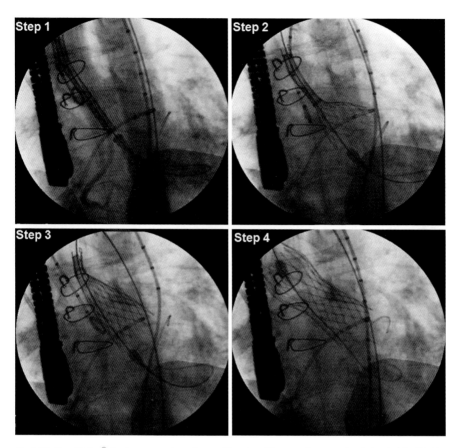

Fig. 3.62 CoreValve® device expansion phases. **Step 1**: self-expanding prosthesis loaded inside the delivery catheter placed across the native aortic valve. **Step 2**: device expansion by one-third; at this point, neither the prosthetic valve nor the native valve work, so this phase must be carried out as quickly as possible. **Step 3**: two-thirds of the prosthesis are expanded, the prosthesic valve is already working. **Step 4**: final release

system (Angio-Seal™ 6 Fr, St Jude Medical), while the temporary pacemaker is maintained for 24–48 hours.

The self-expansion mechanism of the CoreValve® device offers many potential advantages compared to devices requiring a balloon to be positioned (e.g. the ES system).

The first and most important is the device's ability to self-expand, which makes it possible to reduce the incidence of peri-prosthetic leak (failure) to a minimum, and to treat patients with AR, as opposed to the experience reported with percutaneous aortic valve mounted on an expandable balloon. Second, by avoiding the trauma caused by the balloon on the prosthetic valve leaflets, the

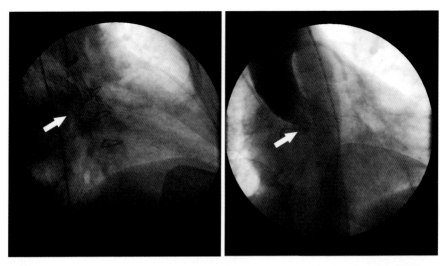

Fig. 3.63 Aortogram performed at the end of the device release (*white arrow*) and after retracting the guidewire

self-expanding mechanism can, in theory, extend the valve's life. Third, the upper self-expanding segment of the valve allows for secure fastening on the ascending aorta.

The CoreValve® design also offers many other advantages in terms of device positioning:

- the possibility of a certain margin of error in releasing the device without negatively affecting device function
- longitudinal self-alignment of the stent
- the possibility to recover the device after partial exposure of the distal two-thirds of the stent (Fig. 3.66)
- the possibility to also reposition the device after some time if it is released in a suboptimal position (low).

The possibility of recovering the device is very important for correct positioning: once the distal two-thirds of the device are expanded, the valve works almost adequately, while the stent it is mounted on can be further adjusted or even pulled back completely. If the device is not perfectly expanded, especially when it is placed in extremely calcified valves, the valve can be further dilated using a valvuloplasty balloon without damaging the biological valve sewn on the inside (Fig. 3.67). Transapical implantation has also been described for the CoreValve® device; due to technical issues related to the release of the device by the release catheter when using this approach, it has now been abandoned [73].

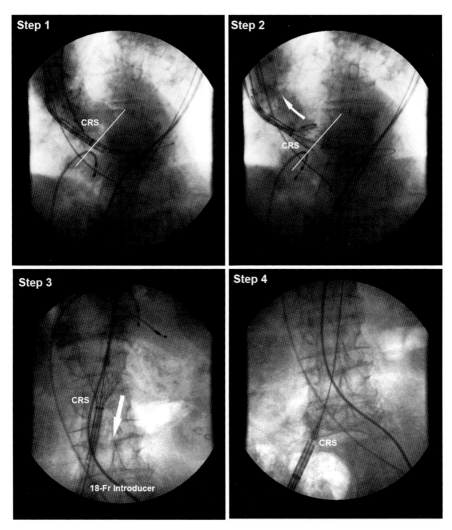

Fig. 3.66 Step 1: CRS placed across the aortic annulus (*white line*). **Step 2**: prosthesis jumped inside the sinus of Valsalva (*white arrow*). **Step 3**: The one-third-expanded CRS and the guidewire are withdrawn with the delivery catheter in the descending aorta (*white arrow*). **Step 4**: the CoreValve® frame is inserted inside the 18 Fr introducer. *CRS*: CoreValve® Revalving System

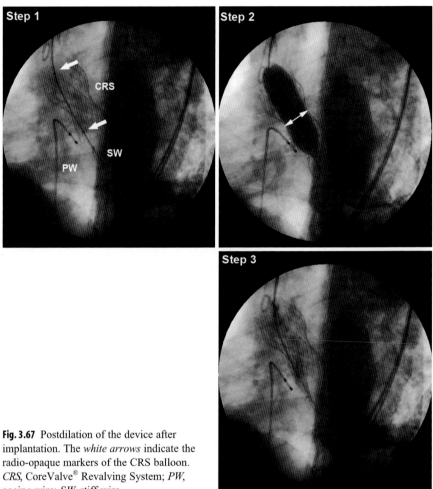

Fig. 3.67 Postdilation of the device after implantation. The *white arrows* indicate the radio-opaque markers of the CRS balloon. *CRS*, CoreValve® Revalving System; *PW*, pacing wire; *SW*, stiff wire

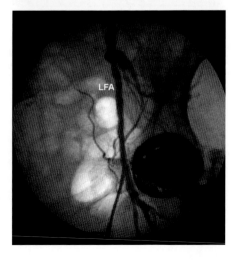

Fig. 3.68 Peripheral angiogram showing small-diameter femoral arteries (<6 mm) and diffuse vasal atheromatosis. *LFA*, left femoral artery

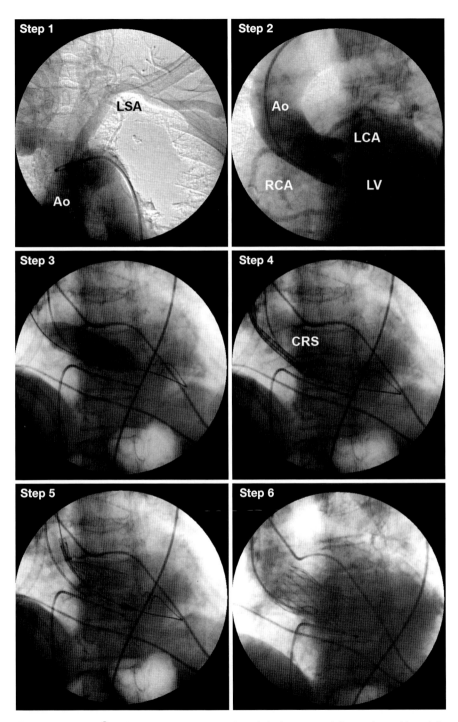

Fig. 3.69 CoreValve® device implantation phases by subclavian approach in a patient with peripheral accesses not suitable for the transfemoral procedure. *Ao*, aorta; *CRS*, CoreValve® Revalving System; *LCA*, left coronary artery; *LSA*, left subclavian artery; *LV*, left ventricle; *RCA*, right coronary artery

3.1.5.2.3
Essential Bibliography

The first data published on the CoreValve® device are those relating to the first experience using the 24 Fr and 21 Fr devices. Grube et al [68] described the results of 25 high-risk patients with severe AS; they were mainly women, with a mean age of 80 years and various comorbidities. Acute device success, understood as effective device implantation, was 88%. The success of the procedure, defined as device success and no MACCEs at 48 h, was 68%. The mean aortic gradient acutely dropped from 44.24 ± 10.79 mmHg to 12.38 ± 3.03 mmHg and remained unchanged at 30 days [68]. Two patients required immediate surgical conversion for device malapposition. Intrahospital MACCEs were observed in 32% of cases and included 20% of mortality and 24% of major bleeding. In all patients in whom circulatory support systems were used, thrombocytopenia occurred. The use of extracorporeal circulation support systems was soon abandoned with the introduction of smaller diameter catheters, which have led to a drastic reduction in episodes of thrombocytopenia and bleeding. The number of MACCEs also dropped with the progression in the learning curve. The following case history published by Grube et al on 86 patients used 21 Fr and 18 Fr devices [69]. The acute device success was 88% and the success of procedure at 48 h was 74%. Two patients needed the implantation of a second device to reduce the degree of peri-prosthetic failure. The aortic valve area was drastically improved, and post-procedure peri-prosthetic leak improved or did not vary in 66% of cases. The close link between the improvement in outcomes and in materials and experience was examined in a study published in 2008 [70]; it showed that procedural success rose from the first/second generation to the third generation of devices from 70.0/70.8% to 91.2% ($P = 0.003$). The composite of death/stroke/myocardial infarction at 30 days was 40.0/20.8/14.7% for the first, second, and third generation respectively, with no intraprocedure death in the third-generation group. In 2008, the results of the expanded evaluation registry [71] on 646 patients, all treated with the 18 Fr device, were published and showed a procedural success of 97% with an intraprocedure mortality of 1.5%. Mortality at 30 days for all causes of death was 8%, and the composite of death, stroke and myocardial infarction was 9.3%; in 9.3% of cases, the implantation of a permanent pacemaker was needed. Tamburino et al [72] reported a single-center experience on 30 patients in whom procedural success was achieved in 93% of cases and 30-day mortality was 7%. In all patients, there was a substantial improvement in the functional class. A paper published in 2009 by Ussia et al [75] showed for the first time that the improvement in the functional class and hemodynamic and echocardiographic parameters of the TAVI patients was matched by a substantial improvement in quality of life. More recently, Buellesfeld et al [76] sought to identify the procedural success predictors of TAVI in a population of 168 patients. Acute and in-hospital procedural success rates were 90.5% and 83.9%, respectively, with in-hospital mortality, myocardial infarction, and stroke rates of 11.9%, 1.8%, and 3.6%, respectively. This study showed that at univariate analysis the predictors of in-hospital procedural success were the type of access (odds ratio [OR] 0.33 in favour of the femoral over the iliac and subclavian access, 95% confidence interval [CI] 0.13–0.82, $P = 0.017$), prior coronary angioplasty (OR 5.3, 95% CI 1.20–23.41, $P = 0.028$), and the pre-procedural functional performance status of the patient, as expressed by the Karnofsky index; the latter was the only independent predictor in the multivariate analysis (OR 1.04, 95% CI 1.00–1.08, $P = 0.032$).

3.1.5.3
Other Devices

The devices described above are the only ones that are widely applied today in clinical practice. However, new generations of devices are being experimented. In addition to the features already offered by current devices, they also offer a lower profile and the possibility of being repositioned, and they reduce the occurrence of peri-prosthetic leaks.

The *Lotus™ percutaneous aortic valve* (Lotus™ Valve, Sadra Medical, CA, USA) [77] (Fig. 3.70) represents the first example of retrievable and repositioning percutaneous aortic bioprosthesis; it comprises a continuous lengthened nitinol braid frame with a bovine pericardial trileaflet valve and an 18 Fr diameter catheter delivery system (the First-in-Man [FIM] study was carried out using a 21 Fr delivery catheter), which allows the user to advance the prosthesis across the aortic valve and to unsheath it for deployment (Fig. 3.71). The self-expanding nitinol prosthesis passively shortens and self-centers with low radial force, which allows the valve to begin functioning. When it is optimally located, the nitinol frame is actively shortened and locked to its final height (19 mm), which increases the radial force and secures the bioprosthesis. Currently, the frame-valve assembly is attached to the catheter-deployment system by 15 fingers, which make the release procedure extremely complex and challenging; thus a new three-finger design has been projected, which will make the deployment of the prosthesis simpler (Fig. 3.72). The main advantage of this device is that it can be re-elongated, retrieved, and repositioned at any time before final release from the catheter, and this characteristic is one of the most developed in new technologies for a transcatheter aortic valve.

The *Direct Flow valve* (Direct Flow Medical Inc., Santa Rosa, CA, USA) [78] (Fig. 3.73) represents a new-generation of non-metallic, stentless, and repositionable percutaneous heart valve which is composed of three fundamental components: a bovine pericardial tissue heart valve, which is attached to an inflatable framework with a conformable polyester fabric cuff to provide a

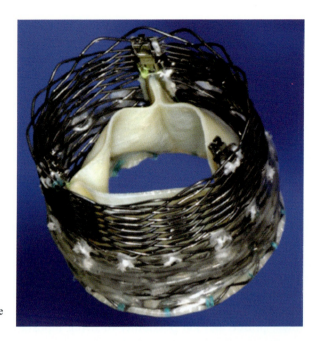

Fig. 3.70 Lotus™ self-expanding and repositionable device, Sadra Medical

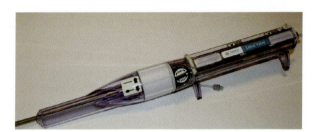

Fig. 3.71 Sadra Lotus™ handle catheter

seal and minimize paravalvular leak (both the upper [aortic] and the lower [ventricular] margin of the cuff consist of an independently inflatable balloon ring), and a 22 Fr delivery system with an integrated recovery system and solidifying inflation media that forms the support structure (Fig. 3.74). Currently the procedure is performed under general anesthesia, without extracorporeal circulation, using TEE guidance. After surgical exposition of a femoral artery, a 22 Fr introducer is inserted; thus, repeated valvuloplasty is performed to obtain a significant improvement of mobility of the leaflets and decrease in transaortic gradient of ~30 mmHg. At this point, the delivery catheter is advanced through the native valve; once the delivery system is entirely inside the LV, firstly the lower part in a subannular position and then the upper part in a subcoronary position are inflated with a 50:50 mixed contrast media and saline solution injection; thus, function and sealing are checked with

3.1 Aortic Stenosis

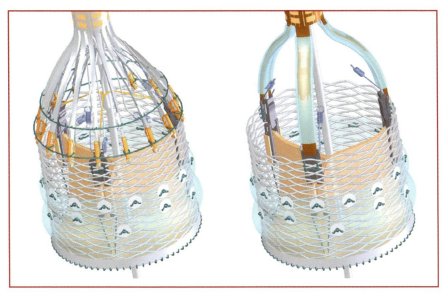

Fig. 3.72 Development of the Lotus™ release system. **Left**, schematic image of the 15-finger design; **right**, scheme for the new 3-finger device

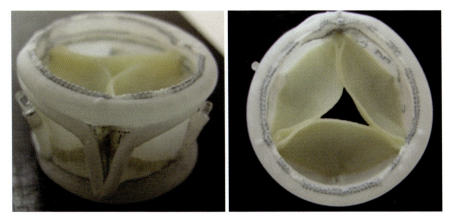

Fig. 3.73 Direct Flow stentless percutaneous device (courtesy of Direct Flow Medical Inc.)

contrast injection, and at this stage the valve can be recovered and repositioned in the case of suboptimal deployment. Once the optimal position has been achieved, contrast and saline solution are replaced with permanent polymer and the device is disengaged from catheter.

In the FIM experience [79], of the 15 patients enrolled, implantation was acutely successful in 12 patients (80%) in whom a considerable increase in AVA and a concomitant decrease in the mean transvalvular pressure gradient was

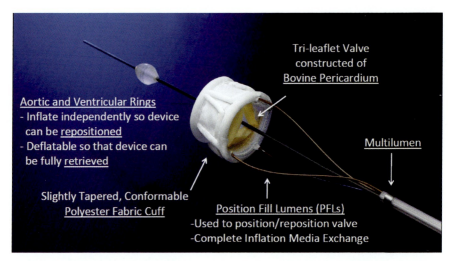

Fig. 3.74 The Direct Flow valve is attached to the delivery system by three catheter lumens that are used to position the valve and fill the supporting ventricular and aortic rings (courtesy of Direct Flow Medical Inc.)

reached. One patient had to undergo surgical conversion at day 2, and 11 patients (73%) were discharged with a permanent implant. At 30 days, one cardiac death (6.7%) and one major stroke were observed. The 10 patients surviving 30 days with a permanent implant showed marked hemodynamic and clinical improvement. The main benefit of the highly flexible prosthesis is that it gives the operator unprecedented freedom of handling the device during implantation; it can be easily settled even through a calcified aortic arch, allows repeated advancement and retraction across the native annulus for correct positioning, and functions immediately upon expansion.

The *AorTx* percutaneous aortic valve (Hansen Medical, Mountain View, CA, USA) consists of a low-profile, folded, metallic frame that incorporates a pericardial tissue valve (Fig. 3.75). The frame is positioned, sprung open to unfold the trileaflet valve, and with high radial force is securely implanted. As with the previously discussed designs, the system is fully retrievable and can be repositioned before final detachment from the catheter-delivery system. The prosthesis was tested in the laboratory on a billion cardiac cycles, showing excellent performance; eight temporary implants have been performed on humans with a 100% success rate [80]

The *JenaClip*™ (JenaValve Technology GmbH, Munich, Germany) (Fig. 3.76) is a recently designed device made of a porcine valve mounted on a self-expanding nitinol support (Fig. 3.77) whose purpose is to fasten the native aortic valve with hooks to prevent displacement. This allows the stent to be very

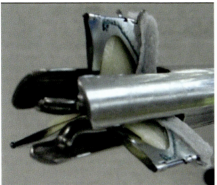 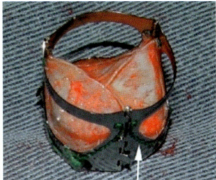

Fig. 3.75 AorTx percutaneous aortic valve

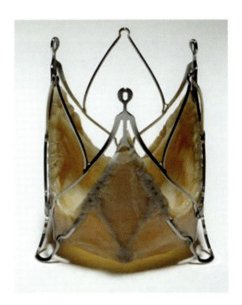

Fig. 3.76 JenaValve prosthesis (courtesy of JenaValve Technology GmbH, Munich, Germany)

short. Transfemoral and transapical implantation is currently envisaged (Fig. 3.78); in the latter case, four device sizes are available (21 mm, 23 mm, 25 mm, and 27 mm) to cover a range of annuli from 18 mm to 26.6 mm [81]. It is a device with a very low profile and it offers the possibility of being repositioned in case of non-optimal release. The device has been tested on animal models with excellent results and important implications for the treatment of AR, considering the high anchoring capacity also seen in animal models of elastic and scarcely calcified aortas (Fig. 3.79) [82].

The *Ventor Embracer*™ Transcatheter Aortic Valve Bioprosthesis (Medtronic Inc. MN, USA) (Fig. 3.80) is a new-concept self-expandable nitinol device,

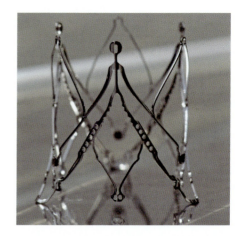

Fig. 3.77 JenaClip™ stent (courtesy of JenaValve Technology GmbH, Munich, Germany)

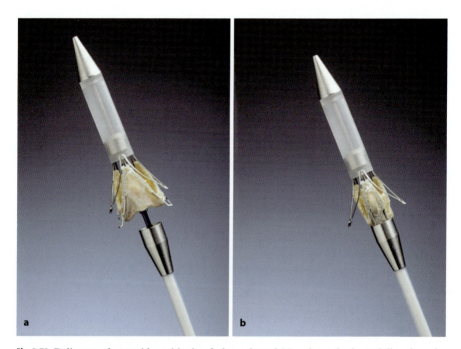

Fig. 3.78 Delivery catheter with positioning feelers released (**a**) and prosthesis partially released (**b**). (Courtesy of JenaValve Technology GmbH, Munich, Germany)

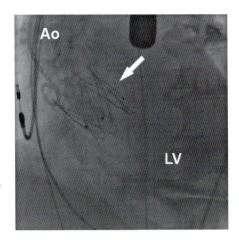

Fig. 3.79 JenaValve prosthesis deployed at the aortic annulus. *Ao*, aorta; *LV*, left ventricle (courtesy of JenaValve Technology GmbH, Munich, Germany)

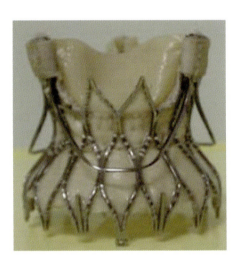

Fig. 3.80 The Ventor Embracer™ Transcatheter Aortic Valve Bioprosthesis (courtesy of Medtronic Inc. MN, USA)

which has a design with an anatomic orientation that creates an optimal anatomic fit, facilitating intuitive deployment and axial fixation. The stent is composed of two parts: the outer frame, modeled similarly to a stent frame for surgical bioprosthesis, and the inner frame which determines the general shape of the prosthesis. On this frame, scalloped bovine pericardial leaflets are mounted. The FIM study using the transapical approach has already been reported [83].

3.1.5.4
Procedural Complications

The potential acute complications of this procedure related to the device used are [84]:

- *periprosthetic regurgitation*: this is definitely the most frequent condition, although most of the time it is mild and well tolerated without any hemodynamic repercussions; when the valve is placed at the right height, it is generally located posteriorly, along the tract involving the non-coronary cusp and the left coronary artery, and it is assessed and quantified thanks to angiography or echocardiography (either transthoracic or transesophageal) immediately after device placement, but especially at catheterization, measuring the differential aortic pressure, which is the best index of the hemodynamic impact of regurgitation. In addition, in the case of the self-expanding device, it has been seen that it tends to reduce over time. If the leak is persistently severe, with hemodynamic instability, alternatives to cardiac surgery can be: (1) in cases of device hypo-expansion, post-dilation with valvuloplasty balloon; (2) in cases of suboptimal device position (too low or too high), implantation of a new device inside the previous one (*"valve-in-valve" technique*) [85, 86]
- *intraprosthetic regurgitation*: this may occur when a device that is undersized compared to the actual dimensions of the aortic annulus is placed, or when the device was post-dilated with an oversized balloon. In most cases, central intraprosthetic regurgitation is caused by the persistence of the guidewire inside the device; in these cases, retracting the guidewire eliminates this kind of failure. More rarely, intravalve regurgitation can arise due to the failure of one of the prosthetic valve's cusps to close: this may occur when the native aortic valve's cusps overhang on the stent, causing pressure that is inadequate to close the cusp. This involves a generally non-tolerated failure, which requires the implantation of a second device, as post-dilation seldom helps in redirecting the native cusp and improving device performance
- *intra-procedural valve migration*: this is a rare event typically occurring within a few cardiac cycles; it is a more frequent complication in the procedure using the ES device compared to the CRS device; the latter's self-expanding characteristics and the greater frame height allow anchoring of the device to the aortic annulus and ascending aorta. More commonly, distal embolization occurs; in these cases, the valve can be recaptured and released in the descending aorta. Proximal migration into the LV requires surgery to remove the device
- *obstruction of the coronary ostia by the device, or displacement of large calcified cusps*: this complication too is very rare and observed above all in patients with heavily calcified native valves
- *interference of the biological prosthesis with the mitral valve's anterior*

leaflet: this occurs mainly when the device is implanted too low in the left ventricular outflow tract; this is most often the case with the CRS device; if interference with the mitral valve causes a defect that is not hemodynamically tolerated, a valid approach is to carry out a maneuver to hook the device's aortic portion with a "*loop catheter*" and pull it back towards the ascending aorta

- *development of advanced atrioventricular conduction disorders* requiring the implantation of a permanent pacemaker: this is also one of the most frequent complications of this procedure and is due to the close proximity of the atrioventricular node to the aortic valve annulus [87–90]
- *introducer access site complications* (pseudoaneurysm, femoral occlusion, dissection, avulsion): in these cases, aortography and selective injection are of crucial importance to obtain an early diagnosis and conduct staging of the lesion's severity
- *cerebrovascular events (stroke and transient ischemic attack)* following calcium fragment mobilization during catheter advancement through a heavily calcified aorta or during valvuloplasty or device expansion due to the embolization of calcium from the native valve cusps
- *aortic dissection*: this is a rare complication, which mainly occurs when various attempts are made to cross the stenotic native valve with the device
- more rarely, *ventricle or interventricular septum perforation* by the stiff guidewire [91] may occur: this is a dramatic event often requiring urgent surgical treatment, and it often leads to death.

3.2
Aortic Regurgitation

3.2.1
The Pathophysiology of Aortic Regurgitation

Aortic regurgitation (AR) is marked by blood regurgitation from the aorta into the LV, due to failure of the valve leaflets to close during the diastolic phase of the cardiac cycle. Valve failure can develop progressively, leaving the ventricle time to compensate for the defect (chronic regurgitation), or acutely (acute regurgitation), often causing an emergency.

It is usually an acquired valve disease, while congenital origin is rare. Acquired AR can be caused by alterations of the valve leaflets only, which can lead to diverse pathologies, more often of calcific-degenerative nature, as the result of acute or chronic endocarditic valve processes, or due to myxomatous degeneration of the leaflets. There has been a progressive reduction in primary valve disease of rheumatic origin, which is now a rare event. Systemic arterial hypertension, aortic dissection, connectivopathies like Marfan's syndrome, Reiter's syndrome, Ehlers–Danlos syndrome, or rheumatoid arthritis alter the aortic root, leading to dilation and valve dysfunction [92].

The pathophysiological alterations resulting from AR are correlated to the degree of regurgitation and take different forms in chronic AR and acute AR. Chronic AR is a progressive condition involving several compensatory mechanisms [93]. In AR the overall systolic output volume comprises the antegrade output and the regurgitant volume. In AR the LV pumps the total volume into the aorta against high systemic impedance. The main compensatory mechanism is the rise in telediastolic volume (increase in preload) caused by regurgitation. The LV manages to compensate the volume overload by progressively dilating. The rise in preload involves in a first phase, according to Starling's law, an increase in ventricular contractile efficiency. On the other hand, according to Laplace's law, LV dilation leads to an increase in wall systolic tension, which is addressed by the ventricle, with eccentric hypertrophy of the walls to normalize the systolic stress. As a consequence, in AR hypertrophy and dilation are combined.

The valve defect can be well tolerated for a long time due to the compensatory mechanisms implemented. As the pathology progressively evolves, due to the effects of chronic volume overload, hypertrophy can prove to be inadequate for dilation, thus leading to structural alterations of ventricular myocardium. This brings about an increase in telediastolic pressure and a reduction in systolic output, thus increasing left atrial and pulmonary vein and capillary pressure and eliciting the clinical manifestations of heart failure. The worsening in ventricular function is favored by the development of ischemic damage secondary to inadequate coronary artery perfusion due to reduced aortic diastolic pressure.

In acute AR, the inability of the LV to adapt to the sudden volume overload leads to a rapid increase in ventricular diastolic pressure. This involves a sharp increase in atrial and pulmonary vein and capillary pressure, which elicits the clinical manifestations of acute heart failure such as orthopnea and pulmonary edema [92–94].

3.2.2
Diagnosis

3.2.2.1
Non-invasive Diagnosis

In chronic AR patients, the symptoms due to reduced cardiac or coronary reserve, such as effort dyspnea and angina pectoris, have a late onset. Sudden dyspnea at rest and low-flow symptoms characterize the clinical course of acute

AR patients. Some of the objective signs typical of chronic AR are a wide and fast arterial pulse, increased differential pressure, decreasing aortic diastolic murmur, best audible in the third to fourth intercostal space on the left of the sternum in expiratory apnea, click and systolic ejection murmur, and telediastolic murmur of mitral origin (so-called Austin–Flint murmur). In acute AR the peripheral signs are missing, diastolic murmur is usually short, and there is a prevalence of the signs typical of low cardiac output and pulmonary venous congestion.

With regard to the instrumental examinations, standard ECG can show the signs of left ventricular hypertrophy, left ventricular overload, or left bundle branch block (Fig. 3.81); these signs are not present in acute AR, where sinus tachycardia and aspecific disorders in ventricular repolarization may occur.

Chest x-ray can show an increase in the volume of the LV and, at times, of the thoracic aorta, especially in the ascending tract.

However, the staple examination for non-invasive diagnosis of AR is TTE with color-Doppler.

This method consists of:
- assessing the anatomy and structural alterations of the aortic valve and the presence and severity of aortic root dilation
- estimating the presence and severity of AR
- assessing the structural adaptations and degree of left ventricular impairment
- studying the anatomy of the valve apparatus.

TTE provides very accurate morphological and functional information on the aortic valve and root, identifying, for instance, the presence of bicuspid aortic valve disease, the thickening and reduced mobility of the cusps in the

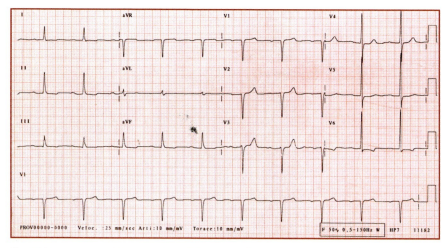

Fig. 3.81 ECG picture of hypertrophy and left ventricular overload in patient with aortic regurgitation

degenerative or post-rheumatic forms, thickened and redundant leaflets in myxomatosis, erosion and perforation of the cusps in the forms secondary to endocarditis, and aortic ectasia in Marfan's syndrome. In addition, AR can also be secondary to degenerative processes affecting the biological valve devices; in this case, TTE diagnosis uses the techniques applied for native valve disorders with small expedients [95].

M-mode examination can show the distance of the mitral-interventricular septum E, high-frequency diastolic fluttering of the anterior mitral leaflet, inverse diastolic doming of the anterior mitral leaflet and, in acute AR, early diastolic closing of the mitral valve.

The color-Doppler technique shows blood regurgitation through the aortic valve during diastole and allows estimation of the severity, assessing the following parameters [96] (Fig. 3.82):
- width and area of the regurgitant jet cross-section
- vena contracta
- effective regurgitant orifice area (EROA) by the proximal isovelocity surface area (PISA) method.

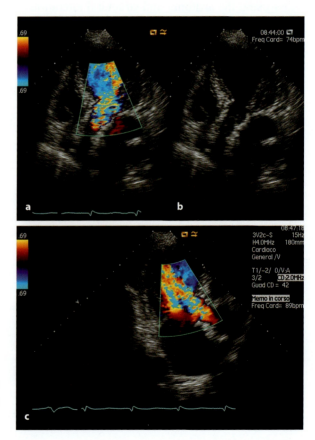

Fig. 3.82 a, b Color-Doppler ECG in apical four-chamber view; c three-chamber view, showing severe aortic regurgitation

3.2 Aortic Regurgitation

The width and cross-sectional area of the regurgitant jet must be measured in parasternal view, right below the aortic valve (within 1 cm from the valve). The relationship between the maximum width of the proximal jet and the left ventricular outflow diameter, measured in parasternal long-axis view, or the relationship between the jet cross-sectional area and the LVOT, measured in parasternal short-axis view, make it possible to estimate the severity of regurgitation [97]; AR is defined as severe if the relationship between the jet widths is ≥65%, or the relationship between the jet areas is ≥60% [1, 3] (Table 3.4).

Accurate measurement of the width and area of the regurgitant jet depends on the shape of the regurgitant orifice and jet direction; by occupying a small portion of the outflow tract, eccentric jets can lead to underestimation of the severity of the valvulopathy, while central jets, by contrast, can overestimate it.

Measurement of the vena contracta, at the aortic valve, in parasternal long-axis view, makes it possible to distinguish between severe forms, if it is >0.6 cm, and mild forms, if <0.3 cm [15, 96] (Table 3.4). In order to obtain accurate measurement of the vena contracta, the convergence flow, vena contracta, and jet should be clearly visible. The use of this parameter, though, is indicated in the presence of multiple jets.

The PISA method is based on the concept that the quantity of regurgitant flow through the aortic valve is obtained from the flow quantity of a proximal surface area with a known flow velocity, and calculates the EROA [98].

Table 3.4 Criteria for the definition of aortic regurgitation severity

Parameters	Mild	Moderate	Severe
Doppler parameters			
Jet width in LVOT – color-flow	Small in central jets	Intermediate	Large in central jets
Jet deceleration rate – continuous wave Doppler (pressure half-time, ms)	>500	500–200	<200
Diastolic flow reversal in descending aorta – pulsed wave Doppler	Brief, early diastolic reversal	Intermediate	Holodiastolic reversal
Quantitative parameters			
Jet width/LVOT width, %	<25	25–64	≥65
Jet CSA/LVOT CSA, %	<5	5–59	≥60
Vena contracta width, cm	<0.3	0.3–0.6	>0.6
Regurgitant volume, ml/beat	<30	30–59	≥60
Regurgitant fraction, %	<30	30–49	≥50
Effective regurgitant orifice area, cm^2	<0.10	0.10–0.29	≥0.30
Structural parameters			
Left ventricular size	Normal	Normal or dilated	Usually dilated

CSA, cross-sectional area; *LVOT*, left ventricular outflow tract

Imaging of the proximal flow convergence region by TTE is performed from the apical, and para-apical views, or the upper right-sternal border. This method cannot be used in the case of multiple jets and it is less accurate for eccentric jets. In addition, the presence of an aneurysm of the ascending aorta, which deforms the valve plane, can lead to an underestimation of the degree of AR. AR is defined as severe when the EROA is ≥ 0.30 cm^2 [15, 96] (Table 3.4).

PW Doppler allows quantification of AR by calculating the regurgitant volume (RV) and regurgitant fraction (RF). Aortic RV is obtained by subtracting the systolic volume crossing the LVOT from the mitral inflow or pulmonary outflow volume. RF is obtained from the equation:

$$RF = (aortic\ RV/LVOT\ systolic\ volume) \times 100\ \%.$$

The EROA can be calculated this way as well, since the flow volume is given by the product of the area by the velocity–time integral of the regurgitant jet at CW Doppler [99]. This method applies to multiple and eccentric jets, but it cannot be used in the presence of MR of a degree worse than mild, except for those cases in which pulmonary output is used as reference. A RV ≥ 60 ml and EROA ≥ 0.30 cm^2 are consistent with severe AR [15, 96] (Table 3.4).

PW Doppler also allows the observation of a diastolic Doppler signal due to aortic diastolic flow reversal in either the ascending or descending aorta. With increasing AR, the duration and velocity of the reversal increase (Figs. 3.83 and 3.84).

CW color-Doppler recording of the flow velocity–time curve of AR with an apical approach is marked by a rapid increase in velocity during isovolumetric relaxation, followed by a gradual slowdown during diastole and a sudden drop during isovolumetric contraction. As the degree of severity of AR worsens, left ventricular diastolic pressure rises, and the pressure half-time (PHT) of the regurgitant flow and the deceleration time of the mitral protodiastolic flow velocity become shorter [100]. A PHT >500 ms is usually compatible with mild

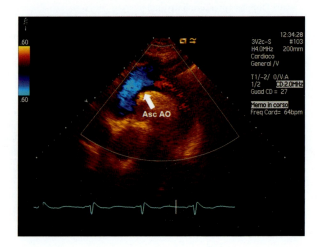

Fig. 3.83 Transthoracic echocardiogram: color Doppler image of an aortic regurgitation jet recorded in the ascending aorta (*Asc AO*)

AR, whereas a value <200 ms is considered consistent with severe AR [15, 96] (Table 3.4) (Fig. 3.85). This technique has some limitations, though, as it is affected, for instance, by LV compliance, which, if reduced, leads to a shortening of PHT, due to the faster rise in LV pressure. The density of the CW Doppler spectral display of the AR jet reflects the volume of regurgitation, even if is an imperfect indicator of the severity of AR.

TEE is seldom used in the assessment of AR, but it may be needed if there is a poor acoustic window, or if accurate assessment of aortic valve anatomy or Doppler scans is not possible.

Finally, in the overall assessment of a patient, an assessment of the LV is also needed for therapeutic and prognostic purposes; in particular, the increase in its telesystolic diameter to over 55 mm, without any other causes for volume overload, is an indication of severe ventricular function impairment.

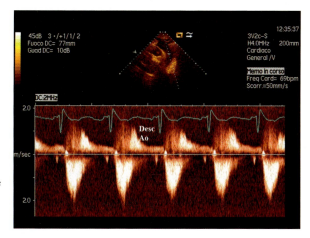

Fig. 3.84 Transthoracic echocardiogram: PW Doppler of the flow in the descending aorta in patient with aortic regurgitation. The reverse diastolic flow can be seen during diastole. *Desc Ao*, descending aorta

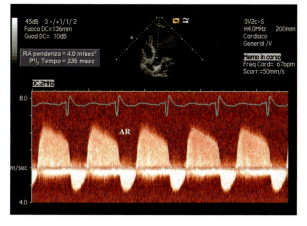

Fig. 3.85 Transthoracic echocardiogram: CW Doppler recording in a patient with aortic regurgitation showing how to measure the diastolic gradient of the regurgitant signal (*AR*) and the pressure half-time (P1/2 tempo)

The effort test in severe AR patients has not been validated.

Cardiac MRI is recommended when the quality of the echo images is not good, or, together with MSCT, for an assessment of the aorta when the echo shows that it is dilated.

3.2.2.2
Invasive Diagnosis

The role of invasive diagnosis in AR is rather limited, since TTE and TEE provide an extensive and accurate analysis of the degree of regurgitation [15].

Cardiac catheterization may be useful in assessing differential pressure in the ascending aorta, but aortography with rapid injection of contrast in the aortic root (25–35 ml/s) is particularly successful in quantifying the degree of regurgitation (Fig. 3.86). In the percutaneous treatment of degenerated biological devices, aortography is complementary to angio-CT and echo to study the interaction of the device with the aortic apparatus and to achieve optimal implantation of the percutaneous device.

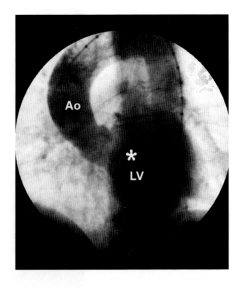

Fig. 3.86 Aortogram in left anterior oblique view showing major regurgitation (*) with contrast medium in the left ventricle (*LV*). *Ao*, aorta

3.2.3
Timing of Interventions

Moderate or severe AR is generally associated with a favorable prognosis for many years. Among asymptomatic subjects with severe AR and normal left ventricle ejection fraction (LVEF), more than 45% of patients maintain this condition and normal ventricular function at 10 years [101–103], with a percentage of <6% a year developing left ventricular dysfunction [15].

The risk of sudden death in these patients is less than 0.5% a year. However, as for AS, once the patient becomes symptomatic, there is rapid and progressive worsening. Heart failure may occur along with episodes of pulmonary edema, or cases of sudden death, usually among previously symptomatic patients with major LV dilation. Pre-surgery data show that death in non-operated patients usually occurs within 4 years from the onset of angina pectoris and within 2 years from the onset of heart failure [104]. Over the past 20 years, many surgical case histories have shown that a low LVEF is one of the most important determinants of mortality after valve replacement, especially when ventricular dysfunction is irreversible and does not improve after surgery [15].

It is more likely that left ventricular dysfunction is reversible if diagnosed early on, before the LVEF becomes so low that the ventricle dilates greatly and develops significant symptoms; therefore, surgical intervention is important before these alterations become irreversible [15].

AR can also be a condition with an acute development; in these cases urgent surgery is clearly indicated.

When speaking of chronic AR, considering the excellent prognosis in the short and medium term, surgical repair must be delayed in patients with severe AR who are asymptomatic, and have a good tolerance to effort and a LVEF >50% without marked LV dilation (i.e. a telediastolic diameter <70 mm and a telesystolic diameter <50 mm). Similarly, without clear contraindications or associated pathologies, surgery is indicated in symptomatic patients with severe AR and asymptomatic patients with LVEF <50% and marked left ventricular dilation (telediastolic diameter >70 mm and telesystolic diameter >50 mm). Since serious symptoms (NYHA class III or IV) and left ventricular dysfunction with LVEF <50% are independent risk factors for a worse post-operative survival, surgery must be performed in NYHA class II patients before they develop severe left ventricular dysfunction [15] (Table 3.5). Finally, valve replacement must be performed regardless of the symptoms in cases of severe AR in patients who must undergo surgery for other contingent conditions (Table 3.5).

Indications for surgery in patients with severe AR secondary to aortic root dilation are similar to those for patients with primary valve disease. However, progressive expansion of the aortic root and/or a diameter greater than 45 mm at echo (in the case of Marfan's syndrome), greater than 50 mm (in the case of

Table 3.5 Indications for valve replacement in aortic regurgitation, adapted from 2007 European guidelines for the treatment of valve diseases

Indication	Recommendation
Severe aortic regurgitation	
Symptomatic patients (dyspnea, NYHA class II, III, IV, or angina)	IB
Asymptomatic patients with resting LVEF <50%	IB
Patients undergoing coronary artery bypass, graft surgery of the ascending aorta, or another valve	IC
Asymptomatic patients with resting LVEF >50% with severe left ventricular dilation IIaC	IIaC
Whatever the severity of aortic regurgitation	
Patients who have aortic root disease with maximal aortic diameter	
≥45 mm for patients with Marfan's syndrome	IC
≥50 mm for patients with bicuspid valves	IIbC
≥55 mm for other patients	IIbC

LVEF, left ventricular ejection fraction; *NYHA*, New York Heart Association

bicuspid valve), and greater than 55 mm (in all other cases) with any other degree of regurgitation is also an indication for surgery [15] (Table 3.5).

The role of the percutaneous approach to AR treatment is rather marginal and currently consists of "*off-label*" application in patients for whom cardiac surgery is an absolute contraindication; this is also because the devices used are designed for the treatment of AS, to be implanted in heavily calcified and degenerated valves. There are also reports of cases of transcatheter valve implantation in patients who have previously undergone surgical aortic valve replacement with now degenerated biological valves and for whom reintervention is at extremely high risk. However, these are anecdotal cases and it is not possible to conclude whether this procedure is a real alternative to surgery [105–110].

3.2.4
Patient Selection

The gold standard for treating AR is surgical valve replacement [15]. Unlike the treatment of AS, in which the transcatheter approach is emerging as a valid alternative [40], the same cannot be said for AR. There are no percutaneous devices specifically designed for this pathology, and the few cases described have been performed on native valves and on degenerated biological devices [105–110] using devices created for implantation on stenotic valves. In this regard, patient selection from a clinical and anatomical perspective is more or less the same as the selection of AS patients to undergo percutaneous replacement, although though there are no data systematically documenting and confirming it.

3.2.5
Percutaneous Therapy

As already stated, at present, the treatment of AR and regurgitation due to degenerated biological devices falls solely within the realm of cardiac surgery [15].

The percutaneous technique is almost identical to the one used to treat AS, but some clarifications need to be made:
- valvuloplasty before implantation is not performed
- in treating AR of a native valve (Fig. 3.86) or a degenerated stentless biological device (Fig. 3.87) [106], there are generally no annulus calcifications: while on the one hand, this reduces the incidence of complications due to the embolization of the calcium fragments during device expansion, on the other hand, an important fluoroscopic point of marker is lost during valve release, which may paradoxically prove to be more challenging and lead to major perivalvular leaks (Fig. 3.88)
- valve calcifications are an effective structure on which percutaneous biological devices can be anchored with a high radial force, reducing the risk of its migration and peri-prosthetic leaks to a minimum; for this reason, the implantation of a self-expanding CRS device in a diseased aortic valve may

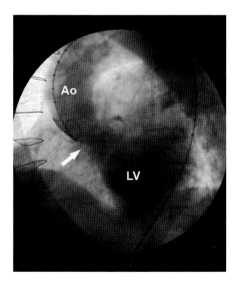

Fig. 3.87 Aortogram in left anterior oblique view showing major regurgitation of contrast medium in the left ventricle through a degenerated Biocor 21 stentless aortic biodevice (*white arrow*) (St Jude Medical, St Paul, MN, USA). *Ao*, aorta; *LV*, left ventricle

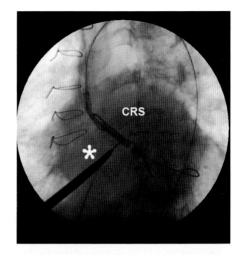

Fig. 3.88 Fluoroscopy in left anterior oblique view. The marker (*) shows the position of the stentless biodevice, which cannot be visualized. *CRS*, CoreValve ReValving® System

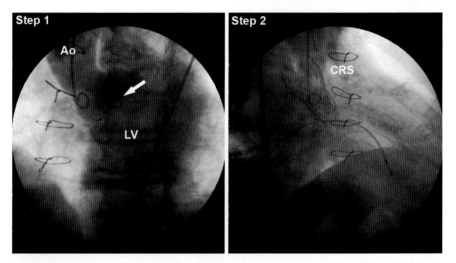

Fig. 3.89 Angiogram showing a degenerated stented aortic biodevice (*white arrow*), treated by implantation of a CoreValve® self-expanding transcatheter device. *Ao*, aorta; *CRS*: CoreValve ReValving® System; *LV*, left ventricle

require ventricular pacing during release of the device to ensure that it is placed as accurately as possible
- in the treatment of degenerated stented biological devices, placement is favored by the presence of a radio-opaque device ring, which is a precise marker for device release [105] (Fig. 3.89).

References

1. Rahimtoola SH. Aortic valve disease. In: Fuster V, Alexander RW, O'Ruourke RA (eds) Hurst's the heart (11th edn). New York: McGraw Hill, 2004; pp 1987–2000.
2. Alpert JS. Aortic stenosis: a new face for an old disease. Arch Intern Med 2003;163:1769–1770.
3. Bonow RO, Carabello BA, Chatterjee K et al. ACC/AHA 2006 guidelines for the management of patients with valvular heart disease. J Am Coll Cardiol 2006;48:1–148.
4. Tobin JR Jr, Rahimtoola SH, Blundell PE et al. Percentage of left ventricular stroke work loss: a simple hemodynamic concept for estimation of severity in valvular aortic stenosis. Circulation 1967;35:868–879.
5. Hess OM, Villari B, Krayenbuehl HP. Diastolic dysfunction in aortic stenosis. Circulation 1993;87:73–76.
6. Braunwald E, Fraham CJ. Studies on the Starling's law of the heart. IV. Observations on hemodynamic functions of the left atrium in man. Circulation 1961;24:633–642.
7. Ross J Jr. Afterload mismatch and preload reserve: a conceptual framework for the analysis of ventricular function. Prog Cardiovasc Des 1976;18:255–264.
8. Johnson LL, Sciacca RR, Ellis K et al. Reduced left ventricular myocardial blood flow per unit mass in aortic stenosis. Circulation 1978;57:582–590.
9. Marcus ML, Doty DB, Horatzka LF et al. Decreased coronary reserve. A mechanism for angina pectoris in patients with aortic stenosis and normal coronary arteries. N Engl J Med 1982;46:1362–1366.
10. Gould KL, Carabello BA. Why angina in aortic stenosis with normal coronary arteriograms? Circulation 2003;107:3121–3123.
11. Chambers BJ. Aortic stenosis. Eur J Echocardiogr 2009;10:i11–i19.
12. Baumgartner H, Hung J, Bermejo J et al. Echocardiographic assessment of valve stenosis: EAE/ASE reccomandations for clinical practice. Eur J Echocardiogr 2009;10:1–25.
13. Smith MD, Kwan OL, DeMaria AN. Value and limitations of continuous-wave Doppler echocardiography in estimating severity of valvular stenosis. J Am Med Assoc 1986;255:3145–3151.
14. Bonow RO, Carabello BA, Chatterjee K et al. ACC/AHA 2006 guidelines for the management of patients with valvular heart disease. J Am Coll Cardiol 2006;48:e1–e148.
15. Vahanian A, Baumgartner H, Bax J et al, Task Force on the Management of Valvular Heart Disease of the European Society of Cardiology; ESC Committee For Practice Guidelines. Guidelines on the management of valvular heart disease. Eur Heart J 2007;28:230–268.
16. Otto CM, Pearlman AS, Comess KA et al. Determination of the stenotic aortic valve area in adults using Doppler echocardiography. J Am Coll Cardiol 1986;7: 509–517.
17. Razzolini R, Tarantini G. Quando è critica una stenosi valvolare? Ital Heart J Suppl 2002;3:767–769.
18. Otto CM, Pearlman AS, Kraft CD et al. Physiologic changes with maximal exercise in asymptomatic valvular aortic stenosis assessed by Doppler echocardiography. J Am Coll Cardiol 1992;20:1160–1167.
19. Oh JK, Taliercio CP, Holmes DR Jr et al. Prediction of the severity of aortic stenosis by Doppler aortic valve area determination: prospective Doppler–catheterization correlation in 100 patients. J Am Coll Cardiol 1988;11:1227–1234.
20. De Filippi CR, DuWayne LW, Brickner ME et al. Usefulness of dobutamine echocardiography in distinguishing severe from non severe valvular aortic stenosis in patients with depressed left ventricular function and low transvalvular gradients. Am J Cardiol 1995;75:192–194.

21. Takeda S, Rimington H, Chambers J. The relation between transaortic pressure difference and flow during dobutamine stress echocardiography in patients with aortic stenosis. Heart 1999;82:11–14.
22. Otto MC. Valvular aortic stenosis. Disease severity and timing of intervention. J Am Coll Cardiol 2006;47:2141–2151.
23. Monin JL, Quere JP, Monchi M et al. Low-gradient aortic stenosis. Operative risk stratification and predictors for long-term outcome: a multicenter study using dobutamine stress hemodynamics. Circulation 2003;108:319–324.
24. Das P, Rimington H, Chambers J. Exercise testing to stratify risk in aortic stenosis. Eur Heart J 2005;26:1309–1313.
25. Popoviç AD, Thomas JD, Neskoviç AN et al. Time-related trends in the preoperative evaluation of patients with valvular stenosis. Am J Cardiol 1997;80:1464–1468.
26. Baim DS. Grossman's cardiac catheterization, angiography and intervention (7th edn). Philadelphia: Lipincott Williams and Wilkins, 2006.
27. Hakke AH. A simplified valve formula for the calculation of stenotic valve areas. Circulation 1981;63:1050–1055.
28. Bache RJ, Jorgensen CR, Wany Y. Simplified estimation of aortic valve area. Br Heart J 1972;34:408–411.
29. Freeman RV, Otto CM. Spectrum of calcific aortic valve disease: pathogenesis, disease progression, and treatment strategies. Circulation 2005;111:3316–3326.
30. Otto CM, Burwash IG, Legget ME et al. A prospective study of asymptomatic valvular aortic stenosis: clinical, echocardiographic, and exercise predictors of outcome. Circulation 1997;95:2262–2270.
31. Rosenhek R, Klaar U, Schemper M et al. Mild and moderate aortic stenosis. Natural history and risk stratification by echocardiography. Eur Heart J 2004;25:199–205.
32. Pellikka PA, Sarano ME, Nishimura RA et al. Outcome of 622 adults with asymptomatic, hemodynamically significant aortic stenosis during prolonged follow-up. Circulation 2005;111:3290–3295.
33. Chart Ross J Jr, Braunwald E. Aortic stenosis. Circulation 1968;38(Suppl 1):61–67.
34. Lancellotti P, Lebois F, Simon M et al. Prognostic importance of quantitative exercise Doppler echocardiography in asymptomatic valvular aortic stenosis. Circulation 2005;112:I377–1382.
35. Astor BC, Kaczmarek RG, Hefflin B, Daley WR. Mortality after aortic valve replacement: results from a nationally representative database. Ann Thorac Surg 2000;70:1939–1945.
36. Culliford AT, Galloway AC, Colvin SB et al. Aortic valve replacement for aortic stenosis in persons aged 80 years and over. Am J Cardiol 1991;67:1256–1260.
37. Shroyer AL, Coombs LP, Peterson E et al. The Society of Thoracic Surgeons: 30-day operative mortality and morbidity risk models. Ann Thorac Surg 2003;75:1856–1865.
38. Roques F, Nashef SA, Michel P et al. EuroSCORE study group. Risk factors for early mortality after valve surgery in Europe in the 1990s: lessons from the EuroSCORE pilot program. J Heart Valve Dis 2001;10:572–577.
39. Iung B, Baron G, Butchart EG et al. A prospective survey of patients with valvular heart disease in Europe: The Euro Heart Survey on valvular disease. Eur Heart J 2003;24:1231–1243.
40. Vahanian A, Alfieri O, Al-Attar et al. Transcatheter valve implantation for patients with aortic stenosis: a position statement from the European Association of Cardio-Thoracic Surgery (EACTS) and the European Society of Cardiology (ESC), in collaboration with the European Association of Percutaneous Cardiovascular Interventions (EAPCI). Eur Heart J 2008;11:1463–1470.
41. Descoutures F, Himbert D, Lepage L et al. Contemporary surgical or percutaneous management of severe aortic stenosis in the elderly. Eur Heart J 2008;29:1410–1417.

42. Tops LF, Wood DA, Delgado V et al. Noninvasive evaluation of the aortic root with multi-slice computed tomography implications for transcatheter aortic valve replacement. JACC Cardiovasc Imaging 2008;1:321–330.
43. Ng AC, Delgado V, van der Kley F et al. Comparison of aortic root dimensions and geometries before and after transcatheter aortic valve implantation by 2- and 3-dimensional transesophageal echocardiography and multislice computed tomography. Circ Cardiovasc Imaging. 2010;3:94-102.
44. Delgado V, Ng AC, Van de Veire NR et al. Transcatheter aortic valve implantation: role of multi-detector row computed tomography to evaluate prosthesis positioning and deployment in relation to valve function. Eur Heart J 2010; 19 Feb, epub ahead of print.
45. Messika-Zeitoun D, Serfaty JM, Brochet E et al. Multimodal assessment of the aortic annulus diameter: implications for transcatheter aortic valve implantation. J Am Coll Cardiol. 2010;55:186–194.
46. Cribier A, Sabin T, Saoudi N et al. Percutaneous transluminal valvuloplasty of acquired aortic stenosis in elderly patients: an alternative to valve replacement? Lancet 1986;1:63–67.
47. McKay RG, Safian RD, Lock JE et al. Balloon dilatation of calcific aortic stenosis in elderly patients: post mortem, intraoperative, and percutaneous valvuloplasty studies. Circulation 1986;74:119–125.
48. Block PC, Palacios IF. Clinical and hemodynamic follow-up after percutaneous aortic valvuloplasty in the elderly. Am J Cardiol 1988;62:760–763.
49. Otto CM, Mickel MC, Kennedy JW et al. Three-year outcome after balloon aortic valvuloplasty. Insights into prognosis of valvular aortic stenosis. Circulation 1994;89:642–650.
50. NHLBI Balloon Valvuloplasty Registry Participants. Percutaneous balloon aortic valvuloplasty: acute and 30-day follow-up results in 674 patients from the NHLBI Balloon Valvuloplasty Registry. Circulation 1991;84:2383–2397.
51. Zimrin DA, Reyes PA, Miller KL et al. Heart failure and "inoperable" aortic stenosis: staged balloon aortic valvuloplasty and aortic valve bypass. Congest Heart Fail 2008;14:211–213.
52. Iung B, Cachier A, Baron G et al. Decision-making in elderly patients with severe aortic stenosis: why are so many denied surgery? Eur Heart J 2005;26:2714–2720.
53. Andersen HR, Knudsen LL, Hasenkam JM. Transluminal implantation of artificial heart valves. Description of a new expandable aortic valve and initial results with implantation by catheter technique in closed chest pigs. Eur Heart J 1992;13:704–708.
54. Cribier A, Eltchaninoff H, Bash A et al. Percutaneous transcatheter implantation of an aortic valve prosthesis for calcific aortic stenosis: first human case description. Circulation 2002;106:3006–3008.
55. Grube E, Laborde JC, Zickmann B et al. First report on a human percutaneous transluminal implantation of a self-expanding valve prosthesis for interventional treatment of aortic valve stenosis. Catheter Cardiovasc Interv 2005;66:465–469.
56. Cribier A, Eltchaninoff H, Tron C et al. Early experience with percutaneous transcatheter implantation of heart valve prosthesis for the treatment of end-stage inoperable patients with calcific aortic stenosis. J Am Coll Cardiol 2004;43:698–703.
57. Cribier A, Eltchaninoff H, Tron C et al. Treatment of calcific aortic stenosis with the percutaneous heart valve: mid-term follow-up from the initial feasibility studies: the French experience. J Am Coll Cardiol 2006;47:1214–1223.
58. Webb JG, Chandavimol M, Thompson CR et al. Percutaneous aortic valve implantation retrograde from the femoral artery. Circulation 2006;113:842–850.
59. Webb JG, Pasupati S, Humphries K et al. Percutaneous transarterial aortic valve replacement in selected high-risk patients with aortic stenosis. Circulation 2007;116:755–763.
60. Webb JG, Altwegg L, Boone RH et al. Transcatheter aortic valve implantation: impact on clinical and valve-related outcomes. Circulation 2009;119:3009–3016.
61. Webb JG, Altwegg L, Masson JB et al. A new transcatheter aortic valve and percutaneous valve delivery system. J Am Coll Cardiol 2009;53:1855–1858.

62. Nietlispach F, Wijesinghe N, Wood D et al. Current balloon-expandable transcatheter heart valve and delivery systems. Catheter Cardiovasc Interv 2010;75:295–300.
63. Lichtenstein SV, Cheung A, Ye J et al. Transapical transcatheter aortic valve implantation in humans: initial clinical experience. Circulation 2006;114:591–596.
64. Ye J, Cheung A, Lichtenstein SV et al. Six month outcome of transapical transcatheter aortic valve implantation in the initial seven patients. Eur J Cardiothorac Surg 2007;31:16–21.
65. Walther T, Simon P, Dewey T et al. Transapical minimally invasive aortic valve implantation. Multicenter experience. Circulation 2007;116(Suppl I):1240–1245.
66. Svensson LG, Dewey T, Kapadia S et al. United States feasibility study of transcatheter insertion of a stented aortic valve by the left ventricular apex. Ann Thorac Surg 2008;86:46–55.
67. Ye J, Cheung A, Lichtenstein SV et al.Transapical transcatheter aortic valve implantation: 1-year outcome in 26 patients. J Thorac Cardiovasc Surg 2009;137:167–173.
68. Grube E, Laborde JC, Gerckens U et al. Percutaneous implantation of the CoreValve self-expanding valve prosthesis in high-risk patients with aortic valve disease: the Siegburg first-in-man study. Circulation 2006;114:1616–1624.
69. Grube E, Schuler G, Buellesfeld L et al. Percutaneous aortic valve replacement for severe aortic stenosis in high-risk patients using the second- and current third-generation self-expanding CoreValve prosthesis: device success and 30-day clinical outcome. J Am Coll Cardiol 2007;50:69–76.
70. Grube E, Buellesfeld L, Mueller R et al. Progress and current status of percutaneous aortic valve replacement: results of three device generations of the CoreValve Revalving System. Circ Cardiovasc Interv 2008;1:167–175.
71. Piazza N, Grube E, Gerckens U et al. On the behalf of the clinical centres who actively participated in the registry. Procedural and 30-day outcomes following transcatheter aortic\valve implantation using the third generation (18 Fr) CoreValve ReValving System: results from the multicentre, expanded\evaluation registry 1-year following CE mark approval. EuroIntervention 2008;4:242–249.
72. Tamburino C, Capodanno D, Mulè M et al. Procedural success and 30-day clinical outcomes after percutaneous aortic valve replacement using current third-generation self-expanding CoreValve prosthesis. Journal Invasive Cardiol 2009;21:93–98.
73. Bleiziffer S, Ruge H, Mazzitelli D et al. Results of percutaneous and transapical transcatheter aortic valve implantation performed by a surgical team. Eur J Cardiothorac Surg 2009;35:615–620.
74. Fraccaro C, Napodano M, Tarantini G et al. Expanding the eligibility for transcatheter aortic valve implantation: the trans-subclavian retrograde approach using the III generation CoreValve Revalving System. J Am Coll Cardiol Intv 2009;2;828–833.
75. Ussia GP, Mulè M, Barbanti M et al. Quality of life assessment after percutaneous aortic valve implantation. Eur Heart J 2009;30:1790–1796.
76. Buellesfeld L, Wenaweser P, Gerckens U et al. Transcatheter aortic valve implantation: predictors of procedural success – the Siegburg-Bern experience. Eur Heart J 2009; 27 Dec, epub ahead of print.
77. Buellesfeld L, Gerckens U, Grube E. Percutaneous implantation of the first repositionable aortic valve prosthesis in a patient with severe aortic stenosis. Catheter Cardiovasc Interv 2008;71:579–584.
78. Low RI, Bolling SF, Yeo KK, Ebner A. Direct flow percutaneous aortic valve: proof of concept. Eurointerventions 2008;4:256–261.
79. Schofer J, Schlüter M, Treede H et al. Retrograde transarterial implantation of a nonmetallic aortic valve prosthesis in high surgical-risk patients with severe aortic stenosis: a first-in-man feasibility and safety study. Circ Cardiovasc Interv 2008;1;126–133.

80. Cannon LA. AorTx: the low profile self-expanding valve. Presented at Transcatheter Cardiovascular Therapeutics (CTC) Congress, 2008, Washington DC, USA, October 13. 2008. http://www.tctmd.com/.
81. Figullas HR: The jena valve aortic leaflet clip concept. Presented at Transcatheter Cardiovascular Therapeutics (CTC) Congress, September 25, 2009, San Francisco. http://www.tctmd.com/.
82. Lauten A, Ferrari M, Petri A et al. Experimental evaluation of the JenaClip transcatheter aortic valve. Circ Cardiovasc Interv 2009;74:514–519.
83. Falk V, Schwammenthal EE, Kempfert J et al. New anatomically oriented transapical aortic valve. Ann Thorac Surg 2009;87:925–926.
84. Masson JB, Kovac J, Schuler G et al. Transcatheter aortic valve implantation: review of the nature, management, and avoidance of procedural complications. J Am Coll Cardiol Interv 2009;2:811–820.
85. Ussia GP, Mulè M, Tamburino C. The valve-in-valve technique: transcatheter treatment of aortic bioprosthesis mal position. Catheter Cardiovasc Interv 2009;73:713–716.
86. Piazza N, Schultz C, de Jaegere P, Serruys PW. Implantation of two self-expanding aortic bioprosthesis valves during the same procedure? Insight into valve-in-valve implantation ("Russian Doll" concept). Catheter Cardiovasc Interv 2009;73:530–553.
87. Piazza N, Onuma Y, Jesserun E et al. Early and persistent intraventricular conduction abnormalities and requirements for pacemaking after percutaneous replacement of the aortic valve. JACC Cardiovasc Interv 2008;1:310–316.
88. Sinhal A, Altwegg L, Pasupati S et al. Atrioventricular block after transcatheter balloon expandable aortic valve implantation. JACC Cardiovasc Interv 2008;1:305–309.
89. Calvi V, Puzzangara E, Pruiti GP et al. Early conduction disorders following percutaneous aortic valve replacement. Pacing Clin Electrophysiol 2009;32(Suppl 1):S126–130.
90. Jilaihawi H, Chin D, Vasa-Nicotera M et al. Predictors for permanent pacemaker requirement after transcatheter aortic valve implantation with the CoreValve bioprosthesis. Am Heart J 2009;157:860–866.
91. Tzikas A, Schultz C, Piazza N et al. Perforation of the membranous interventricular septum after transcatheter aortic valve implantation. Circ Cardiovasc Interv 2009;2:582–583.
92. Braunwald E, Goldman L. Primary Cardiology (2nd edn). New York: Elsevier Science, 2003.
93. Mihaljevic Ti, Sayeed MR, Stamou SC, Paul S. Pathophysiology of aortic valve disease. In: Cohn LH, ed. Cardiac surgery in the adult. New York: McGraw-Hill, 2008, pp 825–840.
94. Braunwald E, Fauci AS, Kasper DL et al. Harrison's principles of internal medicine (15th edn). New York: McGraw Hill, 2002.
95. Zoghbi WA, Chambers JB, Dumesnil JG et al. Recommendations for evaluation of prosthetic valves with echocardiography and Doppler ultrasound. J Am Soc Echocardiogr 2009;22:975–1014.
96. Zoghbi WA, Eriquez-Sarano M, Foster E et al. Recommendations for evaluation of the severity of native valvular regurgitation with two-dimensional and Doppler echocardiography. J Am Soc Echocardiogr 2003;16:777–802.
97. Perry GJ, Helmcke F, Nanda NC et al. Evaluation of aortic insufficiency by Doppler color flow mapping. J Am Coll Cardiol 1987;9:952–959.
98. Tribouilloy CM, Enriquez-Sarano M, Fett SL et al. Application of the proximal flow convergence method to calculate the effective regurgitant orifice area in aortic regurgitation. J Am Coll Cardiol 1998;32:1032–1039.
99. Enriquez-Sarano M, Bailey KR, Seward JB et al. Quantitative Doppler assessment of valvular regurgitation. Circulation 1993;87:841–848.

100. Teague SM, Heinsimer JA, Anderson JL et al. Quantification of aortic regurgitation utilizing continuous wave Doppler ultrasound. J Am Coll Cardiol 1986;8:592–599.
101. Bonow RO. Chronic aortic regurgitation. Role of medical therapy and optimal timing for surgery. Cardiol Clin 1998;16:449.
102. Borer JS, Hochreiter C, Herrold EM et al. Prediction of indications for valve replacement among asymptomatic or minimally symptomatic patients with chronic aortic regurgitation and normal left ventricular performance. Circulation 1998; 97:525–534.
103. Tarasoutchi F, Grinberg M, Spina GS et al. Ten-year clinical laboratory follow-up after application of a symptom-based therapeutic strategy to patients with severe chronic aortic regurgitation of predominant rheumatic etiology. J Am Coll Cardiol 2003;41:1316–1324.
104. Dujardin KS, Enriquez-Sarano M, Schaff HV et al. Mortality and morbidity of aortic regurgitation in clinical practice. A long-term follow-up study. Circulation 1999;99:1851–1857.
105. Wenaweser P, Buellesfeld L, Gerckens U, Grube E. Percutaneous aortic valve replacement for severe aortic regurgitation in degenerated bioprosthesis: the first valve in valve procedure using the Corevalve Revalving System. Catheter Cardiovasc Interv 2007;70:760–764.
106. Ussia GP, Barbanti M, Tamburino C. Treatment of severe regurgitation of stentless aortic valve prosthesis with a self-expandable biological valve. J Invasive Cardiol 2009;21:E51–54.
107. Attias D, Himbert D, Brochet E, Laborde JC, Vahanian A. "Valve-in-valve" implantation in a patient with degenerated aortic bioprosthesis and severe regurgitation. Eur Heart J 2009;30:1852.
108. Kelpis TG, Mezilis NE, Ninios VN, Pitsis AA. Minimally invasive transapical aortic valve-in-a-valve implantation for severe aortic regurgitation in a degenerated stentless bioprosthesis. J Thorac Cardiovasc Surg. 2009;138:1018–1020.
109. Bruschi G, Demarco F, Oreglia J et al. Transcatheter aortic valve-in-valve implantation of a CoreValve in a degenerated aortic bioprosthesis. J Cardiovasc Med (Hagerstown) 2010;11:182–185.
110. Maroto LC, Rodríguez JE, Cobiella J, Marcos P. Transapical off-pump aortic valve-in-a-valve implantation in two elderly patients with a degenerated porcine bioprosthesis. Eur J Cardiothorac Surg 2010;37:738–740.

Tips and Tricks and Management of Complications in Valvular Interventional Cardiology

4

Transcatheter treatment of acquired valve diseases, and especially aortic stenosis (AS) and mitral regurgitation (MR), is a recent and super-specialized branch of interventional cardiology, which is still undergoing further refinement.

Growing experience gained in the field, along with the continual exchange of information and ideas among interventional cardiologists, is today the only strategy to shorten the learning curve and provide patients with effective and safe procedures, as guidelines are still lacking.

There are three essential prerequisites to start a program for the transcatheter treatment of valve diseases:
- adequate experience in the transcatheter treatment of congenital and structural heart diseases and coronary and peripheral circulation pathologies
- adequate training in the transcatheter treatment of valve diseases under the guidance of qualified and expert personnel
- in-depth knowledge of techniques and materials, in order to ensure appropriate use, and knowledge of possible unexpected events associated with these procedures, and of the devices necessary for treatment in order to achieve success.

The use of inappropriate instruments or alternative materials can make these already complex procedures a genuine nightmare for the interventional cardiologist, the back-up team, and the patient (Box 4.1).

Knowledge of therapeutic devices for the management of complication also makes it possible for the catheterization laboratory to be duly equipped with an appropriate emergency kit, always available for use by trained personnel (Box 4.1).

These three prerequisites associated with the theoretical and hands-on training of the medical team are absolutely necessary, but are not enough to guarantee procedural success. The fourth prerequisite is adequate selection of patients for treatment.

> **Box 4.1 Materials for bailout procedures during transcatheter aortic valve implantation**
> - Snare catheter
> - Balloon catheter for peripheral angioplasty
> - Self-expandable covered stent
> - Self-expandable stent
> - Balloon catheter for aortic occlusion
> - Percutaneous pericardiocentesis kit
> - Guiding catheters and wires for peripheral vascular interventions

Considering these prerequisites, there are five critical elements to the transcatheter treatment of valve diseases:
- patient selection and, above all, the anatomical typing of the valve disease
- work-up for the procedure
- the procedure itself
- post-procedure management
- follow-up.

The purpose of this chapter is to provide experience-based tips on the first three factors (selection, work-up and procedure), as the post-procedure management and follow-up are discussed in the next chapter.

4.1
Patient Selection and Work-up

4.1.1
Anatomical Typing

In patient selection, a thorough description of the anatomy of the patient's cardiovascular system is of the utmost importance, especially with regard to the valve to be treated and the vascular accesses.

Therefore, various imaging techniques are needed in order to integrate the information they provide, predict any procedural problems associated with cardiovascular anatomy, and plan possible solutions in advance.

The basic anatomical features for patient selection have already been described. What follows is an overview of those aspects that are deemed to be of greater importance to operators.

4.1.2
Valve and Heart Anatomy

The anatomical criteria determining the feasibility of transcatheter aortic valve implantation (TAVI) and the choice of device type have already been described.

This section provides some tips derived from hands-on experience with TAVI using the CoreValve® device.

As already discussed, the choice of the valve size for an annulus with borderline dimensions (23 to 24 mm) is quite difficult. In this case the entire valve apparatus, understood as the whole structure formed by the left ventricular outflow tract (LVOT)/annulus/sinuses of Valsalva/sinotubular junction/ascending aorta, should be assessed, and not just the valve ring. In the case of a 23 mm annulus with a diameter of the sinuses of Valsalva greater than 30 mm and/or a height greater than 12 mm, a 29 mm CoreValve® device is recommended, despite the greater mechanical compression force in the LVOT and hence a greater incidence of advanced atrioventricular block. In these cases, the benefit of an "oversized" device is a greater stability of the system during implantation, associated with a minor incidence of peri-prosthetic leaks.

The use of an oversized device is also possible in the presence of a "horizontal aorta" (Fig. 4.1), as in these cases the implantation of a large device reduces the disadvantages associated with an unfavorable aortic angle, thus ensuring greater implant stability and reducing the likelihood of intraprocedural malpositioning to a minimum.

Valves with a 27 mm annulus are just as challenging, as the expanded distal part is difficult to position in the outflow tract below the left coronary cusp during the release of the first one-third of the device (step 1).

Implantation requires a certain degree of skill to release at least a mesh of the distal one-third of the device below the native left coronary cusp; in these cases,

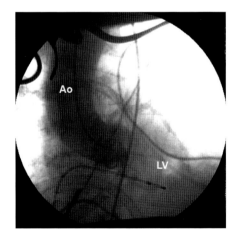

Fig. 4.1 Aortography in right anterior oblique view. The ascending aorta has a horizontal pattern compared to the left ventricle. *Ao*, aorta; *LV*, left ventricle

the procedure is as follows: during step 1, adequate expansion of the distal one-third of the device should be obtained; then, during step 2, the device should be slowly and gradually pulled back, straightening it while leveraging on the left side. Therefore, it is always recommended to use a good cranial or caudal left anterior oblique view to align the three native cusps.

Another technical expedient in the case of large annuli is to perform valvuloplasty using an undersized balloon so the annulus has greater support on the calcified cusps for release and, if necessary, to dilate the device with an adequately sized balloon after implantation.

Furthermore, with regard to the heart's structural and functional anatomy, the morphofunctional alterations often associated with AS, which can prejudice the procedure's outcome, are briefly illustrated next. In the concomitant presence of moderate-to-severe- functional MR, pulmonary hypertension, or reduced ejection fraction, bridge valvuloplasty with a balloon having a diameter smaller than that of the annulus (ratio 0.6–0.8) can be a useful maneuver to assess the reduction in the MR and pulmonary hypertension or the increase in left ventricle ejection fraction (LVEF).

The concomitant presence of coronary artery disease is not a contraindication to the procedure, but the coronary artery revascularization strategy can be difficult at times. Type A and B critical stenoses always need to be revascularized; in the case of type C or multivessel lesions, the procedure's risk/benefit ratio needs to be considered. At times, incomplete revascularization can actually be the most appropriate choice.

4.1.3
Vascular Anatomy

Another important step in patient selection based on the anatomical criteria is the typing of the aorto-iliac-femoral axis, since these procedures require the use of large-diameter catheters.

Besides angiography, which provides useful information on the inner diameter of the vessels and presence of wall calcifications, contrast-enhanced multi-slice computed tomography (MSCT) gives much more accurate information on wall calcifications and the tortuosity of the aorto-iliac-femoral axis.

MSCT, too, measures the inner diameter, which needs to be over 6 mm in these procedures. Calcifications around the entire diameter or just a part of it, as well as the presence of calcified focal stenosis in large-diameter vessels, should be carefully sought and assessed for potential problems associated with the insertion of the introducers and guiding catheter in the vascular axis.

4.1.3.1
Femoral Arteries

In assessing the femoral artery access, the position of the femoral bifurcation should be well identified: for proper preimplantation of the percutaneous suture device in the vascular access, the proper artery puncture site should be at least 5–10 mm above the bifurcation (Fig. 4.2).

In obese or short patients, the bifurcation can be located at a higher level. In these cases, angiographic reference is useful and, without moving the table, the relationship between the bifurcation and the underlying femoral head is used as an anatomical marker (Fig. 4.3).

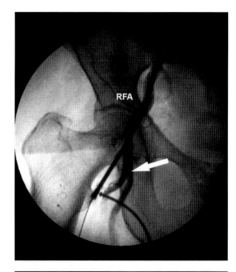

Fig. 4.2 Angiography of the right femoral artery *(RFA)* after 9 Fr introducer placement. The femoral bifurcation (*white arrow*) is 10 mm lower than the artery access

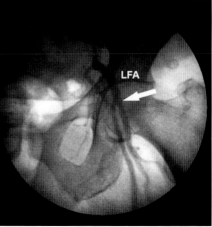

Fig. 4.3 Angiography of a left common femoral artery (*LFA*). Note the very high femoral bifurcation (*white arrow*), compared to Fig. 4.2

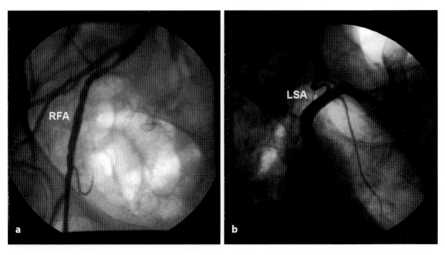

Fig. 4.4 Selective angiography of right femoral artery (*RFA*) shows a diameter <6 mm (**a**). In this case the left subclavian artery (*LSA*) was used for the 18 Fr introducer (**b**)

In femoral arteries with a diameter of less than 6 mm, the left subclavian artery can be used by surgically exposing the vessel (Fig. 4.4).

Calfications and/or stenosing plaques should be avoided, if possible, during the vessel puncture phase to ensure a better suture and reduce complications to a minimum.

4.1.3.2
Iliac Arteries

The choice of the vascular access must take into account the stenoses, calcifications, atheromatous plaques, and tortuosity of the iliac arteries.

In the case of major calcifications, the possibility that the arterial introducer does not advance should be considered; in these cases, preliminary balloon dilation can be performed or the introducer can be left in the iliac artery without necessarily inserting it in the aorta (Fig. 4.5).

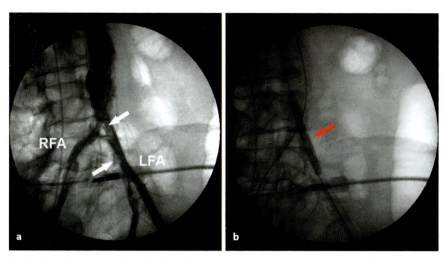

Fig. 4.5 Selective angiography of the left iliac-femoral artery. The severe stenosis (*white arrows*) of both common iliac arteries have been treated with balloon angioplasty (*red arrow*) before delivery-catheter insertion. *LFA*, left femoral artery; *RFA*, right femoral artery

4.1.3.3
Abdominal Aorta

Major atheromatosis or calcification should be assessed, especially if the CoreValve® device is to be retrieved after partial expansion, with possible mobilization of plaque material and peripheral embolization of atheromatous debris (Fig. 4.6).

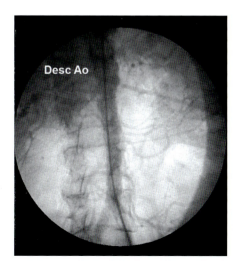

Fig. 4.6 Angiography of the abdominal aorta. Severe calcification and diameter reduction of the abdominal aorta. *Desc Ao*, descending aorta

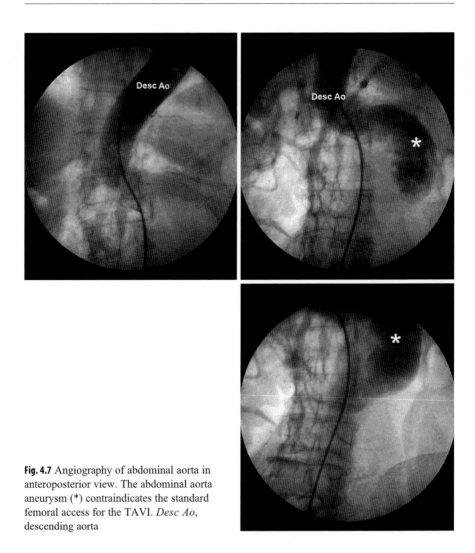

Fig. 4.7 Angiography of abdominal aorta in anteroposterior view. The abdominal aorta aneurysm (*) contraindicates the standard femoral access for the TAVI. *Desc Ao*, descending aorta

The presence of abdominal aneurysm is a contraindication to femoral access; in these cases, an alternative access like the subclavian or axillary artery is recommended (Fig. 4.7).

4.1.3.4
Thoracic Aorta

Calcified walls, acute angle, and endoluminal calcified plaques are factors that increase the risk of brain ischemia and peripheral embolism, due to the possible mobilization of plaques protruding in the lumen. The diagnostic catheters must be maneuvered according to the state of the art using J tip guides, and the delivery catheter should be placed with caution, trying not to adhere to the wall and pulling out the super-stiff guidewire a few millimeters if necessary.

During assessment, it is always recommended to perform selective angiography of the left and right subclavian artery. This is a very useful alternative route in case of difficult femoral access or unexpected delivery-catheter navigation problems during the procedure.

4.2
Procedure

The procedure can be performed under general anesthesia or deep sedation with local anesthesia. Generally speaking, the second option is to be preferred, as patients with a clinical indication for TAVI who have been rejected for surgery or are considered at high risk often have a serious respiratory deficit.

The pre-procedural placement of a central venous catheter in the internal jugular or subclavian vein, although associated with a few complications linked to the cannulation procedure, is very useful in cases in which the urgent administration of inotropic or antiarrhythmic drugs is necessary, or, especially during the first 24 hours after the procedure, for the monitoring of central venous pressure and the adjustment of serum electrolytes, if needed.

4.2.1
Vascular Access

Two arterial accesses, one for the 18 Fr catheter, the other for the diagnostic catheter, are needed, along with a venous access for insertion of the temporary pacemaker.

The choice of the optimal vascular access has already been discussed. The introducers currently used have an inner diameter of 18 Fr and an outer diameter of 21 Fr. The access that should be preferred for the diagnostic catheter is the contralateral femoral artery, as it can be rapidly utilized for emergency maneuvers in case of peripheral vascular complications or problems during device implantation.

Arterial puncture should be performed at least 5–10 mm above the bifurcation, on the vessel's anterior wall, with an angle of 45–60° compared to the plane of the vessel wall, in order to allow proper preimplantation of the percutaneous suture device in the vascular access. For an optimal puncture, angiography of the artery selected should be used to visualize the anatomical markers, especially with regard to the femoral head, and to perform the puncture with the help of small puffs of contrast medium (Fig. 4.8). Another possible technique is to insert a 5 Fr pigtail through the contralateral artery and use the pigtail's eyelet to guide puncture.

Once the artery is cannulated with a 9 Fr catheter, angiography is recommended to check the introducer's position and record the image to obtain information on the anatomy in case of subsequent vessel rupture or hematomas.

The Prostar™ device requires a few minor expedients: the cutaneous incision must be horizontal and at least 8–10 mm wide; the subcutaneous tissue should be dissected with Klemmer forceps with rounded tips, both above and below the introducer mounting the dilator and guidewire (Fig. 4.9 step 1). When inserting the Prostar™, make sure that the tip does not engage a renal artery. Therefore, this maneuver should be performed under fluoroscopy.

Once the Prostar™ is inserted, make sure that the blood jet exiting the posterior straight cannula is pulsatile (Fig. 4.9, step 2), also during needle extraction. It is recommended to make sure that the system rests against the artery wall using your left hand, and to pull back the needles with your right hand (Fig. 4.9, step 3). If one or more needles do not come out, check that they have not deviated into the subcutis (Fig. 4.10).

There are two possible ways to proceed:
- maneuver A - using a Klemmer forceps, reinsert the central steel barrel making sure not to bend it, and try to fit the needles completely into their lodging. This maneuver can be long and cumbersome (Fig. 4.11)
- maneuver B - pull out the needles, duly extracted, cut them off the wire, and reinsert the misaligned needle with the steel sheath as described above. In this case, inserting a single needle is much easier (Fig. 4.12).

Once the needles are reinserted, pull back the Prostar™ to the guide-insertion hole, reinsert the guide, and remove the system leaving the guide in the artery.

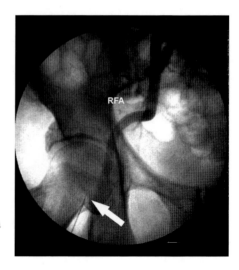

Fig. 4.8 A small injection of contrast helps in a correct puncture (*white arrow*) of the right femoral artery (*RFA*)

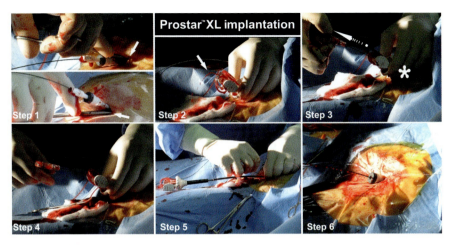

Fig. 4.9 Prostar™ insertion. After dissecting the subcutaneous upper and lower part of the introducer (*white arrow*) (**Step 1**), the Prostar™ is inserted until a pulsatile blood flow comes out from the straight tube (*white arrow*) (**Step 2**), maintaining the position using the left hand (**Step 3**, *) and using the right hand to pull out the needles (**Step 4**) and, once removed, the suture lines are cut (**Step 5**); at this point the Prostar™ is pulled out and the guidewire reinserted, with repositioning of the 9 Fr introducer (**Step 6**)

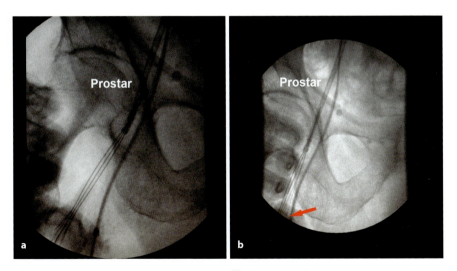

Fig. 4.10 Maneuver of needle retraction of Prostar™ XL 10 Fr. **a** The correct position of the four needles; **b** deviation of one of the medial needles (*red arrow*), which is in the subcutaneous tissue

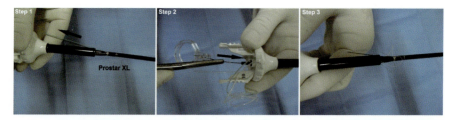

Fig. 4.11 Needle deviation during extraction. One of the needles can be deviated by a calcification or an incorrect position of the Prostar™. The first maneuver is to reinsert all the needles with the help of a Klemmer, in order to retract the entire system

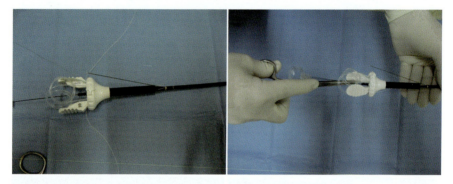

Fig. 4.12 To facilitate reinsertion of the deviated needles, extract and cut the correct needles, then reinsert the last one as in Fig. 4.11

Now reimplant the other Prostar™. When performing maneuver B (see page 224), the sutures should be removed by pulling one end.

Once the Prostar™ is implanted, reposition a 9 or 10 Fr introducer on the standard guide and, using a diagnostic catheter, place the Amplatz Super Stiff (ASS) guidewire in the descending aorta and the 18 Fr introducer on it.

4.2.2
Choosing the Introducer

The ideal introducer must have a low profile and be sheathed and equipped with an effective hemostasis valve to avoid bleeding when inserting the guide. There is no ideal introducer though. The 18 Fr Cook introducer is the one most widely used because it has a very efficient hemostasis valve and is sturdy enough for valve recovery. The main disadvantage is its wide outer diameter, which is about 21 Fr.

Other introducers have a lower outer profile and a less efficient hemostasis valve and are less stiff, so there is actually the risk that they can curl up when trying to recover the device (Fig. 4.13).

The introducer must always be inserted on a long stiff guide and advanced slowly under fluoroscopy to identify the reasons for any obstacles, such as calcified plaques or severe artery tortuosity.

In the case of vascular stenoses, balloon dilation can be performed to facilitate introducer navigation (Fig. 4.14). Stent implantation for a better result is not recommended at this stage, as it may hinder introducer insertion, but the stent should be implanted at the end of the procedure.

If the introducer does not advance, it can be left it in the iliac or even femoral artery. The CoreValve® delivery catheter has an outer diameter of 18 Fr, is more flexible than the introducer, and can also pass along a stiff guide in segments, opposing resistance to the introducer. In this case, however, it must be consid-

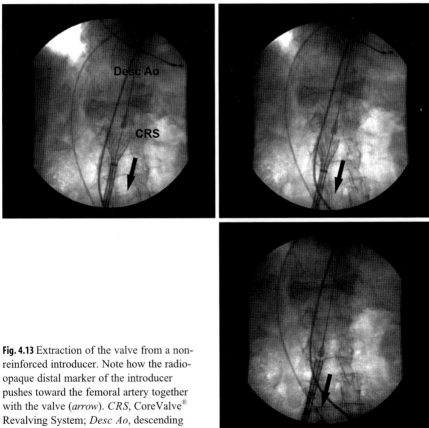

Fig. 4.13 Extraction of the valve from a non-reinforced introducer. Note how the radio-opaque distal marker of the introducer pushes toward the femoral artery together with the valve (*arrow*). *CRS*, CoreValve® Revalving System; *Desc Ao*, descending aorta

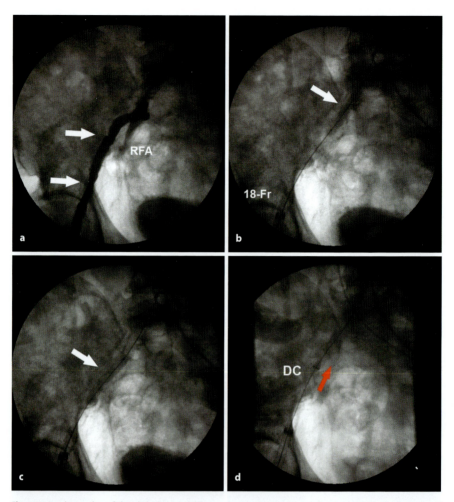

Fig. 4.14 Angiography of the right internal iliac artery and right femoral artery (*RFA*). Despite the 7 mm diameter of the arterial axis, there are three points (**a**, *white arrows*) of calcific stenosis. After balloon angioplasty (**b**, **c**, *white arrows*), it is still impossible to advance the 18 Fr introducer; then a trial of passage is performed using an empty catheter. **d** The introducer (*red arrow*) is left a few centimeters in the femoral artery and the procedure is performed uneventfully. *DC*, delivery catheter

ered that valve retrieval can be more cumbersome, as it should reach the iliac artery before entering the introducer; otherwise, there is the risk of iliac artery dissection.

When the introducer is partially inserted, make sure to hold the outer part firmly during all pushing operations.

It is also important to make sure to flush each time a catheter is changed in the introducer, as its diameter may lead to clot formation.

4.2.3
Passing the Aortic Valve

There are various techniques to pass the native aortic valve, and each varies depending on operator experience.

Generally speaking, the most widely used materials are the soft tip straight standard guide with an Amplatz catheter for the left coronary artery (AL-1 or AL-2), a Judkins catheter for the right coronary artery (JR), or a multipurpose catheter (MP) (Fig. 4.15).

In left anterior oblique view, the catheter tip is pointed to the valve orifice. Probe delicately with the guide while rotating the catheter clockwise. Cusp calcifications help to find the orifice, while an orthogonal view helps to guide the catheter, especially in bicuspid valves.

One technique for passing the valve consists of delicately probing the valve plane with catheter AL-1, using a straight guide with mobile core in order to adjust the guide system's stiffness and change the direction of the diagnostic catheter. After positioning the catheter on the valve plane, rotate it clockwise and probe using the guidewire, then pull it out a few millimeters.

During this maneuver, you need to watch out not to accidentally puncture the cusps, as this may complicate the deployment of the delivery catheter and hinder complete device expansion.

Another situation to be avoided is insertion of the guidewire in the left main coronary artery. In order to avoid incorrect guide insertion in the left main coronary artery or aortic cusp perforation, the use of hydrophilic guidewires should be avoided.

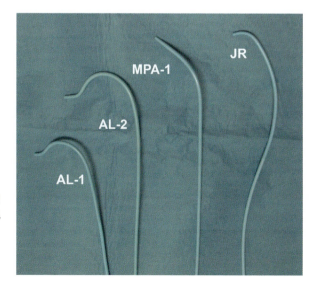

Fig. 4.15 The catheter most often used for passage through a stenotic aortic valve. *AL-1*, Amplatz Left 1 for small aortic valve; *AL-2*, Amplatz Left 2 for large aortic valve; *MPA-1*, multipurpose A1; *JR*, Judkins right catheter

Once the catheter is inserted in the left ventricle (LV), it is good practice to measure left ventricular pressure, both to confirm the transvalvular pressure gradient and to register the protodiastolic and telediastolic pressure of the LV. This information is very useful at the end of the procedure, to assess whether the implantation is hemodynamically effective. The diagnostic catheter is advanced in right anterior oblique view, to place the catheter at the apex of the ventricle (Fig. 4.16a) and position the back-up ASS guidewire. (Fig. 4.16b).

This is a very important step in the procedure, requiring the utmost attention. The back-up guidewire we recommend is the super-stiff Amplatz with 10 mm and soft distal segment. This way it is possible to shape the distal part like a pigtail, with a curve angle adapted to the size of the LV (Fig. 4.17). The smaller and more hypertrophic the LV is, the smaller the curve's radius should be.

Using this guidewire offers two advantages: low arrhythmogenicity thanks to the small soft distal segment positioned in the ventricle, and system stability during device release thanks to the stiff proximal segment). Moreover, a stable guidewire in the ventricle avoids movements of the delivery catheter in the ventricle and reduces the risk of LV perforation and tearing.

If the guidewire's position in the LV is not deemed optimal, a pigtail catheter can be used for repositioning.

In addition, it is important not to pass between the papillary muscles or trabeculae of the mitral subvalvular apparatus. During implantation of the

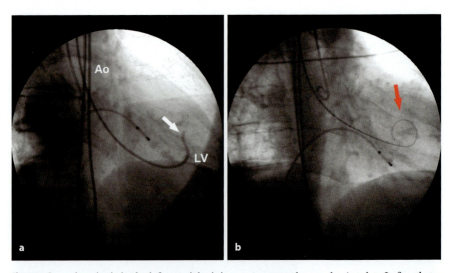

Fig. 4.16 Once the wire is in the left ventricle, it is necessary to advance the Amplatz Left catheter (*white arrow*) and, using the right oblique view, place it in a way that it adapts the curve to the left ventricular apex. Then it is necessary to change the straight wire with a J tip standard wire (**a**). When the catheter position is considered optimal, the Amplatz Super Stiff 260 cm has to be placed, with the 1 cm straight soft tip wire with a handmade J in the ventricle (*red arrow*) (**b**)

CoreValve® device, the guidewire may distort the apparatus and cause acute MR, with subsequent hemodynamic instability.

As already mentioned, one possible complication that may occur during deployment through the native valve is cusp perforation. Diagnosing cusp perforation is not simple, but some signs and maneuvers can be useful.

First of all, it should be noted that this occurrence is more frequent in all cases in which valve anatomy is so distorted that probing the native valve to find the stenotic orifice is difficult. Extremely calcified valves with an eccentric orifice, or bicuspid valves, are typical examples.

Some signs can help detect a suspicion of perforation. An unmistakable sign of cusp perforation is difficult deployment of the device's delivery catheter; you should avoid reaching as far as this phase of the procedure, since in these cases any maneuver, and especially exerting force on the delivery catheter, is contraindicated due to the risk of aortic root dissection and annulus tear.

The following signs are useful in the preliminary phases: abnormal resistance of the diagnostic catheter placed in the LV, abnormal course of the diagnostic catheter (Fig. 4.18), excessively acute angle of the catheter in the section

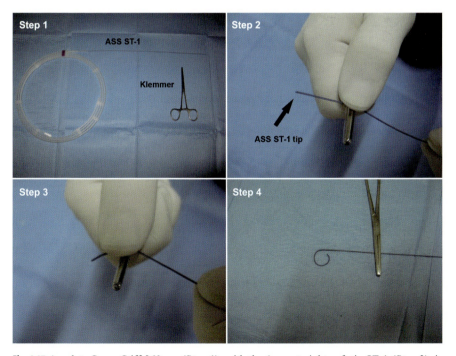

Fig. 4.17 Amplatz Super Stiff 260 cm (**Step 1**), with the 1 cm straight soft tip ST-1 (**Step 2**), is remodeled using a Klemmer (**Step 3**) obtaining a J pigtail-like shape, changing the radius if the left ventricle is small or large (**Step 4**)

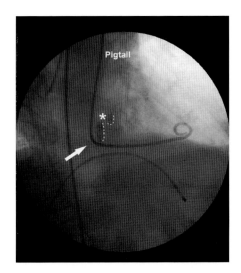

Fig. 4.18 Right anterior oblique view. The pigtail is clearly passing through the posterior cusp (*white arrow*), far from the native orifice (*), delineated by calcific cusps (*dotted lines*)

between the valve plane and the ventricle's base and body, and difficult maneuvering of the Amplatz or pigtail catheter inside the LV.

Another major sign is unusual resistance to valvuloplasty balloon deployment, especially when using low-profile balloons.

A handy maneuver is to inflate the balloon in the descending aorta to increase the profile and give a greater degree of certainty that you have passed the native orifice.

Another sign is an excessive degree of waist at the center of the balloon, visible once it is inflated, with excessive recoil during deflation (Fig. 4.19).

If there is a suspicion of perforation, angiography should be performed with the guide inserted through the tear to distinguish the native orifice from the tear.

At this point, one tip is to try crossing the stenotic orifice (in left or right anterior oblique view) leaving the super-stiff guidewire or a diagnostic catheter in the LV through the perforated cusp, to serve as reference for crossing the orifice and not re-entering the tear (Fig. 4.20). Once the native orifice has been crossed, the different course taken by the guidewires will be clear (especially in right oblique view).

Once the native orifice has been passed, the catheter or guidewire can be pulled out of the perforation and standard maneuvers can be started again.

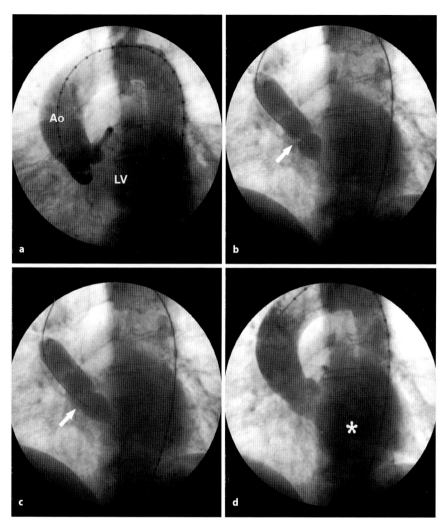

Fig. 4.19 Left anterior oblique view. A very tight balloon waist (**b, c** *white arrow*) during valvuloplasty can be a marker of cusp perforation. **d** Severe aortic regurgitation (*) caused by leaflet perforation. *Ao*, aorta; *LV*, left ventricle

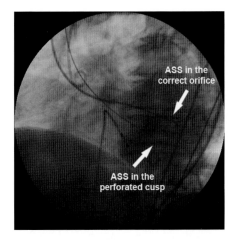

Fig. 4.20 The first wire is left in a perforated cusp, as a marker to cross the native orifice. *ASS*, Amplatz Super Stiff

4.2.4
Valvuloplasty

The operator is free to choose the type and brand of the valvuloplasty balloon, but it must be always borne in mind that the ratio between the balloon diameter and aortic annulus must be 1:1.

Balloons of two sizes are generally used to implant a CoreValve® device: a 22 mm balloon for patients in whom a 26 mm device is to be implanted; a 25 mm balloon for 29 mm devices. The balloon must be at least 40 mm long; as a rule, the longer the balloon, the greater the stability during inflation. During balloon valvuloplasty, the pigtail diagnostic catheter in the aorta should be pulled back over the balloon, as it may mobilize atheromatous/calcified material if it is pressed by the inflated balloon against the aortic wall.

4.2.5
CoreValve® Revalving System Delivery and Implantation

Once the optimal view offering perfect aligment of the three cusps on the same plane has been chosen, the pigtail catheter is positioned on the right coronary or non-coronary cusp, and optimal positioning of the super-stiff guidewire in the LV has been assessed, the delivery catheter with valve can be deployed in the aorta.

It is highly recommended to always flush the introducer before inserting the catheter, and make it advance gently on the duly positioned super-stiff guidewire.

It is recommended not to keep the CoreValve® device out of the low-temperature solution or inside the vascular system for too long, as nitinol tends to self-expand at high temperatures, making release difficult.

Deployment through the aortic arch should be done gently, as the delivery catheter, while being adaptable to various arch angles and being able to advance without any trouble up to the ascending tract, may scratch the atheromatous aortic wall and mobilize atheromata, leading to the risk of brain ischemia. If the guidewire is too close to the aortic wall, it can be pulled back slightly and the delivery catheter can be advanced under fluoroscopy.

Once on the valve plane, the valve is crossed and the distal radio-opaque marker is placed on the valve plane. Angiography with low contrast volume (e.g. 10 ml at a rate of 10 ml/s at 900 PSI) makes it possible to check the ratio between the distal part of the delivery catheter and the aortic valve plane.

At this point, the second operator starts to slowly unscrew the posterior knob; once the first 8 mm are exposed, he stops the maneuver and readjusts the position slowly, pulling back the delivery catheter system without easing tension. Another 4 mm should be exposed and flaring can be started; once flaring is completed, it should be adjusted compared to the left side using a left anterior oblique view. Then move to the next step. The second operator slowly exposes the medial third without stopping, while the first operator pulls back the catheter by a few millimeters to avoid it moving forward; during this phase the heart is under flow arrest, because neither the native valve nor the biological valve are working. Once the pressure wave appears on the monitor again, the maneuver is stopped, the second operator holds the sliding knob with a finger, and the first operator applies minor force to prevent the valve from being pulled into the ventricle. An angiogram is performed and, if the position is deemed optimal, the last part of the device is released (step 3). If the angiogram shows that the device's position is too low, try pulling the device slightly back before moving on to step 3.

Since device exposure is basically correlated with the forward push of the delivery catheter out of the plastic sheath, the most frequent cause of a low implant is a lack of coordination between the first and second operator, because the second operator unscrews too fast while the first does not manage to recover the valve. It is hence recommended to unscrew the device slowly enough.

On the other hand, if the position is too high above the valve plane, the device is completely retrieved in the introducer to prevent the risk of coronary artery occlusion caused by the distal part of the device covered with porcine pericardium.

Retrieval of the valve partially attached to the delivery catheter is possible using the braided 18 Fr introducer; even if the medial and distal thirds of the device are expanded, the device can be collapsed inside the 18 Fr and extracted. Use your thumb to hold the macro-slide to avoid it accidentally slipping off during retrieval. If the device comes off the delivery catheter during retrieval, it can be left in the descending or even the ascending aorta; in this case, it should be positioned so that it does not interfere with the epiaortic vessels and leaves a distance of at least 40–50 mm from the valve plane to give enough space for the implantation of a second device (Fig. 4.21). If the device has completely come off, all you need to do is to grip it firmly with a snare on one of the two proximal hooks. Of course, these maneuvers increase the risk of scratching the aortic wall and hence the risk of transient ischemic attack (TIA)/stroke or peripheral emboli.

Step 3 consists of releasing the valve. Once the distal two-thirds of the device are optimally positioned, the pigtail is pulled back and the last one-third is released while maintaining the entire system slightly taut.

Complete valve exposure consists of expansion of the terminal part and freeing of the distal hooks. Sometimes these hooks used to load the valve cannot be freed immediately, so it is important to check, in two orthogonal views, that they have been completely released before the delivery catheter is pulled back.

A deformed device profile is a sign that it is still hooked; in these cases, proceed as follows: pull back the super-stiff guidewire by 1 cm to reduce the system's tautness, and perform small rotary or push-and-pull movements, and wait patiently for the device to be released. Sometimes it might be necessary to advance the delivery catheter's sheath by a centimeter, using the macro-slide to force release.

Delayed delivery-catheter release is more frequent with 29 mm valves, as loading can be slightly more difficult, or in the case of pulling maneuvers to reposition the valve during step 2: these maneuvers require pulling on the metal hooks on the delivery catheter's plastic supports.

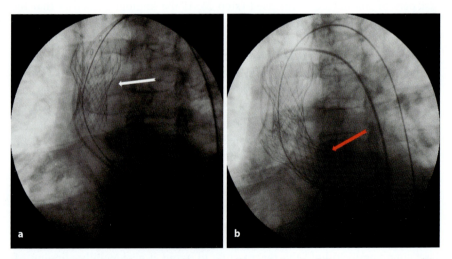

Fig. 4.21 The valve, jumped in the ascending aorta, still attached to the delivery system at one of the hooks, is left in the higher part of the ascending aorta (*white arrow*) (**a**) in order to have enough space to implant a second valve (*red arrow*) (**b**)

Once the device is completed, the delivery catheter should be pulled back delicately: the ASS-ST1 guidewire is pulled back by about a centimeter, keeping it in the LV, and the delivery catheter is pulled into the descending aorta. The distal cone is closed at this point, under fluoroscopy, to make sure that the delivery catheter and introducer are perfectly aligned to avoid any difficulties in pulling out the introducer, which may damage and break the delivery catheter. Rotary movements of the delivery catheter during withdrawal help to obtain optimal adhesion.

4.2.5.1
Check on Implantation

Once the device is implanted, check the following:
- aortic pressure, especially the diastolic and differential pressure
- systolic left ventricular pressure, together with aortic pressure to assess the gradient, and telediastolic pressure
- aortogram in two orthogonal views to assess proper device position and expansion, the presence of intraprosthetic or paravalvular regurgitation, and the ascending aorta (Figure 4.22).

Hemodynamic assessment plays an even more important role compared to angiography and echocardiography in assessing device malpositioning.

Evidence of a low aortic diastolic pressure (<40 mmHg), with a high differential pressure, can be a sign of aortic regurgitation of major hemodynamic relevance.

In these cases, possible errors in measurement should be ruled out by reassessing the pressure values after zeroing the pressure. The same applies to other causes like hypotension due to anesthetic drugs, or hypovolemia.

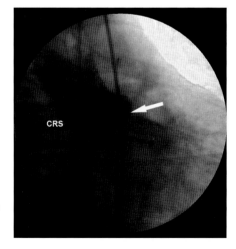

Fig. 4.22 Final arteriography in left anterior oblique view. The valve is well expanded, but a paraprosthetic leak is present due to incomplete apposition of the prosthesis to the calcified annulus (*white arrow*). *CRS,* CoreValve® Revalving System

The latter case is rather common among TAVI patients in whom major hypotension occurs often in the early phases following implantation. It can be solved by administering fluids up to about 1000 ml/h. Central venous pressure and urine output should be carefully monitored and fluids or plasma expander administered. The hemodynamic response to this treatment is usually very rapid.

If hypovolemia or iatrogenic vasoplegia is ruled out, a suspicion of device failure can be confirmed hemodynamically by recording the aortic pressure and left ventricular pressure simultaneously: if aortic diastolic pressure tends to be equal to the LV's telediastolic pressure, then there is a device failure.

Aortography in two orthogonal views (left and right anterior oblique) gives information on the valve expansion profile (Fig. 4.23), namely whether it is circular or oval, and on the presence of intra- and paraprosthetic failure.

Intraprosthetic failure is a rare occurrence and it is due occasionally to the ASS guidewire; in these cases, the best thing to do is remove the guide and replace it with a pigtail catheter.

Paraprosthetic leak is caused, instead, by incomplete apposition of the device's distal third, or it can be secondary to an excessively low implant or to a lack of sealing of the device inflow into the LVOT, with regurgitation above the device cusps.

The maneuver recommended in these cases is adjustment of the device by positioning using a snare (Fig. 4.24). The technique consists of snaring one of the two hooks of the prosthesis, and slowly but firmly pulling the valve, in a step-by-step manner: (a) pull, (b) maintain the position with tension, (c) wait, (d) fill the release of tension, then repeat the steps millimeter by millimeter,

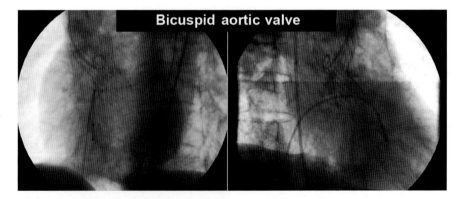

Fig. 4.23 Final arteriography after TAVI. The valve seems well expanded in left anterior oblique view (**left image**), but it is clearly underexpanded in the right anterior oblique view (**right image**) because of bicuspid valve

using the aortic diastolic pressure as a marker of maneuver efficacy. When the valve moves higher into the correct position, aortic diastolic pressure suddenly increases.

Another cause for paraprosthetic leak is the presence of calcifications preventing proper device placement in the LVOT and/or on the annulus. This may be due to ineffective preparatory valvuloplasty or to major calcifications.

In these cases, post-dilation is recommended using a 25 or 28 mm balloon diameter, for the 26 mm or 29 mm valve respectively, positioned in the lower part of the valve with careful right ventricular pacing to lower left ventricular systolic pressure. Balloon stability during valvuloplasty is crucial, in order to avoid potential damage of the prosthetic leaflets (Fig. 4.25).

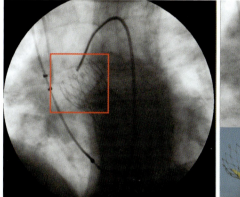
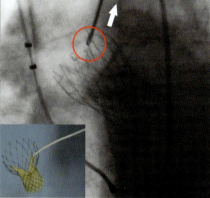

Fig. 4.24 The valve is placed in a lower position, causing paraprosthetic leak with hemodynamic burden (**left**). With the help of a snare, one hook is caught and gently, but firmly, pulled until the aortic diastolic pressure rises (**right**). The insert in the right panel shows an off-patient picture of the snare eatheing one of the two hooks

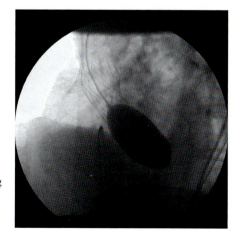

Fig. 4.25 Balloon valvuloplasty of the lower part of the prosthesis for incomplete apposition of the valve to the annulus causing severe paravalvular leak. A 28 mm large-diameter, 50-mm-long balloon is inflated during right ventricular pacing at 180 bpm

Prosthesis jumping in the aortic root while it is deployed can happen in the so-called borderline annulus, namely the gray zone between 23 and 24 mm. It is recommended to use the small 26 mm valve for annuli below 23 mm, and the larger valve in annuli over 24 mm, but it should be borne in mind that the measure variation is of one millimeter, and even with the most accurate echocardiographic and computed tomography (CT) scan measurements, there can be some errors.

4.2.6
Closing the Arterial Breach with the Prostar™ Device

Closing the arterial breach using the preimplanted Prostar™ device is a crucial moment in the procedure. Effective closing requires optimal Prostar™ implantation.

In order to implant a second Prostar™ at the end of the procedure, the problem is that the hole is too large, so I suggest the following maneuver: remove the 18 Fr introducer and place a 10 Fr introducer on the stiff wire. Tighten the knots on the 10 Fr introducer to reduce the hole diameter, then implant a second Prostar™, rotating from 45° to 90° compared to the first.

To summarize, the following steps must be performed for effective hemostasis:
- optimal arterial puncture under angiographic monitoring, at least 5–10 mm from the femoral bifurcation
- angiography after placing the 9 Fr introducer, to examine the anatomy of the iliac-femoral axis and detect any criticalities (calcified stenoses, major tortuosity, etc)
- placement of a pigtail catheter in the abdominal aorta after implanting the device
- pull back the introducer on the standard guidewire, downstream of the iliac bifurcation and rule out any ruptures by angiography
- pull back the introducer downstream of the emergence of the hypogastric artery and performing another angiogram using the pigtail catheter, while simultaneously opening the introducer's valve or the introducer to determine whether the artery is intact
- wash the sutures and breach removing any clots or fragments of subcutaneous tissue, which may prevent the knots from sliding
- tie the knots correctly by tying the ends of the white thread on top of the introducer, and then the green threads
- check that the knot slides and, if necessary, use the knot pusher; if the suture does not slide on the artery, do not force it, as it may damage the artery wall
- pull back the introducer and tighten the knots starting first from the white and then the green

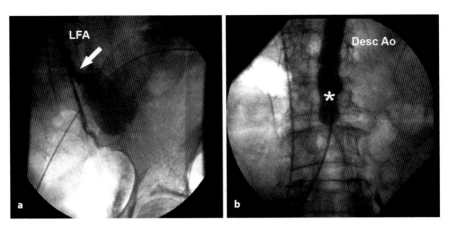

Fig. 4.26 Rupture of the left femoral artery (*LFA*) during retrieval of the 18 Fr introducer (*arrow*, **a**). Hemostasis is obtained in few minutes, using a large-diameter balloon (*) placed in the abdominal aorta under the take-off of the renal arteries (**b**). *DescAo*, descending aorta

- before tightening the knots, remove the guidewire and perform angiography
  - in the case of incomplete hemostasis with minor pulsatile extravasation, applying a compressive dressing or inflating the balloon in the controlateral artery is enough
  - in the case of uncontrollable extravasation, a coated self-expanding stent with access through the contralateral artery is necessary
  - in the case of artery rupture, a compliant balloon should be promptly positioned in the subrenal abdominal aorta; once bleeding has been stopped and hemodynamic stability has been achieved, the patient should be transferred to the operating room for surgical hemostasis (Fig. 4.26).

4.2.7
Miscellaneous

In addition to the material needed for the procedure, special catheters are needed as well, since these can be handy in case of bailout.

The snare is a useful tool. It is typically used in structural interventional cardiology, and knowledge of its possible uses can be useful to solve problems that, at times, may seem to be insurmountable.

There are several types of snares with different diameters, and the choice depends on the vessel you are working on. For the aorta, diameters of 25 or 30 mm are typically more convenient.

In our case history, there have been several cases, reported next, in which these tools have been used.

4.2.7.1
Difficult Navigation of the Delivery Catheter in the Aortic Arch

The snare can be used to straighten the delivery catheter in the case of difficult navigation in the aortic arch, or when it is necessary to center the delivery catheter to avoid knocking against obstacles such as, for instance, a valve that is already implanted (Fig. 4.27).

In these cases, the contralateral femoral artery can be used to insert the snare. In order to perform this maneuver, replace the stiff guidewire with a standard guidewire, which should be hooked by the snare in the descending aorta. Once the system is hooked with the snare, cross the native valve as you would do with the Amplatz catheter. At this point, position the stiff guidewire, remove the Amplatz, and advance the delivery catheter. Once the distal part of the delivery catheter in the descending aorta is hooked with the snare, slide the snare to the beginning of the aortic arch and then start to exert force gradually to narrow the delivery catheter's curve and align it to the aorta.

Another option is to insert the snare from the tail of the delivery catheter and insert it in parallel in the 18 Fr introducer. Bear in mind that the body of the delivery catheter has a diameter of 12 Fr, while a 5 Fr catheter can be used for the snare.

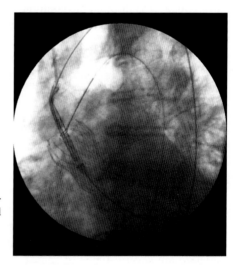

Fig. 4.27 Because of the high position of the first valve causing severe aortic regurgitation, a second valve is implanted with the valve-in-valve technique. The navigation of the second valve is hindered by the first valve, but using a snare the valve is re-oriented and easily placed in the correct position

4.2.7.2
Recovery of Catheter Fragments

In another case, the snare was used to recover the distal part that broke off the introducer still placed on the guidewire.

In the case of a fracture of the distal part of an 18 Fr introducer, it can be recovered by inserting the snare coaxially to the guidewire in the 18 Fr, pulling it upstream of the fragment, and blocking it to avoid losing it. Finally, using a 7 mm balloon inside the fragment, pull out the system composed of the snare, fragment, and balloon from the artery without damaging it, while keeping the stiff guidewire and using the same access for the placement of a second introducer (Fig. 4.28).

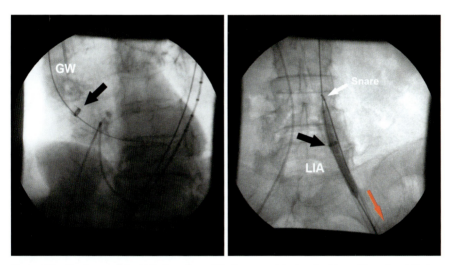

Fig. 4.28 The distal part of the 18 Fr introducer (*black arrow*, **a**) is detached but still on the stiff wire. With the help of a 6 mm balloon and a snare (*white arrow*), the ring is caught and retrieved through the femoral artery (*red arrow*), maintaining the wire in place for the second introducer (**b**). *LIA*, left iliac artery; *GW*, guidewire

4.2.7.3
Balloon Valvuloplasty Trapping

It may be necessary to post-dilate the device after valve implantation. When the guidewire is pulled back from the ventricle, it may be difficult to pass the valve. Although a pigtail is used, it may happen that you pass by mistake through the large mesh of the valve's distal portion. The problem can be detected by performing a check using two views. Otherwise, the width of the mesh of the proximal third allows the deflated balloon to pass, while it is trapped when removing it after valvuloplasty (Fig. 4.29).

In these cases, since the system cannot be forced due to the risk of displacing the device, the following method can be used. Cut the tail of the balloon catheter removing the thicker part (Fig. 4.30a, b) and use the snare as an extension to

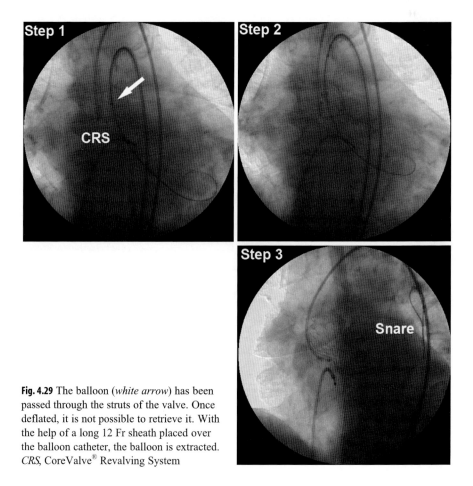

Fig. 4.29 The balloon (*white arrow*) has been passed through the struts of the valve. Once deflated, it is not possible to retrieve it. With the help of a long 12 Fr sheath placed over the balloon catheter, the balloon is extracted. *CRS*, CoreValve® Revalving System

insert a 12 Fr introducer in the system composed of the stiff guidewire, balloon catheter, and snare (Fig. 4.30c, e). The 12 Fr catheter is then placed on the valve and the balloon is easily pulled back (Fig. 4.30d, f).

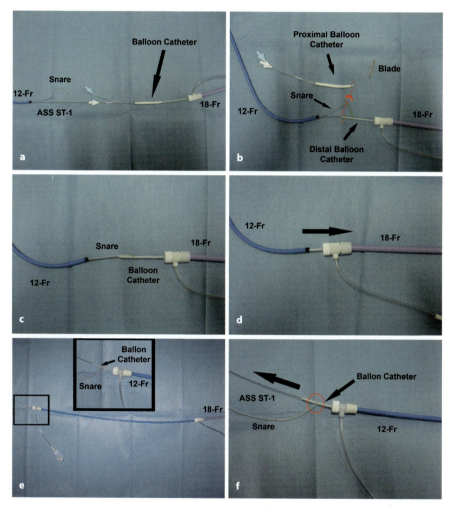

Fig. 4.30 Off-patient reproduction of the system used for recapture of the jailed balloon. **a** A snare is introduced in 12 Fr long sheath, coaxial to the ASS wire to check that the system works; **b** the tail of the balloon via the catheter is cut and removed, and the snare is caught on the proximal edge of the cut catheter; **c, d** the 12 Fr sheath is advanced over the system in the 18 Fr introducer until it touches the prosthesis struts; **e, f** the system of snare/balloon is retracted, and maintained firmly in the 12 Fr. In this way, the balloon goes through the struts and is retrieved in the 12 Fr sheath

4.2.7.4
Cardiac Perforation

The first hours after the procedure can be complicated by right ventricular perforation by the pacemaker lead. A sudden bradycardia with hypotension can be the very first sign of perforation, confirmed by echocardiography. At this point, give protamine sulfate to antagonize heparinazation; start pericardiocentesis with placement of a pigtail in the pericardium; place a second pacemaker lead from the contralateral vein; then remove the first pacemaker lead and continue aspiration until the end of bleeding. Apply a drain to the pigtail for 24 hours and replace the blood lost with transfusion.

4.2.7.5
Introducer Replacement

If it is necessary to remove the 18 Fr introducer, for any reason at all, before transcatheter aortic valve implantation, it is possible to puncture the introducer sheath just before it enters the cutis and insert a parallel wire, in order to maintain the arterial access (Fig. 4.31)

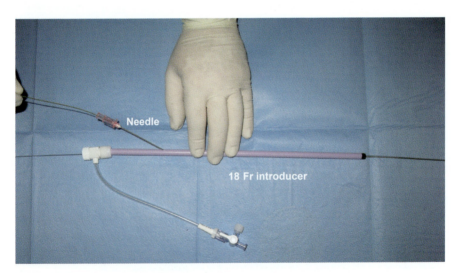

Fig. 4.31 Puncture of the 18 Fr introducer

4.3 The MitraClip®

The only commercially available device for transcatheter mitral valve repair is the MitraClip® system (Abbott Vascular Device, Redwood City, California, USA). It received the CE mark in 2008, and clinical experience, though limited to few centers, is exponentially increasing.

4.3.1 Device and Technique

The MitraClip® System (Fig. 4.32) consists of a catheter-based device designed to perform, on a beating heart, an edge-to-edge reconstruction of the insufficient mitral valve as an alternative to the conventional surgical approach.

The cardiovascular valve repair system (CVRS) includes a 24-Fr steerable guide catheter (SGC), and a delivery catheter system (DCS), with a clip mounted on its tip, which allows placement of the clip on the mitral valve leaflets.

Maneuvers of opening, closing, locking, and clip-detaching are controlled by the delivery catheter handle mechanism, which is firmly lodged on a metal sterilized external support (stabilizer) placed outside of the patient, on the bottom of a small table, above the upper leg.

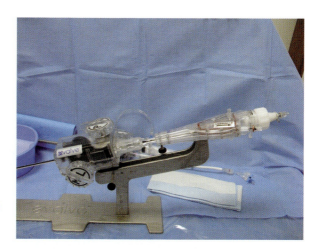

Fig. 4.32 Preparation of the MitraClip® Delivery System is easier using the stabilizer or the prep table

4.3.2 Procedure

The procedure is performed under general anesthesia, because transesophageal echocardiographic (TEE) guidance is needed.

For better monitoring of cardiopulmonary hemodynamics during the procedure, it is preferable to insert a central venous catheter and an arterial line; moreover, before covering the patient with the sterile drape, the dedicated small table must be placed over the patient's legs, maintaining a distance of 80 cm from the heart.

A sterile long table of 150 cm, and pressurized bags with heparin solution for continuous flushing, are needed to prepare the SGC and DCS. Our suggestion is to heparinize 1000 ml of saline solution with 5000 IU of heparin sulfate only, in order to avoid excessive anticoagulation of the patient in case of long procedures.

While the nurse is preparing the system, the interventional cardiologist starts the procedure.

A right common femoral vein is cannulated with a 7 Fr introducer, and a 5 Fr introducer is placed in the left femoral artery.

Complete right heart catheterization can be useful to assess the capillary wedge pressure (CWP) and the V wave on the CWP traces, a typical sign of severe MR, although it should be borne in mind that pressures are underestimated in this setting because of general anesthesia.

At this stage, a trans-septal puncture is performed using a Brockenbrough needle under TEE guidance. This maneuver is crucial for the outcome of the procedure, because the puncture has to be located in the posterosuperior part of the inter-atrial septum (Fig. 4.33) in order to obtain enough room in the left atrium for safe and optimal orientation of the steerable distal part of the DCS.

In our opinion, the best TEE views to guide the puncture are the bicaval

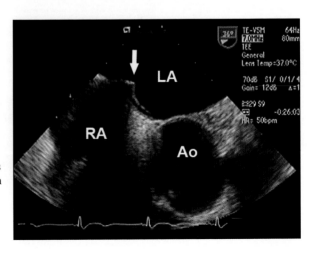

Fig. 4.33 Transesophageal short-axis view, the trans-septal sheath (*white arrow*) is tenting the inter-atrial septum and helps to point out the correct location for puncture. *Ao*, aorta; *LA*, left atrium; *RA*, right atrium

view, to assess puncture height, and the short-axis view, to evaluate posteriority. The four-chamber view is useful for measuring the distance between the tenting and annular plane.

Usually, the catheter tip is directed anteriorly: with gentle clockwise torsion it is possible to direct the needle and the Mullins catheter posteriorly. In this setting, it is desirable to have a less pronounced catheter curve, withdrawing the dilator by 2 cm and placing the needle a few millimeters before the catheter tip to confer rigidity to the system.

During these maneuvers, fluoroscopy is useless, as the catheter is directed toward an unusual position compared to the standard trans-septal puncture (Fig. 4.34). Before crossing the septum, it is better to check the distance between the tenting of the septum, caused by the needle, and the mitral annular plane: it should be between 3.5 and 4 cm.

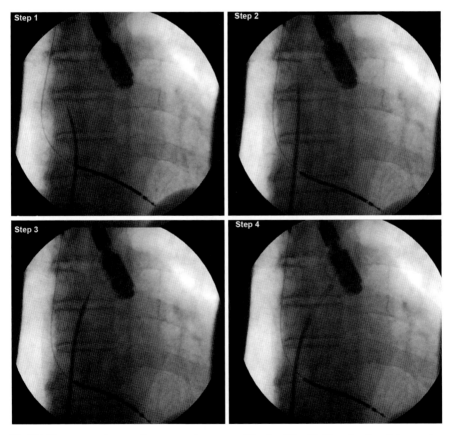

Fig. 4.34 Fluoroscopy image of trans-septal puncture. The tip of the Mullins sheath points superior and posterior of the septum. Under transesophageal echocardiography guidance, during entry in the left atrium, the catheter is rotated counterclockwise to avoid the roof of the atrium and place the catheter at the center of the left atrium

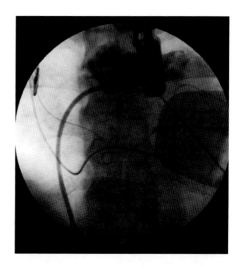

Fig. 4.35 Angiography of the left atrium to confirm the correct position of the catheter

While crossing the septum, a 30° counterclockwise rotation is preferable, to avoid the posterior wall of the left atrium and place the catheter tip at the center of the left atrium. Contrast injection is useful to document the correct position of the catheter in the left atrium (Fig. 4.35).

Once the septum is crossed, unfractioned heparin 100 IU/kg is administered.

Then a 6 Fr MP-A2 catheter is inserted into the 8 Fr Mullins catheter and, with the help of a standard J tip wire, selective cannulation of the left pulmonary veins is attempted.

The withdrawal of the 8 Fr Mullins catheter a few millimeters inside the right atrium, with a consensual clockwise rotation of both the 8 Fr Mullins catheter and the 6 Fr MP-A2 catheter will help to center the left pulmonary vein. Once the pulmonary vein is cannulated, contrast injection for confirmation of positioning is needed (Fig. 4.36).

When the catheter tip is placed in the pulmonary vein, a 260 cm ASS with a 10 mm floppy straight tip is inserted into the MP-A2 catheter; the 24 Fr SGC is placed over this wire in the left atrium.

Sometimes it is not possible to place the stiff wire in the left pulmonary veins; in this case I place the ASS wire with a hand-modeled pigtail in the LV (Fig. 4.37) to have enough stiff wire in the left atrium, and pass the interatrial septum with the 24 Fr guiding catheter (Fig. 4.37).

A horizontal skin incision of 10 mm is recommended for smoother insertion of the hydrophilic-coated SGC. The tip of the white dilator must be straightened and placed 5–8 cm over the distal part of the SGC to allow smooth crossing through the skin and vein. The curve of the tip must be restored in the right atrium.

Once the SGC tip is placed in the left atrium for at least 2–3 cm, the dilator and ASS wire are slowly withdrawn. At this stage the DCS can be inserted into the SGC.

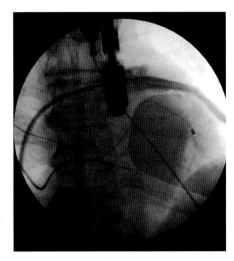

Fig. 4.36 Elective angiography of the left upper pulmonary vein before insertion of the super-stiff guidewire

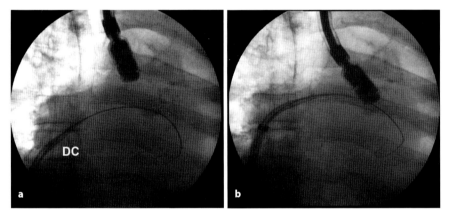

Fig. 4.37 The patients have had left pneumonectomy and ligation of the left pulmonary veins. In this case the Amplatz Super Stiff ST-1 wire has been modified with a pigtail-like shape and placed in the left ventricle (**a**). In this way, it is possible to safely advance the guiding catheter through the inter-atrial septum (**b**). *DC*, delivery catheter

In our opinion, it is better to place the entire DCS, connected to a 50 ml syringe full of saline solution, under the heart level. In this way, the formation of large air bubbles, due to negative pressure when delivery is above the level of left atrium, can be avoided. However, to lower the risk of air embolization, it is preferable to aspire blood and check back-bleeding and hemostatic valve efficiency.

At this point, the SGC is placed on the stabilizer and the DCS is inserted, with the blue line aligned with the SGC blue line. During these maneuvers, spontaneous torsion of the DCS into the SGC must be avoided, because of excessive and undesired torsion tension conferred to the system.

Once the DCS tip is aligned with the SGC tip, the guiding catheter is withdrawn by a few millimeters, in order to maintain its distal part 1.5–2 cm in the left atrium; the correct position must be checked by TEE. Sometimes after this maneuver, the system is placed against the atrial wall; this suspicion can be confirmed by trying to aspirate blood from the GCS: if the blood is not coming, the likelihood of contact with the atrial wall is high. In these cases, a slight counterclockwise rotation of the SGC is useful to fix the problem.

At this stage, the DCS must be inserted until its two proximal markers are on the saddle of the distal SGC marker. At this point, the mediolateral knob is rotated in the medial direction and the catheter is retrieved, while continuously checking that the MitraClip® tip does not touch the left atrial wall. With clockwise and counterclockwise rotation maneuvers, it is possible to move the DCS posteriorly and anteriorly for better orientation of the clip above the valve.

Occasionally, it is crucial to use the anteroposterior knob of the SGC and DCS, especially in those patients with unusual orientation of the heart due to comorbidities (i.e. previous lung resection, severe scoliosis).

When the clip orientation is satisfactory, with the clip within the regurgitant jet and its arms perpendicular to the mitral coaptation line, it is time to grasp.

The grasping technique consists of:
- slowly retracting the clip to or just above the level of the mitral annulus
- partially closing the clip (~120°)
- unhooking the grippers, and
- closing both arms.

During these maneuvers, it is crucial to be focused on inserting the arms on the leaflets, especially when there is not enough leaflet tissue between the arms of the clip: with very careful clockwise and counterclockwise rotations, it is possible to catch more anterior or posterior leaflet tissue, respectively.

Another maneuver, learned by experience, consists of leaving the arms opened at 180°, retracting the clip till the leaflets are caught, unhooking the grippers, and slowly closing the arms.

If substantial catheter repositioning is indicated for better grasping (e.g. if the DCS is not properly aligned, the clip is not sufficiently perpendicular to the line of coaptation, etc), the arms must be inverted, and the clip and DCS must be withdrawn into the left atrium, where manipulations and adjustments can be performed distant from the valve leaflets and *chordae tendineae*.

When a double orifice has been created with a stable grasp of both leaflets, and there is a satisfactory decrease in MR, the clip is closed in a locked position and detached. In cases of suboptimal decrease in MR, for example in degenerative mitral valve disease or in ruptured *chordae*, a second clip can be implanted. After the withdrawal of the DCS, a final right cardiac catheterization is done to record post-procedural pressures. Then, the SGC is removed and the venous femoral access is closed using a "figure-of-eight" subcutaneous stitch (Fig. 4.38) [1].

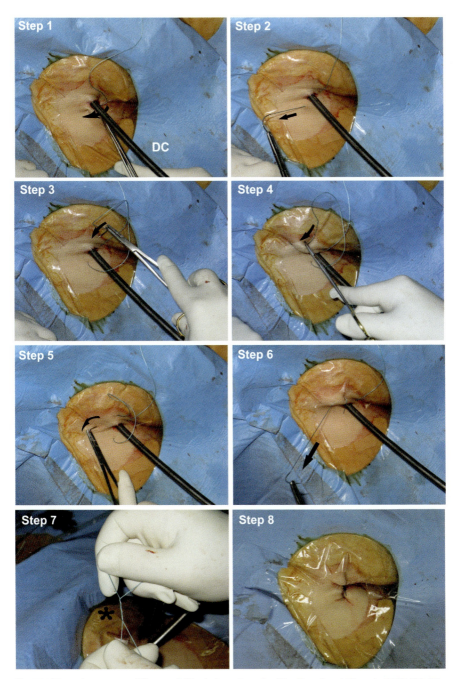

Fig. 4.38 The subcutaneous "figure-of-8" stitch as described by Bagai and Zhao in 2008 [1]. The 0-0 silk suture line is passed in the subcutaneous tissue under the 24 Fr catheter (**Steps 1** and **2**) from left to right, including a certain amount of tissue. Then the needle is passed over sheath and sewn again from left to right (**Steps 3–5**), a knot with three passages (*) of the suture line is performed (**Steps 6** and **7**) in order to have a self-blocking knot, then the knot is tightened (**Step 8**). In this way, the vein access is compressed and the risk of bleeding is reduced

Reference

1. Bagai J, Zhao D. Subcutaneous "figure-of-eight" stitch to achieve hemostasis after removal of large-caliber femoral venous sheaths. Cardiac Inteventions Today 2008;July/August:22–23 http://bmctoday.net/citoday/2008/08/article.asp?f=CIT0808_02.php (accessed 17 March 2010).

Transcatheter Valve Treatment: Peri-procedural Management

5

Progress in the field of interventional cardiology today allows percutaneous treatment of various valve diseases. A growing population of elderly and/or high-risk patients can benefit from a non-surgical approach, with limited peri-procedural risk and a minor incidence of adverse events compared to surgery. However, the severity of the clinical picture of these patients and the greater invasiveness and complexity of these procedures compared to conventional interventional cardiology procedures require a higher level of attention to detect and manage an ever growing number of "new" complications accompanying these innovative techniques. Therefore, all physicians involved in the management and care of these patients need to have adequate knowledge and be frequently updated on the pre- and post-procedural management, based on the experience gained day to day. This chapter illustrates various aspects relating to the diagnosis, management, and care of patients before and after novel aortic valve implantation procedures to treat aortic stenosis (AS) and mitral valve repair procedures using the MitraClip® device to treat mitral regurgitation (MR). Special attention will be focused on the general and specific principles of each technique and the hemodynamic impairment model associated with each valve disease. Table 5.1 summarizes the components of routine care before and after transcatheter aortic valve implantation (TAVI) and MitraClip® device implantation.

Table 5.1 Peri-procedural management

Time	Tests and procedure
Pre-procedure/baseline	Informed consent (at any time pre-procedure) History, physical examination and vital signs (temperature, heart rate, systemic blood pressure and respiratory rate) Transthoracic echocardiogram (TTE) Transesophageal echocardiogram (TEE) prior to treatment for MitraClip® 12-Lead ECG (within 24 hours of procedure) Chest x-ray NYHA functional status Quality of life measure Lab work: complete blood count (CBC), creatinine, blood urea nitrogen, creatine kinase (CK), CK-MB, liver enzymes, clotting parameters, electrolytes, inflammation markers, urine exam, ABO and Rh typing Estimation of creatinine clearance and pretreatment of case if high risk of contrast induced nephropathy (CIN) Request concentrated red blood cells Holter ECG in TAVI procedures Prophylactic antibiotic therapy
After procedure	Vital signs (temperature, heart rate, systemic blood pressure and respiratory rate) Cardiovascular and neurological evaluation Lab work: CBC, creatinine, blood urea nitrogen, CK, CK-MB, liver enzymes, clotting parameters, electrolytes Oxygen saturation pulse oximetry Monitoring of central venous pressure and input/output: fluid infusion for CIN or dehydration Check of vascular accesses and color-Doppler in case of suspicion of hematoma 12-Lead ECG Removal of temporary pacemaker within 24 h and implantation of permanent pacemaker if necessary (complete atrioventricular block) in TAVI Holter ECG in TAVI procedures TTE Low molecular weight heparin until deambulation, acetylsalicylic acid, clopidogrel Prophylactic antibiotic therapy
30 Days after hospital discharge	Brief physical exam, including vital signs Cardiac health status including NYHA functional status CBC, creatinine, blood urea nitrogen TTE 12-Lead ECG Quality-of-life measure Endocarditis prophylaxis Document adverse events

(cont. →)

Table 5.1 (*continued*)

Time	Tests and procedure
3 Months, 6, 12, 18, 24 months and yearly after 24 months	Brief physical exam, including vital signs Cardiac health status including NYHA functional status CBC, creatinine, blood urea nitrogen TTE 12-Lead ECG Quality-of-life measure (at 12-month follow-up only) Endocarditis prophylaxis Document adverse events

5.1 Pre-procedural Care

Patients should be admitted to hospital about two days before the scheduled date of the procedure, after undergoing various screening examinations to assess the feasibility of the procedure and diagnose or rule out any concurrent pathology that may affect the procedural and post-procedural outcome. Therefore, a thorough clinical examination is important to assess the patient's New York Heart Association (NYHA) functional class and quality of life.

During this phase, a routine check of laboratory examinations is also necessary and these include a complete blood count, liver and kidney function indices, creatine kinase (CK) and CK-MB, clotting parameters, electrolytes, urine exam, urine culture, if needed, inflammation markers, and ABO and Rh (D) blood typing. The creatinine clearance rate should be estimated from the serum creatinine level according to the Cockcroft–Gault formula to identify more accurately those patients with values below 60 ml/min, who are at increased risk for contrast-induced nephropathy (CIN) [1, 2]. A simple CIN risk score may be applied to assess the cumulative risk of several variables on renal function, such as older age, pre-existent renal insufficiency, and diabetes mellitus [1]. High-risk patients for CIN should receive adequate hydration with intravenous (IV) infusion of isotonic solution, and adjunctive therapies such as *N*-acetyl cysteine [3–5].

Chest x-ray and respiratory function tests, if needed, should be performed to assess overall anesthesia risk. More invasive examinations, such as esophagogastroduodenoscopy or colonoscopy, should be performed in patients for whom there is a suspicion of gastrointestinal bleeding; the administration of unfractionated heparin (UFH) during the procedure, and low molecular weight heparin (LMWH), acetylsalicylic acid (ASA), and clopidogrel after the procedure may actually worsen or upset the latency of an already existing situation.

In the case of a prior event of cerebrovascular ischemia, brain magnetic resonance imaging (MRI) may be performed, both in TAVI procedures, where ischemic risk seems to be mainly associated with the maneuvering of the catheters and guidewires especially in heavily calcified aortic vessels, and in MitraClip® device implantation procedures for possible episodes of thromboembolism or gas embolism secondary to the crossing of the catheters in the left atrium after trans-septal puncture. Holter electrocardiogram (ECG) monitoring is also recommended before TAVI to identify existing rhythm disorders.

In addition to ASA 100 mg once a day, medical therapy should include a loading dose of clopidogrel 300 mg before the procedure, and antibiotic prophylaxis for the risk of bacterial endocarditis and/or sepsis one hour before the procedure (cephalosporin or vancomycin).

Finally, at least two units of concentrated red blood cells should be available during the procedure in case of complications with bleeding; in TAVI procedures, major bleeding is not a rare event, while during MitraClip® implantation, the use of large-gauge introducers (24 Fr) is associated with a higher risk of inguinal hematomas.

5.2
Post-procedural Management

5.2.1
ICU Care

After the procedure, generally performed under sedation or general anesthesia with extubation following the procedure in the catheterization laboratory, a short period of observation (about 48 hours) is needed in an intensive care unit (ICU). Careful monitoring of vital signs and an accurate clinical examination are absolutely necessary to detect, early on, the onset of complications and to diagnose or rule out any states of heart failure or neurological impairment. For instance, the sudden onset of hypotension and signs of peripheral hypoperfusion can point to a diagnosis of cardiogenic shock secondary to valve malfunction, ventricular dysfunction, cardiac tamponade, retroperitoneal hematoma, arrhythmia, or myocardial infarction; signs of neurological impairment, such as aphasia, hyposthenia, confusion, or memory deficit, point instead to a suspicion of brain ischemia, which must be carefully investigated by complete neurological examination and a brain computed tomography (CT) scan, if need be.

Special attention must also be paid to:
- laboratory tests
- renal function and fluid balance

- vascular access
- rhythm control
- transthoracic echocardiogram (TTE).

5.2.1.1
Laboratory Tests

A routine check of laboratory examinations is recommended immediately after the procedure and every 24 hours. The blood count is useful for the early detection of anemia secondary to occult bleeding, leukocytosis due to infection, and thrombocytopenia. Thrombocytopenia is a rare side-effect linked to the use of thienopyridines, UFH, and LMWH. For TAVI, it has actually been noted after the first procedures that the administration of a loading dose of clopidogrel 300 mg reduces the risk of thrombocytopenia, probably because it inhibits platelet activation and consumption [6]. Nonetheless, the use of a thienopyridine can be associated with the onset of thrombotic thrombocytopenic purpura, a condition marked by intravascular clotting, thrombocytopenia, and bleeding. In this case, platelet transfusion is contraindicated, except for cases of major bleeding, while plasmapheresis and fresh plasma administration are useful [7]. If there is a suspicion of thrombocytopenia secondary to administration of heparin (either UFH or LMWH), early detection of the form secondary to an immune-type mechanism is necessary; this is known as heparin-induced thrombocytopenia (HIT), and is less common than the non-immune-mediated form, yet more serious because it is associated with a high risk of thromboembolic events. In this case, administration of the drug must be stopped and non-heparin anticoagulants must be used [8].

Blood nitrogen and creatinine values should be monitored to assess kidney function and diagnose the presence of CIN, while careful monitoring of serum electrolytes should be performed frequently over the first 48 hours or in the presence of polyuria for the early detection of a state of depletion and for adequate correction. Other laboratory examinations include the specific cardiac enzymes (CK, CK-MB, troponin-I) necessary to diagnose acute myocardial ischemia, which may be caused after TAVI by embolization of calcific debris, displacement of native aortic leaflets, or large bulky calcium deposits over coronary artery ostia. In this case, an angiogram should be performed to rule out coronary artery obstruction. Liver enzymes and clotting parameters should be monitored frequently.

5.2.1.2
Renal Function and Fluid Balance

CIN is a complex syndrome of acute renal failure subsequent to contrast media administration, and is defined as a relative increase in pre-procedure serum creatinine concentration of >25% or an absolute increase >0.5 mg/dl, occurring within 48 to 72 hours of contrast administration [1]. The pathogenesis of CIN involves the interplay of multiple factors such as a direct toxicity to renal tubular epithelium, oxidative stress, ischemic injury, and tubular obstruction. Serum creatinine peaks in 2–5 days after percutaneous intervention and usually returns to baseline within 2 weeks without specific treatment. Some authors have shown benefits of the use of N-acetyl-cysteine administered 24 hours before the procedure along with adequate hydration in patients with existing kidney failure [3–5]. In the more serious cases one or more dialysis sessions may be needed to restore creatinine values, particularly in patients already affected by chronic kidney failure. The other major but rare differential diagnosis of contrast nephropathy is atheroemboli-induced nephropathy. Renal deterioration in atheroembolic disease usually follows a different time course, with gradual and progressive renal impairment developing in weeks to months. The finding of mottled vasculitic skin changes in the feet strongly supports the clinical diagnosis of atheroembolic disease. The diagnosis can be confirmed with renal or skin biopsy, but this is not usually necessary as the clinical picture is frequently diagnostic. Management of atheroembolic renal impairment is purely supportive.

Careful monitoring of the fluid balance and central venous pressure is necessary to diagnose depleted intravascular volume states, provide adequate hydration, and reduce the risk of CIN. Therefore, a Foley catheter should be retained at least for the first 24 hours after the procedure to facilitate input/output monitoring. It has been observed that after TAVI a significant number of patients with normal kidney function develop acute kidney failure. It is believed that this condition is almost certainly secondary to depleted intravascular volume developing immediately after an intense polyuric phase. It has been hypothesized that polyuria is caused by a sudden and significant rise in cardiac output after valve implantation followed by kidney hyperperfusion. Therapy must be mainly aimed at correcting oliguria, secondary to hypovolemia with an adequate supply of fluids. Diuretic therapy can be useful in patients in whom oliguria persists, even though normovolemia, hemodynamics, and kidney perfusion pressure have been restored.

5.2.1.3
Vascular Access

Vascular complications are frequent in procedures like transfemoral TAVI (about 12%), and many of these are linked to the use of heparin, atheromatosis, calcification, and vascular bed tortuosity in these elderly patients, and the use of large-gauge introducers [9]. These complications include hematomas, pseudoaneurysm, arteriovenous fistulas, embolization, and retroperitoneal bleeding (in the case of transfemoral access). The introducer insertion site and distal pulses should be checked every 15 minutes during the first hour after the procedure and then every hour to detect any signs of bleeding, hematomas, ecchymosis, pulsatile masses, murmurs, weak pulses, or signs of ischemic damage in the limbs. Patients must also be immobilized for 12 hours after arterial hemostasis. Small hematomas and mild murmurs are frequent and do not require any diagnostic investigation or medical treatment. Clinical evidence of a large and progressively growing mass should lead to suspicion of a hematoma or pseudoaneurysm and hence be assessed by color-Doppler ultrasound, especially if it is associated with a sudden development of anemia. Color-Doppler ultrasound also allows the diagnosis of arteriovenous fistulas, which can cause groin pain or new-onset murmurs. Groin hematomas are usually stable and spontaneously vanish without any need for specific treatment. Pseudoaneurysms and arteriovenous fistulas require, as a first therapeutic strategy, ultrasound-guided compression repair (UGCR): the hematoma and the arterial breach should be identified; gradual compression should be applied until the flow from the artery to the hematoma stops; it should then be compressed until an echo-reflecting clot forms inside the hematoma and then a sturdy compressive medication is applied for at least 24–48 hours (Fig. 5.1); if the procedure is ineffective, surgical hemostasis is needed [10].

The diagnosis of retroperitoneal hematoma is more challenging. It is a dangerous complication caused by a high arterial access site, above the inguinal ligament, from which blood exudate flows freely into the retroperitoneum, causing abdominal or back pain without any evidence of groin hematoma. The signs also include bleeding without any apparent origin and no pain, inexplicable hypotension, and recurrent episodes of vagal crisis. Retroperitoneal hematoma is diagnosed by tomography, which should be performed urgently (Fig. 5.2). Most of these cases of bleeding require surgery. The gradual or sudden development of anemia following these vascular complication requires, in many cases, transfusion with concentrated red blood cells.

In the MitraClip® implantation procedure, the venous access may develop hematomas, due either to the large diameter of the guiding catheter or to the use of UFH. Therefore, at the end of the procedure, an activated clotting time (ACT) test should be performed in the catheterization laboratory, and heparin reversal is carried out by administering protamine sulfate. Hemostasis can be

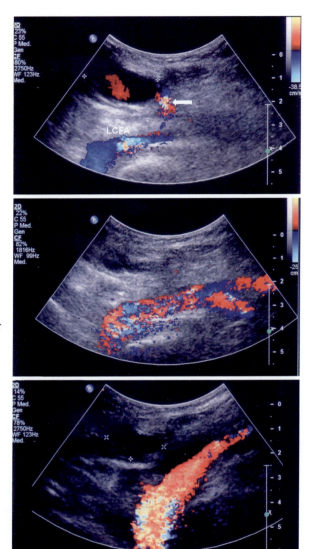

Fig. 5.1 Doppler ultrasound showing the evolution of a pseudo-aneurysm (FAP) after ultrasound-guided compression repair (UGCR) in a patient undergoing transfemoral implantation of an aortic device. The first image shows FAP and blood effusion (*white arrow*) through the left common femoral artery (*LCFA*) 4 hours after the procedure; the second one shows the lack of communicating tract from the LCFA after UGCR; the third one is a pre-discharge check showing complete resolution of FAP

achieved by manual compression or applying sutures at the access site in the skin, by forming a fold in the skin to exert compression on the venous access in a controlled manner. The sutures are removed after 24 hours [11].

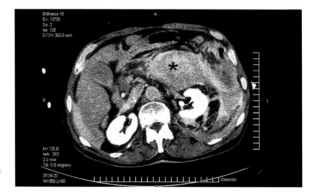

Fig. 5.2 CT scan of the abdomen showing retroperitoneal bleeding originating from the left iliac artery (*)

5.2.1.4 Rhythm Control

Arrhythmias may occur after valve replacement or repair procedures, and continuous ECG monitoring by telemetry is necessary. Atrioventricular or intraventricular conduction disorders are among the most frequent arrhythmic complications in TAVI. Atrial fibrillation secondary to alterations in the electrolyte balance may occasionally characterize the post-procedural course. Percutaneous MitraClip® implantation is not usually affected by arrhythmias, except for atrial fibrillation, which is often a pre-existing condition.

It is known that aortic valvuloplasty is marked by the intraprocedural onset of total left bundle branch block (LBBB) or atrioventricular block (AVB) of various degrees. In the great majority of cases, conduction disorders spontaneously resolve [12, 13]. TAVI has a higher incidence of conduction disorders. Self-expanding valves are marked by the onset of total AVB in about 10–25% of cases [6, 14] versus about 7.5% for balloon-expandable valves [9, 15]. Most of the total AVB and all LBBB cases are intraprocedural; however, there is a small percentage of patients who can develop symptomatic late total AVB between post-procedure day 5 and day 30 (Figs. 5.3 and 5.4).

The predictors of total AVB have not yet been fully defined. Of the risk factors involved in cardiac surgery, the following can be considered: pre-existing bundle branch block (especially of the right branch), pre-procedural aortic regurgitation, prior myocardial infarction, pulmonary hypertension, and electrolyte imbalances [16, 17]. Some authors have suggested, based on the close anatomical relations existing between the atrioventricular conduction system and the aortic valve apparatus, that the expansion of the device may cause mechanical trauma in the conduction system, especially in patients with calcified annulus, worsening pre-existing conduction defects or generating new ones. One study showed that the mean distance from the proximal (or

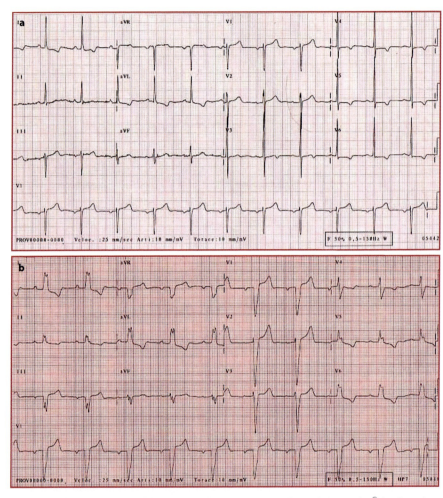

Fig. 5.3 a Baseline ECG recording from a patient prior to transfemoral CoreValve® implantation. **b** 12-lead ECG recording from the same patient immediately after transfemoral implantation of a CoreValve® prosthesis. The patient developed a new left bundle branch block

ventricular) end of the frame of the CoreValve® prosthesis to the lower edge of the non-coronary cusp is significantly greater in patients with new-onset LBBB than patients without new-onset LBBB. Therefore, there exists the possibility of the aortic prosthesis overlapping the left bundle branch with mechanical compression. Better device placement inside the left ventricular outflow tract may limit the risk of developing conduction disorders and hence the need for pacemaker implantation [14, 18]. Other studies have suggested that potential predictors of permanent pacing requirement consist of left axis deviation at

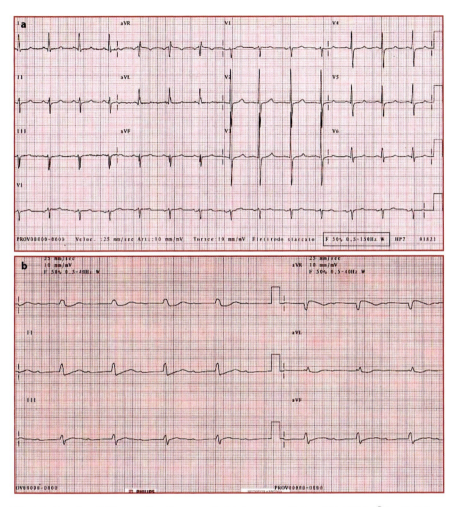

Fig. 5.4 a Baseline ECG recording from a patient prior to transfemoral CoreValve® implantation. **b** 12-lead ECG obtained one day after implantation of the CoreValve® device: identification of a symptomatic, third-degree atrioventricular block led to the implantation of a permanent pacemaker

baseline and LBBB with left axis deviation, the presence of severe septal hypertrophy, and baseline thickness of the native non-coronary cusp [19]. In the case of intraprocedural total AVB, a pacemaker must be implanted within 24 hours, both because it seldom resolves spontaneously and because it is recommended to remove the temporary pacemaker as soon as possible, due to the risk of displacement of the lead inside the right ventricle and hence of perforation and cardiac tamponade. If arrhythmias do not occur in the first 24 hours, the temporary pacemaker should be removed, and rhythm control by telemetry and periodic ECG is recommended over the next 5 days. In the case of an advanced-degree conduction disorder (AVB II type 2 or 3rd degree) within 48 hours of the procedure, permanent pacing, usually dual chamber, is needed. Other conduction defects observed within the first 48 hours after transcatheter aortic valve replacement include: LBBB, 1st-degree AVB, right bundle branch block (RBBB), and atrial fibrillation. Of these, LBBB is definitely the most common and does not require any specific treatment, just regular ECG control at follow-up. Holter ECG monitoring 24 hours before and 48 hours after the procedure can help predict or detect any major arrhythmias. Ventricular arrhythmias or fibrillation seldom appear after these procedures, although they may occur in the presence of ventricular dysfunction, concurrent coronary artery disease, or electrolyte imbalances (e.g. potassium depletion).

5.2.1.5
Transthoracic Echocardiogram

The TTE should be targeted on the procedure performed. In TAVI it allows assessment of the mean transaortic gradient and effective aortic orifice area, the presence and degree of aortic and mitral regurgitation, left ventricular contractility, estimated pulmonary artery pressure, the position of the temporary pacemaker lead in the right ventricle, and pericardial effusion.

The assessment of aortic regurgitation is important. Mild paravalvular leaks secondary to device expansion have no hemodynamic relevance and usually disappear after a few weeks (Fig. 5.5). Multiple or major paravalvular leaks are less common, but they must be detected early, as they may cause heart failure due to volume overload in the left ventricle, especially in the case of reduced contractility. The detection of a high pressure gradient or a diastolic pressure below 50 mmHg can help with recognition of this complication. Aortic regurgitation after TAVI is nearly always paravalvular and may be explained by inadequate sizing of the valve due to inadequate annulus size measurement before

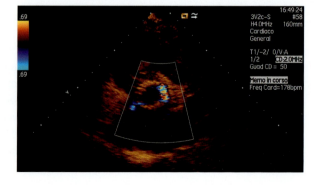

Fig. 5.5 Echocardiographic parasternal short-axis view, showing mild periprosthetic leak after transfemoral implantation of CoreValve® device

TAVI or lack of sufficient ranges of frame sizes, insufficient expansion of the frame due to severe calcification of leaflets and aortic root, leaflets malcoaptation, and malposition of the valve [20]. In the last case, usually, for the CoreValve® Revalving System, the valve is in too low position, the leaks come above the prosthesis skirt which guarantees the sealing of the valve to the annulus, and there are always two jets in symmetrical and opposite locations [21]. In the case of pericardial effusion, it is important to determine whether it is secondary to left ventricle perforation by the stiff guidewire used during the procedure, or to right ventricle perforation by the temporary pacemaker (Fig. 5.6). The former complication is a dramatic event leading to cardiac tamponade. The latter, which occurs after the procedure in most cases, is less serious, yet more difficult to diagnose. In general, it is marked by the onset of unexpected bradycardia and hypotension. Pericardial effusion can also be secondary to bleeding of the access site (apex of the left ventricle) used during transapical implantation. After diagnosing the presence of pericardial effusion, fluids must be administered, concentrated red blood cells should be transfused, heparin should be reversed if the patient is decoagulated, and subxiphoid pericardiocentesis with the positioning of an 8 Fr pigtail should be performed within a short period of time. If complete hemostasis is not achieved following pericardiocentesis, surgical draining and suture are needed.

The systolic pulmonary artery pressure can be a good indirect hemodynamic parameter and it is an index of the degree of impairment of left cardiac function and hence of the overload on the right ventricle.

For the MitraClip® procedure, TTE is performed to assess the degree of residual MR, mitral valve gradient, left ventricular function, derived pulmonary artery pressure, and the presence and degree of left-to-right shunt at the level of trans-septal puncture of the inter-atrial septum, and to rule out pericardial effusion. The MR-reduction goal is defined as MR severity of ≤2+, based on the current guidelines [22]. An overall MR grade is assigned by use of the integrative method defined by the American Society of Ecocardiography guidelines

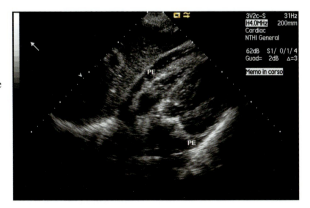

Fig. 5.6 Echocardiographic subcostal view showing the presence of pericardial effusion (*PE*) secondary to puncture of the right ventricle by the temporary pacemaker in a patient undergoing transfemoral implantation of an aortic valve device. Effusion became evident 4 hours after the procedure, and pericardiocentesis was successfully performed

[23]. Vena contracta width and regurgitant orifice area should not be included as parameters for MR assessment because they have not been validated for a double-orifice valve [24]. In order to rule out the onset of mitral stenosis, the mitral valve area by planimetry, the pressure half-time (PHT), and mean and peak transvalvular pressure should be determined. After percutaneous mitral repair, each of the two orifices is planimetered at the level of the clip, and summed to determine the valve area. Pulmonary artery pressure should be monitored and compared to the preoperative value. The inter-atrial shunt usually has no hemodynamic significance and disappears spontaneously within few weeks. Pericardial effusion can be a rare complication of the trans-septal puncture, but it occurs and is detected during the procedure. Although percutaneous mitral repair with the MitraClip® system is a new technique, no clip embolization has been noted, but partial clip detachment, defined as detachment of a single leaflet from the clip has occurred and can be detected by TTE [25]. Therefore, TTE should be performed every 24 hours for the first three days, then, as long as there is no clinical worsening, before discharge.

5.2.2
Medical Treatment and Physical Rehabilitation

In TAVI patients, medical therapy must include LMWH for at least 3 days after the procedure or at least up to complete patient mobilization, ASA 100 mg per day indefinitely, and clopidogrel 75 mg for 3–6 months. After MitraClip® implantation, the length of the dual antiplatelet therapy can be shorter (ASA 100 mg indefinitely and clopidogrel 75 mg for 1 month). Oral anticoagulant therapy must not be suspended in patients affected by chronic atrial fibrillation or with a history of thromboembolism. Therefore, frequent checks of the clotting tests are needed and, in the case of high risk of bleeding, the period of dual antiplatelet therapy should be shortened.

Endocarditis prevention includes antibiotic prophylaxis aimed especially against staphylococci, for three days after the procedure, thorough skin disinfection, thorough care and early removal of the venous accesses and Foley catheter. In the case of signs of infection like leukocytosis or fever, the causes should be thoroughly sought by means of diagnostic examinations such as, for instance, urine culture to exclude an infection of the urinary tract, chest x-ray to detect any pulmonary infections, blood cultures and microbiology examinations of the central catheters. If deemed necessary, targeted antibiotic therapy should be started, while taking into due account the possible risk of sepsis. Hematological parameters should be monitored for evidence of disseminated intravascular coagulation.

Finally, early patient mobilization should be achieved in order to avoid complications like muscular atrophy, constipation, bed ulcers, and thrombophlebitis, and to reduce the length of hospital stay. In some cases, admission to centers specializing in cardiac rehabilitation may be recommended for an earlier recovery of motor functions.

5.2.3
Before Hospital Discharge

Before discharge, a thorough assessment of the cardiac and extra-cardiac status is needed and comprises a clinical examination, ECG, TTE, and blood exams. The vascular accesses, in the case of transfemoral/trans-subclavia TAVI or Mitra-clip® implantation, and the scar, in the case of transapical TAVI, must be accurately examined. Holter ECG monitoring can be indicated after TAVI, in patients at high risk of developing conduction disorders.

5.2.4
Medium-term Management (Out of Hospital)

As there is no standard management after percutaneous valve replacement or repair procedures, given their recent introduction and short follow-up, the management protocols already used in cardiac surgery can be applied [26].

The clinical and ECG follow-up should be scheduled, at least in the early phase, by the cardiology centers where the procedure is performed. The first cardiology visit should be scheduled 4 weeks after discharge if there is no period of cardiac rehabilitation. The next visits should be scheduled at 3, 6, and 12 months from the procedure and then every 6 months, except for cases in which the visit is urgently needed due to a worsening in the patient's clinical conditions.

The first visit must comprise a thorough clinical examination, an assessment of the NYHA functional class and quality of life, an ECG, a control of laboratory examinations, and a TTE to assess ventricular function, valve structure and function, any signs of device displacement or interference with adjacent anatomical structures, the presence of thrombi or vegetation on the device structures and signs of pericardial effusion. If there is a suspicion of valve malfunction, or in case of poor transthoracic acoustic window, a transesophageal echocardiogram (TEE) should be performed, as it allows better definition of the anatomical structures.

Despite the fact that there are no reports in the literature of cases of degenerated biological devices after TAVI, possible reintervention can be considered if a patient is symptomatic and has severe valve dysfunction (severe increase in transprosthetic gradient or severe regurgitation), after carefully assessing the associated risks.

Blood examinations including plasma lactic dehydrogenase (LDH), haptoglobin, and reticulocyte count should be monitored for the risk of hemolysis. Mild paraprosthetic leaks following TAVI can also cause hemolysis. Therefore, in the case of a suspicion of hemolytic anemia, TEE should be performed to rule it out [27]. Current guidelines recommend reintervention only in cases in which paravalvular leak is secondary to endocarditis, is the cause of severe hemolysis requiring repeated blood transfusions, or is associated with a serious symptomatologic picture. If cardiac surgery is contraindicated, medical therapy should comprise iron therapy, beta-blockers, and erythropoietin [26, 27].

The risk of intravalvular thrombosis and thromboembolism in biological valve or clip carriers is low, but it increases in the presence of depressed ventricular function, valve deterioration, or device distortion due to poor positioning [26]. The incidence after TAVI and Mitraclip® implantation is unknown. In any event, in these cases, the clinical suspicion must be confirmed by TTE, TEE, or cinefluoroscopy [28]. Occlusive prosthetic thrombosis should be treated surgically, although in critical and high-risk patients thrombolysis can be a therapeutic alternative [26, 27].

Thromboembolism may have multifactorial causes: thrombi, vegetation on the device, or abnormal flow conditions created by a degenerated prosthesis or other sources. Only after a thorough diagnostic pathway is it possible to start appropriate treatment. In the case of non-occlusive prosthetic thrombosis and thromboembolic events, therapy with vitamin K antagonists (VKAs) should be started, and surgery should be considered as a therapeutic option only if there are large thrombi (>10 mm) or the thrombus persists despite optimization of VKA therapy [27].

The risk of endocarditis is higher in the first 3–6 months after device implantation, although it is constantly present [26]. Just two cases of endocarditis after TAVI have been reported [29, 30]. Therefore, antibiotic prophylaxis should be provided in all conditions at risk, such as dental, endoscopic, and surgical procedures. Antibiotic therapy to prevent endocarditis must be specific to the type of procedure the patient is undergoing, according to standard protocols. If there is a clinical suspicion of endocarditis, the patient must be admitted to hospital and undergo serial blood cultures and TTE to confirm the diagnostic hypothesis. The treatment of endocarditis on valve implants requires a multidisciplinary approach involving the cardiologist, cardiac surgeon, and infectious disease physician. If an early diagnosis is reached and there is no indication for surgical treatment, targeted IV antibiotic therapy for at least 4–6 weeks is sufficient. Surgery is only necessary if appropriate medical therapy is not enough to cure the disease (persistent bacteremia, hemodynamic impairment, embolism) [26].

One case of delayed dislocation of an aortic prosthesis occurring 3 weeks after implantation has been reported [31]. No clip embolization has occurred in Mitraclip® implantation procedures. Only partial detachments have occurred, and they have not required urgent intervention [25].

References

1. Mehran R, Nikolsky E. Contrast induced nephropathy: definition, epidemiology and patients at risk. Kidney Int Suppl 2006;100: S11–15.
2. Cockroff DW, Gault MH. Prediction of creatinine clearance from serum creatinine. Nephron 1976;16:31–41.
3. Mueller C, Buerkle G, Buettner HJ et al. Prevention of contrast media-associated nephropathy; randomized comparison of 2 hydration regimens in 1620 patients undergoing coronary angioplasty. Arch Intern Med 2002;162:329–336.
4. Briguori C, Colombo A, Violante A et al. Standard vs double dose of N-acetylcysteine to prevent contrast agent associated nephrotoxicity. Eur Heart J 2004;25:206–211.
5. Birck R, Kzossok S, Markowetz F et al. Acetylcysteine for prevention of contrast nephropathy: meta-analysis. Lancet 2003;362:598–603.
6. Grube E, Laborde JC, Gerckens U et al. Percutaneous implantation of the CoreValve self-expanding valve prosthesis in high-risk patients with aortic valve disease: the Siegburg first-in-man study. Circulation 2006;114:1616–1624.
7. Bennett CL, Kim B, Zakarija A et al. Two mechanistic pathways for thienopyridine-associated thrombotic thrombocytopenic purpura: a report from the SERF-TTP research group and the RADAR project. J Am Coll Cardiol 2007;50:1138–1143.
8. Shantsila E, Lip GYH and Chong BH. Heparin-induced thrombocytopenia. Chest 2009;135:1651–1664.
9. Webb JG, Pasupati S, Humphries K et al. Percutaneous transarterial aortic valve replacement in selected high-risk patients with aortic stenosis. Circulation 2007;116:755–763.
10. Schaub F, Theiss W, Busch R et al. Management of 219 consecutive cases of postcatheterization pseudoaneurysm. J Am Coll Cardiol 1997;30:670–675.
11. Bagai J, Zhao D. Subcutaneous "figure-of-eight" stitch to achieve hemostasis after removal of large-caliber femoral venous sheaths. Cardiac Interventions Today 2008;July/August:22–23.
12. NHLBI balloon valvuloplasty registry participants. Percutaneous balloon aortic valvuloplasty. Acute and 30-day follow-up results in 674 patients from the NHLBI balloon valvuloplasty registry. Circulation 1991;84:2383–2397.
13. Otto CM, Mickel MC, Kennedy JW et al. Three-year outcome after balloon aortic valvuloplasty. Insights into prognosis of valvular aortic stenosis. Circulation 1994;89:642–650.
14. Piazza N, Onuma Y, Jesserun E et al. Early and persistent intraventricular conduction abnormalities and requirements for pacemaking after percutaneous replacement of the aortic valve. JACC Cardiovasc Interv 2008;1:310–316.
15. Sinhal A, Altwegg L, Pasupati S et al. Atrioventricular block after transcatheter balloon expandable aortic valve implantation. JACC Cardiovasc Interv 2008;1:305–309.
16. Limongelli G, Ducceschi V, D'Andrea A et al. Risk factors for pacemaker implantation following aortic valve replacement: a single centre experience Heart 2003;89:901–904.
17. Koplan BA, Stevenson WG, Epstein LM et al. Development and validation of a simple risk score to predict the need for permanent pacing after cardiac valve surgery. J Am Coll Cardiol 2003;41:795–801.
18. Calvi V, Puzzangara E, Pruiti GP et al. Early conduction disorders following percutaneous aortic valve replacement. Pacing Clin Electrophysiol 2009;32:S126–130.
19. Jilaihawi H, Chin D, Vasa-Nicotera M et al. Predictors for permanent pacemaker requirement after transcatheter aortic valve implantation with the CoreValve bioprosthesis. Am Heart J 2009;157:860–866.
20. De Jaegere PP, Piazza N, Galema TW et al. Early echocardiographic evaluation following percutaneous implantation with the self-expanding CoreValve revalving system aortic valve bioprosthesis. EuroIntervention. 2008;4:351–357.

21. Piazza N, Schultz C, De Jaegere PP, Serruys P. Implantation of two self-expanding aortic bioprosthetic valves during the same procedure—insights into valve in-valve implantation ("Russian doll concept"). Catheter Cardiovasc Interv 2009;73:530–539.
22. Bonow RO, Carabello BA, Chaterjee K et al. ACC/AHA 2006 guidelines for the management of patients with valvular heart disease:a report of the American College of Cardiology/American Heart Association Task Force on Practice Guidelines (writing committee to develop guidelines for the management of patients with valvular heart disease). J Am Coll Cardiol 2006;48:e1–148.
23. Zoghbi WA, Enriquez-Sarano M, Foster E et al. Recommendations for evaluation of the severity of native valvular regurgitation with two-dimensional and Doppler echocardiography. J Am Soc Echocardiogr 2003;16:777–802.
24. Foster E, Wasserman HS, Gray W et al. Quantitative assessment of severity of mitral regurgitation by serial echocardiography in a multicenter clinical trial of percutaneous mitral valve repair. Am J Cardiol 2007;100:1577–1583.
25. Feldman T, Kar S, Rinaldi M et al: for the EVEREST Investigators. Percutaneous mitral repair with the MitraClip system: safety and midterm durability in the initial EVEREST (endovascular valve edge-to-edge repair study) cohort. J Am Coll Cardiol 2009;54;686–694.
26. Butchart EG, Gohlke-Bärwolf C, Antunes MJ et al; Working Groups on Valvular Heart Disease, Thrombosis, Cardiac Rehabilitation, Exercise Physiology and European Society of Cardiology. Recommendations for the management of patients after heart valve surgery. Eur Heart J 2005;26:2463–2471.
27. Vahanian A, Baumgartner H, Bax J et al. Guidelines on the management of valvular heart disease: The Task Force on the management of valvular heart disease of the European Society of Cardiology. Eur Heart J 2007;28:230–268.
28. Montorsi P, De Bernardi F, Muratori M et al. Role of cinefluoroscopy, transthoracic and TEE in patients with suspected prosthetic valve thrombosis. Am J Cardiol 2000;85: 58–64.
29. Webb JG, Altwegg L, Boone RH et al. Transcatheter aortic valve implantation: impact on clinical and valve-related outcomes. Circulation 2009; 119:3009–3016.
30. Comoglio C, Boffini M, El Quarra S et al. Aortic valve replacement and mitral valve repair as treatment of complications after percutaneous CoreValve implantation. J Thorac Cardiovasc Surg 2009; 38:1025–1027.
31. Maroto LC, Rodriguez JE, Cobiella J, Silva J. Delayed dislocation of a transapically implanted aortic bioprosthesis. Eur J Cardiothorac Surg 2009:36:935–937.

Surgical Treatment of Mitral Regurgitation and Aortic Stenosis

6

6.1 Treatment of Degenerative Mitral Regurgitation

6.1.1 Epidemiology and Natural History

The most important objective of modern mitral surgery is to "neutralize" this disease and hence not just correct the valve defect, but also achieve a life expectancy in line with that of the healthy population with normal cardiac function. Disease neutralization is a target that can only be realistically achieved in degenerative mitral regurgitation (MR).

Mitral valve prolapse, secondary to myxomatous degeneration of the valve tissue, can be seen in 4–5% of the general population [1–5] and about 5% of patients with this condition develop severe MR requiring surgical treatment in the course of their life [6, 7]. The mortality of patients with mitral valve prolapse leading to severe MR is about 6–7% a year [8, 9].

The prevalence of MR is rising with age and life expectancy, and this condition will be increasingly frequent in the near future [10, 11]. Recent data show that MR is currently an undertreated pathology, as up to 50% of patients with severe MR are not treated surgically, although they have one or more indications specified in international guidelines [12, 13]. This is often due to advanced age and comorbidities that increase surgical risk. In this context, mitral repair techniques, especially those using the percutaneous approach, are increasingly gaining ground, as they have a minor impact on patients. They also play a major role in the degenerative pathology, but they are not discussed herein.

In many patients, the typical sign of the degenerative pathology is an excess of valve tissue (Barlow's disease), which is the extreme form of myxomatous degeneration (Fig. 6.1). In others, especially in older patients, the valve tissue does not show this alteration, but it is thinner and translucent (fibroelastic deficiency, Fig. 6.2).

MR with a degenerative etiology is the most frequent cause of mitral surgery in the west. Fortunately, about 90% of myxomatous mitral valves can be repaired surgically, without resorting to replacement with a device [14]. However, there is a narrow range of possible anatomical and pathological variants in degenerative MR and, of course, this can increase the complexity of repair.

Anatomical and functional alterations that typically characterize degenerative MR are leaflet prolapse into the atrium during systole, and annular dilation. The *chordae tendineae* can be elongated and thinned, or thickened, and they can even be affected by rupture.

The posterior mitral leaflet and afferent *chordae tendineae* are more frequently affected by the degenerative process compared to the anterior leaflet. The most frequent anatomical and pathological alteration (in about 50% patients

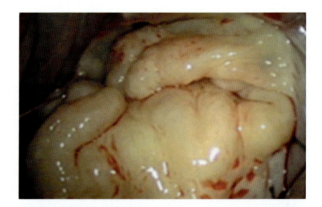

Fig. 6.1 Myxomatous mitral valve ("floppy valve")

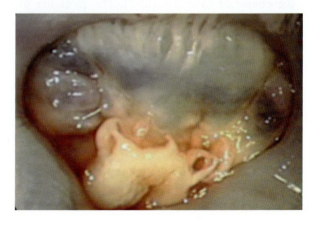

Fig. 6.2 Degenerative mitral regurgitation due to fibroelastic deficiency

with degenerative MR) is elongation or rupture of the *chordae tendineae* of the posterior leaflet. The most frequent consequence is prolapse or isolated flail of the middle scallop of the posterior leaflet [15].

The natural history of mitral valve prolapse is heavily dependent on the extent of MR secondary to it. The mortality of patients with severe degenerative MR is about 6–7% a year and can be even greater depending on how symptomatic the condition is [8, 16, 17]. Many studies, still being debated, have shown that the survival of patients with severe degenerative MR is reduced even in those with no symptoms, compared to healthy individuals of the same age [18–20]. The main clinical consequences of untreated severe MR are the development of left ventricular dysfunction and pulmonary hypertension, and the onset of atrial fibrillation and disabling symptoms.

6.1.2
Diagnosis and Quantification of Degenerative Mitral Regurgitation

Clinical assessment of the patient must take into account any signs and symptoms of heart failure. The instrumental gold-standard examination in diagnosis of MR is color-Doppler ultrasound. The most important prognostic information provided by echocardiogram is determination of the degree of MR. Various quantitative and qualitative parameters are considered by the echocardiographer, to assess the severity of MR. Table 6.1 shows the quantitative variables commonly used in clinical practice to quantify the severity of the defect [3, 21]. The values measured for the effective regurgitation orifice area (EROA) and regurgitant volume (RV) are of great prognostic relevance: it has been proven that patients with an EROA ≥ 0.40 cm^2 and RV ≥ 60 ml/beat have a reduced overall survival rate if left untreated [18]. Other important prognostic factors obtainable from echocardiogram, and which need to be taken into account in determining the timing for surgery, are the left ventricle ejection fraction (LVEF) and the size of the left ventricle (LV) and, in particular, the end-systolic diameter (LVESD) [8, 18–22]. These parameters are the expression of heart failure secondary to valve disease, and they not only negatively affect the

Table 6.1 Assessment of degenerative mitral regurgitation by color-Doppler echocardiography

	Mild	Moderate	Severe
RV (ml/beat)	<30	45–59	≥60
RF (%)	<30	40–49	≥50
EROA (cm^2)	<0.20	0.30–0.39	≥0.40

EROA, effective regurgitation orifice area; *RF*, regurgitant fraction; *RV*, regurgitant volume

natural history of untreated patients, but also have an unfavorable impact on the outcome of patients receiving surgery. Therefore, it is essential that the timing of surgery is correct and that MR is treated before the LV is irreversibly damaged.

Preoperative echocardiogram and, in particular, transesophageal echocardiogram (TEE) also provide a series of essential anatomical and functional information on valve reparability [23].

6.1.3
Surgical Considerations

6.1.3.1
Types of Procedure

There are two possible surgical procedures for the treatment of degenerative MR, each of which has specific advantages and disadvantages and precise indications: mitral valve repair or plasty, and valve replacement with prosthesis.

Mitral repair is the procedure of choice if, at preoperative echocardiogram (more than 90% of cases in high-volume centers), the valve can be repaired and if the procedure is performed at a center with adequate experience in surgical mitral repair. Mitral repair makes it possible to preserve the native valve and avoid anticoagulant therapy and the related risks (bleeding and thrombosis) including device degeneration or malfunction. It has been proven that preserving the native valve apparatus ensures better postoperative systolic function and a better intrahospital and follow-up survival [22]. Despite this evidence, about 50% of patients in Europe still undergo valve replacement with prosthesis, and it is estimated that in at least one-third of cases this is due to a lack of experience with mitral repair surgery [11]. Similarly, in the US just 44.3% of patients referred for MR surgery are treated with valve repair [24]. Mitral repair requires greater experience compared to valve replacement and patients with a mitral valve that is deemed reparable should be referred to centers of referral with a high volume and extensive experience in mitral repair.

Although surgical reintervention is needed in a certain number of cases at a distance of time due to MR relapse after mitral repair, reintervention rates observed in patients who have undergone valve repair are comparable to those of mitral replacement patients. The relapse of post-repair severe MR can be due to a failure of repair or to progression of the degenerative pathology. Patients who have undergone mitral repair due to anterior leaflet prolapse or bileaflet prolapse require reintervention due to MR relapse more frequently than patients with a posterior leaflet lesion [25, 26].

If the valve is deemed not reparable at preoperative examination or surgical inspection (for instance, the presence of extensive annular calcifications), replacement with a device is required.

In this case, mitral replacement with conservation of the subvalvular apparatus offers the advantage of ensuring better postintervention left ventricular performance and better survival compared to cases in which the subvalvular apparatus is removed [27–29].

Mitral repair is the intervention of choice for degenerative MR, both in the case of severe symptomatic MR with associated ventricular dysfunction, as it ensures better postintervention systolic function, and in patients with minimal or no symptoms with severe MR, with conserved systolic function, as it allows prevention of the onset of systolic dysfunction without the disadvantages of prosthetic replacement. The management of asymptomatic patients with severe MR and a morphologically and functionally normal LV is still debated, since there are no randomized trials in this context. A major role in favor in early surgery is played by the excellent results of this approach and the possible presence of an undetected left ventricular dysfunction. On the other hand, a more conservative approach is favored by the fact that there is obviously a low yet ineliminable operative mortality rate related to the surgical procedure.

Enriquez-Sarano et al [18] have reported a greater than expected mortality and incidence of cardiac events in asymptomatic patients with isolated severe MR treated conservatively (5-year survival of 58%). Recently, Montant et al [20] also reported a better outcome at 10 years in terms of survival in the same type of patients treated with early surgery compared to those treated conservatively. By contrast, Rosenhek et al [30] did not see any differences in terms of survival compared to expectations in a cohort of 132 patients followed for 8 years. All the patients in the Rosenhek study were followed with a thorough echocardiographic and clinical follow-up program and sent for surgery at the onset of the symptoms or instrumental evidence of left ventricular dysfunction. However, it should be noted that in the general population it is difficult to conduct such a strict monitoring program and such regular participation by asymptomatic patients.

Regardless of the debate on the optimal strategy to follow for asymptomatic patients with severe MR, the importance of an accurate preoperative determination of the probability that repair will be effective and long-lasting is self-evident.

6.1.3.2
Surgical Indications

According to the latest guidelines of the American College of Cardiology/American Heart Association (ACC/AHA) [31] and the European Society of Cardiology [32], patients with severe MR with symptoms of heart failure or dysfunction (LVEF <60%) or left ventricular dilation (LVESD >40 mm) must be referred for surgery. Surgery should also be offered to patients with severe MR in cases of new-onset atrial fibrillation or pulmonary hypertension. If these conditions are absent, surgery should be considered for patients with a high probability of effective valve repair. Asymptomatic patients with non-severe MR should be subject to close clinical and instrumental monitoring and treated surgically, in case of the onset of symptoms or a worsening of MR. Recent studies have also reported an increased incidence of adverse events in patients with increased left atrium dimensions (left atrium index >60 ml/m^2) and also with moderate MR, thus indicating that atrial dimensions should also be assessed on a routine basis and considered for the timing of surgery.

6.1.3.3
Principles of Mitral Repair Surgery

There are currently several surgical techniques providing effective repair in most patients with degenerative MR. It is of the utmost importance for surgeons to master the various techniques to be able to also repair more complex lesions.

Once an optimal exposure of the mitral valve is achieved, the entire valve apparatus must be carefully examined to identify all the lesions causing the dysfunction and any calcifications not detected during the preoperative examinations that may negatively impact the duration of the repair.

6.1.3.3.1
Posterior Leaflet Prolapse

The technique commonly used to treat posterior leaflet prolapse is *quadrangular resection* of the prolapsing segment [33, 34]. After identifying the segment affected by chordal rupture or elongation, it must be eliminated by performing two incisions running perpendicular to the leaflet's free margin and reaching the annulus. Annulus folding is usually performed at the implantation base of the resected segment to approach the remaining segments, which can hence be sutured directly without exerting excessive tension on them, to restore the continuity of the posterior leaflet (Fig. 6.3).

In many cases, when the tissue is too redundant, as in Barlow's syndrome, there is a high risk of dynamic obstruction to the postoperative left ventricular outflow (known as systolic anterior motion [SAM]), a complication in 5–10% of MR cases treated by simple quadrangular resection [35]. The risk of SAM is also increased in the presence of a small LV. SAM is usually worsened by hypovolemia, vasodilation, and the administration of inotropes. In the case of mild SAM, correcting these factors is enough to achieve complete regression.

The best strategy to avoid SAM in patients at risk is to prevent its onset by reducing the height of the posterior leaflet to less than 15 mm so that the coaptation point of the two valve leaflets can be moved posteriorly. *Sliding plasty* (Fig. 6.4) is the result of the effort to avoid postoperative SAM. It is a variant of conventional quadrangular resection: after resecting the prolapsing segment,

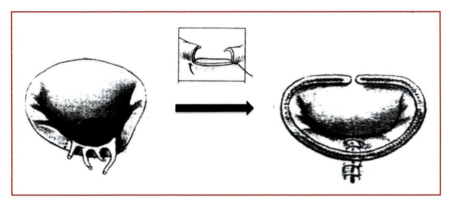

Fig. 6.3 Quadrangular resection of the posterior leaflet due to P2 flail

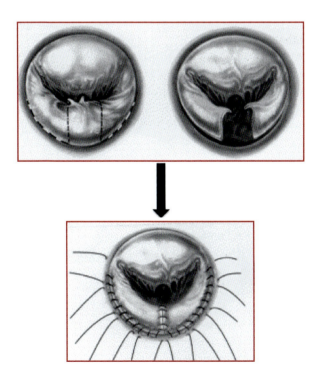

Fig. 6.4 Sliding plasty

the anterior leaflet is detached from both sides of the resection by about 1.5–2 cm, and a triangular portion of tissue is removed at the implantation base of the two portions adjacent to the resection.

The posterior leaflet is then lowered and re-attached to the annulus by means of a 4-0 prolene continuous suture, and the two remaining parts are sutured to fill the gap left by the resected segment by means of a 5-0 continuous suture. If the height of the posterior leaflet is not enough, a variant of sliding plasty called *folding plasty* can be performed. In this case, after conventional quadrangular resection, the portions adjacent to the resected part are detached from the annulus, but no resection is performed at the implantation base. They can be folded and re-attached to the annulus; continuity of the posterior leaflet is then restored by suturing together the parts remaining after quadrangular resection.

Both conventional quadrangular resection and sliding and folding plasty are then completed by implanting a prosthetic ring.

6.1.3.3.2
Anterior Leaflet Prolapse

Several surgical techniques are currently used to correct anterior leaflet prolapse. A short description of the techniques that are currently most widely used follows.

Triangular Resection
A limited prolapse due to tissue in excess can be easily treated by triangular resection of the prolapsing area, followed by direct suture (Fig. 6.5). Resection should never involve an area greater than 10% of the total area of the anterior leaflet, as it may otherwise distort the anatomy, reducing the coaptation surface and impairing its motility. In the case of resections that are too large, there is an

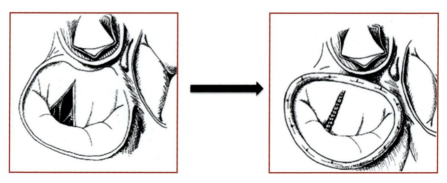

Fig. 6.5 Triangular resection of the anterior leaflet

increased risk of repair failure. Triangular resection is not always applicable, and thorough patient selection based on intraoperative valve inspection is essential. When correctly applied, this technique gives results that are comparable to those of the other repair procedures adopted for anterior leaflet prolapse: Saunders et al [36] have reported at 5 years an overlapping freedom from reintervention (93% versus 94%) using triangular resection and other techniques. One of the advantages of this technique is that it is marked by a low incidence of postoperative SAM [37–40].

Transposition of *Chordae Tendineae*
One of the most widely used techniques to correct anterior leaflet prolapse is transposition of secondary *chordae*, with re-implantation on the free margin of the anterior leaflet. Once a secondary chorda with an adequate length and structure and not affected by myxomatosis is identified, it is detached at about 2 mm from its implantation point on the leaflet's ventricular side. If the chorda is cut at the root, there is a risk of leaflet perforation. The chorda thus prepared is then re-implanted on the free margin of the anterior leaflet near the prolapsing segment (Fig. 6.6). In the case of an extensive prolapse, several *chordae* may have to be transposed, with a distance of no more than 5 mm between two adjacent *chordae*. If there are no secondary *chordae* to the anterior leaflet that are fit for chordal transposition, marginal *chordae* of the segment of the posterior leaflet located in front of the prolapsing one can be used. In this case, a segment of the posterior leaflet with the respective chorda is detached and then re-attached in separate points using a 4-0 prolene suture on the free margin of the prolapsing segment of the anterior leaflet. The defect on the posterior leaflet is then sutured in the same way as a standard quadrangular resection (Fig. 6.7).

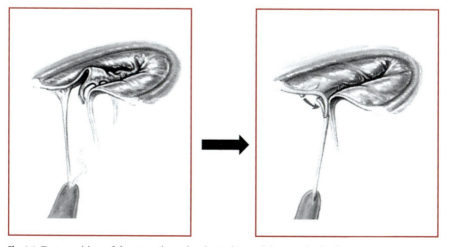

Fig. 6.6 Transposition of the secondary *chorda tendinea* of the anterior leaflet

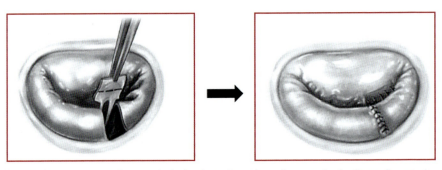

Fig. 6.7 Transposition of the marginal *chorda tendinea* from the posterior leaflet to the anterior leaflet and following repair of the posterior leaflet

The advantage of chordal transposition compared to the use of artificial *chordae* is that the former already have the correct length, while the major challenge for a surgeon when using the latter is to determine the right length. One of the main disadvantages is the fact that a valve segment not affected by the pathology needs to be "tampered with", in order to transpose the *chordae tendineae* of the posterior leaflet.

In the long run, the results of the chordal transposition technique are excellent, with a freedom from reintervention at 5 years of over 95% [41–44]. Technical factors that may lead to the failure of repair are suture dehiscence in the reconstructed posterior leaflet in the case of transposition or detachment of the transposed chorda. This technique has proved to be more effective than shortening of the *chordae tendineae* [41].

Implantation of Artificial *Chordae*

The use of artificial *chordae tendineae* (neochordae) is one of the most widely used techniques to fix anterior leaflet prolapse, and many groups have documented their excellent results. David and colleagues [45, 46] reported a freedom from significant MR at 10 years that was overlapping in patients treated with artificial *chordae* implantation and those treated with other techniques, also including patients undergoing resection due to posterior leaflet prolapse who generally have a less complex valve anatomy. No differences in terms of overall survival, cardiovascular events, or incidence of endocarditis or thromboembolism were reported. As for chordal transposition, the implantation of neochordae has proven to be a more effective technique in the long run, compared to shortening of the *chordae tendineae* [47].

When using this technique, it is essential to comply with the normal anatomy of the mitral subvalvular apparatus and the physiological distribution of the *chordae tendineae*: those originating from the anterior papillary muscle are

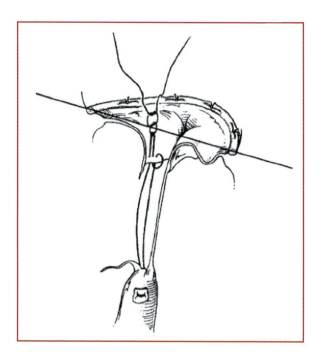

Fig. 6.8 Implantation of artificial *chordae tendineae*

distributed in the lateral half of the anterior and posterior leaflets, while those originating from the posterior papillary muscle anchor the medial half.

The materials most commonly used in surgical practice are the 4-0 or 5-0 PTFE neochordae (suture Gore-Tex®, WL Gore & Associates, Flagstaff, AZ, USA). Artificial *chordae* are fastened to the fibrous portion of the papillary muscle on one end and the anterior leaflet near the prolapsing portion on the other, at a distance that must not exceed 4–5 mm from the leaflet's free margin (Fig. 6.8). In the case of extensive prolapse, several artificial *chordae* are needed.

The main technical difficulty lies in determining the proper length of the neochordae. In the case of isolated prolapse of the anterior leaflet, the best way to determine the correct length is to use the height of the non-prolapsing posterior leaflet as a reference. In the case of bileaflet prolapse or prolapse of several segments, the point of reference to be used is the lateral commissure, unless it is affected by the degenerative process. Modified artificial *chordae* with a premeasured loop have recently been introduced to facilitate the choice of the proper length [48, 49].

When using neochordae, it should be considered that in the case of a very dilated LV there is a higher risk of relapse of prolapse some time after intervention, secondary to inverse geometrical remodeling: the greater vicinity of the papillary muscle to the mitral valve secondary to the reduction in ventricular volume makes the length of the neochorda become too long.

Implantation of artificial *chordae* is also used by many surgeons to fix prolapse of the posterior leaflet, especially if the valve tissue is not too redundant (concept of "respect rather than resect"), with results that overlap with the standard approach in the long run [50].

Edge-to-Edge Technique

The edge-to-edge technique has been proposed as a simple and effective solution to address MR with a complex etiology, as is the case for anterior leaflet prolapse [51–55]. This technique consists of suturing the free margin of the prolapsing segment of the anterior leaflet, with a 4-0 or 5-0 prolene suture, to the free margin of the normal portion opposite the posterior segment, to create a "double-orifice" valve (Fig. 6.9a). In this way, the anterior leaflet is anchored to the posterior leaflet, thus preventing its prolapse into the atrium. The area of the repaired valve orifices is then measured using a Hegar dilator to rule out any stenosis. In the case of fibroelastic deficiency with extremely thin valve tissue, the suture can be reinforced with pledgets. The main advantage of the edge-to-edge technique is that it is technically simple to perform and extremely reproducible. The technique can be used both to fix a central prolapse and to fix a prolapse located at a commissural level (paracommissural edge-to-edge technique, Fig. 6.9b). In patients treated with the edge-to-edge technique to repair anterior leaflet prolapse, freedom from reintervention at 10 years is 96.5%, with no or mild residual MR in 88% of cases. Hemodynamically significant mitral stenosis was not reported in any case [54].

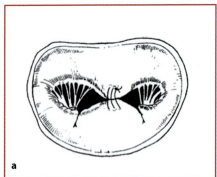 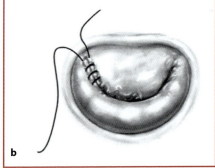

Fig. 6.9 Central (**a**) and paracommissural (**b**) edge-to-edge techniques

Other Techniques

While *shortening of the papillary muscles* is associated with good results in the case of anterior leaflet prolapse [56, 57], *shortening of the chordae tendineae*, by contrast, has been abandoned due to the high failure rate of repair [41, 47].

6.1.3.3.3
Remodeling of the Mitral Annulus by Means of Annuloplasty

Remodeling of the mitral annulus by means of annuloplasty is one of the key concepts in mitral repair surgery. Annular dilation is almost always present in patients with degenerative MR. Dilation typically affects the posterior annulus, since the anterior portion is anchored to the heart's fibrous skeleton.

Besides annular dilation, in degenerative MR there is also an alteration in the shape of the annulus: in physiological conditions, the normal ratio between the anterolateral diameter and the transverse diameter is about 3:4 during systole. This ratio is inverted in myxomatous MR, and the main consequence is a reduced leaflet coaptation surface. Annuloplasty serves not only to restore normal annulus dimensions, but also to restore its physiological shape [58].

All the aforementioned repair techniques are completed by the implantation of a prosthetic ring, as it has been widely proven that annuloplasty increases the repair's duration. The rationale for the implantation of a prosthetic ring is to stabilize the annulus dimensions to prevent further dilation, increasing the coaptation surface of the leaflets, and reducing the stress on the sutures at the leaflets. There are several types of prosthetic rings, which can be classified based on their geometry or structure. In the treatment of degenerative MR, whether complete or incomplete, stiff or flexible rings are used. There are no specific guidelines on the prosthetic ring to be used: the choice is usually based on the operator's preferences.

The suture stitches used to implant the prosthetic ring are passed along the mitral annulus with relatively deep passages, making sure not to damage the circumflex coronary artery, which is in close proximity to the posterior annulus. In cases of use of a complete ring, caution must be used not to damage the aortic valve. It is important that two sutures are placed at the two trigones. The number of remaining sutures varies depending on the ring dimensions (Fig. 6.10) [59]. The ring size is chosen based on the intercommissural distance and the dimensions of the anterior leaflet (Fig. 6.11). In case of doubt between two sizes, the larger ring should generally be used, since small rings increase the risk of postoperative SAM [60, 61].

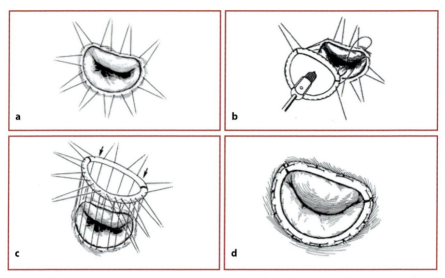

Fig. 6.10 Mitral annuloplasty: the suture stitches are applied first to the mitral annulus (**a**) and then to the prosthetic ring (**b**). The prosthetic ring is lowered on the annulus (**c**) and the sutures are fastened with knots (**d**)

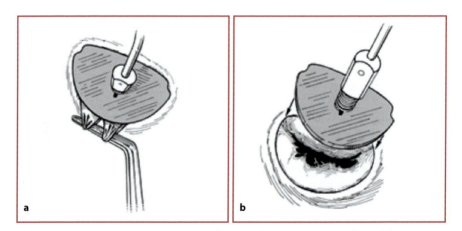

Fig. 6.11 Measurement of the area of the anterior mitral leaflet (**a**) and intertrigonal distance (**b**) to choose the proper size of the prosthetic ring

6.1.3.3.4
Annular Calcifications

In patients with degenerative disease of the mitral valve, there can be calcifications in the annulus. These can cause problems in the implantation of the prosthetic ring and it is essential to perform debridement. If the calcifications are not very extensive, in most cases simple tissue debridement using special calcium forceps can be performed. In the case of extensive and deep calcifications, it may be necessary to detach the posterior leaflet before debriding and then reimplant it as done with sliding plasty. In some cases it may be necessary to reinforce the decalcified area with a patch in the pericardium before reimplanting the leaflet [59].

Extensive calcifications of the valve apparatus can make optimal valve repair technically impossible. In similar cases, it is necessary to resort to valve replacement with a prosthesis.

6.1.3.4
Results

The aforementioned techniques allow repair in more than 90% of degenerative MR.

In a valve with morphology that is deemed satisfactory, the coaptation surface of the leaflets must be adequate and have a coaptation length of at least 5 mm [23]. Of course, residual prolapsing segments are not considered acceptable. In the case of significant residual regurgitation (>2+/4+), cardiopulmonary bypass must be restored and the residual dysfunction mechanism should be corrected. Mild residual regurgitation (1+/4+) can be deemed acceptable only with optimal valve morphology with a large coaptation surface of the leaflets.

Intrahospital mortality due to isolated intervention of mitral repair is less than 1% [26, 46, 61–65]. The low mortality rate of this type of procedure, especially in high-volume centers, has made it possible to extend its indication also to asymptomatic patients, although with a high probability of valve repair.

If the procedure is performed before the onset of the symptoms and left ventricular dysfunction, patient survival after the procedure perfectly matches that of the general population of the same age. By contrast, patient survival is reduced if the procedure is performed after the onset of symptoms of heart failure (New York Heart Association [NYHA] III–IV) [66] and in the presence of a reduced LVEF [67].

With regard to prosthetic replacement, the Society of Thoracic Surgeons (STS) database reports a mortality rate of about 5.5% [68].

Even the incidence of major intrahospital complications (neurological events, acute myocardial infarction [MI], surgical revision for bleeding, infections) is relatively low after isolated mitral repair in elective conditions, amounting to about 1% [61–65, 69].

Many studies have compared the outcome of patients submitted to repair with that of patients submitted to prosthetic replacement, and concluded that mitral repair ensures a better survival at follow-up [22, 28].

The main endpoint to be assessed in the long term, to determine the efficacy of repair, is the echocardiographic recurrence of significant MR and not the freedom from reintervention, which, without any precise echocardiographic reference, tends to underestimate the incidence of failure of repair, since a number of patients are not re-operated despite the recurrence of MR.

The failure rates of mitral repair are mainly affected by the prolapse location and type of technique used. Historically, the best results reported in the literature have been obtained in patients with isolated prolapse of the posterior leaflet treated with quadrangular resection associated with annuloplasty.

The technique for which most long-term data are available in the literature is standard quadrangular resection of the posterior leaflet, with a freedom from reintervention at 20 years of 97%. This percentage drops to 86% due to anterior leaflet prolapse and 83% due to bileaflet prolapse [25]. Other series of patients treated with various techniques, including quadrangular resection and the implantation of artificial *chordae*, report a freedom from reintervention at 12 years of 96%, 88%, and 94% and a freedom from recurrence of MR 3–4+ of 80%, 65%, and 67% for posterior, anterior, and bileaflet prolapse respectively [26]. No differences in terms of MR recurrence are reported, comparing patients with MR secondary to Barlow's disease and patients with fibroelastic deficiency [70].

Flameng et al [71] have reported a recurrence rate of significant MR equal to 3.7% a year. In most cases, MR recurrence has occurred due to progression of the degenerative pathology. Technical errors, too, can cause failure, but these should be reduced to a minimum in expert hands. Surgical factors that may lead to repair failure are failure to implant the prosthetic ring, and recourse to some specific techniques like shortening of the *chordae tendineae*.

6.2
Treatment of Functional Mitral Regurgitation

Surgery for functional MR in patients with chronic heart failure is the challenge of this decade. The mitral valve, initially normal, becomes regurgitant as a consequence of a ventricular disease, due to myopathy – intrinsic or related to coronary artery disease. The mechanism of regurgitation is well known today. Displacement of one (normally the posteromedial) or both papillary muscles accompanies displacement of the left ventricular wall. This mechanism causes traction on the inextensible *chordae tendineae*, particularly the strut chords attached to the body of mainly the anterior leaflet. This pulls the leaflets into the LV, resulting in tenting of the valve below the annulus plane and a reduced area of leaflet coaptation. In turn, reduced coaptation leads to formation of a regurgitant orifice. MR occurring in the setting of LV dilation with structurally normal leaflets is called functional MR.

Displacement involving both papillary muscles, because of tethering effects on both leaflets, is the most complex scenario, as the LV is more globally remodeled, being more spherical, enlarged and dysfunctional. Typically, it is related to anterior acute MI or idiopathic cardiomyopathy.

Recent studies have demonstrated that the assumption that the mitral apparatus is normal, as opposed to MR being organic, is not completely true, as histological and anatomical remodeling of the mitral apparatus is often present. The mitral annulus increases its dimensions and modifies its shape, and the chords are stiffer and less extensible than normal chords. Leaflets show changes in extracellular matrix composition and are stiffer and less viscous. Their extensibility is reduced, but they become more stretched, more redundant and thicker than normal [72, 73]. The anatomical data were confirmed in a three-dimensional (3D) echocardiographic study by Chaput et al [74], which demonstrated that mitral leaflet area increases in response to chronic tethering, and that development of significant MR is associated with insufficient leaflet area relative to that demanded by tethering geometry. Similar data were obtained by Dal Bianco et al [75] in an experimental setting.

Functional MR, when caused by alterations in ventricular geometry and function after acute MI, can itself initiate the remodeling cascade, and cause progressive deterioration of ventricular function at a cellular and molecular level [76–78]. MR increases diastolic wall stress, which can induce eccentric LV hypertrophy and subsequent dilation and failure [79], thereby increasing early systolic wall stress. Although MR allows LV emptying during systole into the lower-pressure left atrium (LA), it has been shown to actually increase end-systolic wall stress and, hence, afterload in patients with chronic MR [80, 81]. Moreover, MR induces further LV dilation due to activation of neurohumoral and cytokine components of the remodeling cascade [82–84]. As MR is both a cause and a result of LV remodeling, it can potentially exacerbate the vicious cycle, spiraling down to cardiac failure unless remodeling or MR is reversed [85–87].

The close relationship between functional MR and LV dilation was confirmed by a sophisticated experimental study by Beeri et al [88], who induced anterior infarction ligating the mid-to-distal left anterior descending artery. An artificial conduit was created between the base of the LV and LA to obtain an LV–LA reflux of 30%. This team of researchers observed that animals with LV–LA reflux incurred a much larger increase in LV volume, as well as more severe systolic and diastolic LV alterations, reduced calcium cycling proteins, activation of prohypertrophic signaling pathways, cellular elongation, and activation of metalloproteinases and their inhibitors in the myocardium remote from the MI. Thus, even a moderate-volume RF, similar to that typically seen clinically with functional MR, is not a bystander from the perspective of progressive LV remodeling, but is directly linked to excess LV remodeling and functional and biochemical markers thereof. Thus, this study establishes a firm link between functional MR and excess LV remodeling, a well-established precursor of clinical events [89]. It can then be deduced that if LV remodeling is due to both functional MR and ventricular injury, as in acute MI, elimination of functional MR stops part of the chain of events that lead to progressive impairment of function and symptoms.

The goal of functional MR surgery is reshaping of the mitral annulus in such a way that the septolateral distance is reduced to allow the anterior leaflet to cover the entire surface of the mitral valve, changing a bileaflet valve into a unileaflet one.

The mitral annulus is a dynamic structure, which changes its shape and dimensions during the cardiac cycle. In systole, the muscular portion of the annulus reduces its size, due to the contraction first of the LA (which accounts for roughly 80% of the reduction) and then of the basal portion of the LV (sinospiral and bulbospiral muscles; accounting for the remaining 20% of reduction). At the same time the muscular annulus displaces toward the apex, and the anterior horn of the saddle moves toward the LA. These modifications of shape and dimensions cause a reduction in mitral size (with consequent increase of coaptation between the leaflets) and an increase of the aortic area, while, at the same time, anterior leaflet insertion is moved away from the left ventricle outflow tract (LVOT). As a consequence, the anterior leaflet is in a pre-opening position (from 20° to 25°), which increases the opening velocity and contributes to further reducing the atrioventricular gradient. In diastole, opposite changes occur. Relaxation of the atrial and ventricular musculatures increases the dimension of the posterior annulus, which moves again toward the LA. At the same time, the anterior horn of the mitral saddle moves toward the LVOT. These changes increase the reciprocal decrease in aortic area.

Surgical implications of the aforementioned are the following: (a) maintaining the systo-diastolic narrowing of the annulus reduces the gradients in diastole and increases the coaptation in systole; (b) maintaining the saddle shape reduces the stress on the leaflets and keeps the anterior leaflet in a pre-opening position; (c) maintaining the saddle shape allows the reciprocal changes of mitral and aortic areas, moving the anterior leaflet insertion away from the LVOT. This latter mechanism seems to be abolished when a complete ring, even if saddle shaped, is used [90].

In patients with symptoms of heart failure, ventricular dilation and MR are both typically present. Although the degree of functional MR can be reduced in some cases by optimizing medical therapies (afterload reduction and treatment of fluid overload), many patients persist with significant functional MR. In the clinical setting, however, it is usually difficult, if not impossible, to identify the relative contributions of primary pump dysfunction and functional MR to LV remodeling and patient symptoms. Consequently, it is not known for a given patient whether fixing functional MR will improve symptoms or play any role in reversing ventricular dilation and pump dysfunction [91]. As a consequence, indications for mitral valve surgery are not well defined.

The guidelines of the European Society of Cardiology [92] are detailed only for patients with chronic ischemic MR. Surgery is indicated in patients with severe MR, LVEF >30% undergoing coronary artery bypass grafting (CABG) (level of evidence IC); in patients with moderate MR undergoing CABG if repair is feasible (level of evidence IIaC); in symptomatic patients with severe MR, LVEF <30% and option for revascularization (level of evidence IIaC); and in patients with severe MR, LVEF >30%, no option for revascularization, refractory to medical therapy, and low comorbidity.

The AHA/ACC guidelines [93] are less clear, as functional MR is considered together with organic MR. Mitral valve surgery is beneficial for patients with chronic severe MR and NYHA functional class II, III, or IV symptoms in the absence of severe LV dysfunction (severe LV dysfunction is defined as LVEF <30%) and/or end-systolic dimension greater than 55 mm (level of evidence: IB). Mitral valve repair may be considered for patients with chronic severe secondary MR due to severe LV dysfunction (LVEF < 30%) who have persistent NYHA functional class III–IV symptoms despite optimal therapy for heart failure, including biventricular pacing (level of evidence IIbC). In the subchapter on ischemic MR the guidelines refer only to patients who undergo CABG with mild to moderate MR: "indication for MV [mitral valve] operation is still unclear, even if there are data to indicate benefit of MV repair in such patients".

Globally, these guidelines reflect the uncertainty that exists today in this domain.

MR is often present in patients with heart failure and is associated with poor outcome [94–97]. Mitral valve surgery in these patients in whom the causes of regurgitation are inside a remodeled ventricle can restore valve competency, but the mid-term and long-term results are not predictable, as the ventricular component can continue to remodel. In the past, surgery for mitral valve regurgitation in advanced heart failure was traditionally considered to be not only ineffective, but also to carry a high or prohibitive risk. Even recent reports underscore that patients with significant MR and LV dysfunction are under-referred for surgery.

Bach et al [98] reported that 84% of patients with moderate-to-severe or severe functional MR (both ischemic and non-ischemic) were not operated, even though accepted guidelines for intervention were present in the great majority of the patients. The experience of Bolling et al [99] showed not only that the early risk was acceptable, but also that survival could be satisfactory. The same team, however, was not able to show any improvement in survival compared to surgically untreated patients in a propensity-matched study [100]. This study included patients with and without coronary artery disease with LVEF ≤30% and at least 3+ or 4+ MR.

However the recent report on the Acorn clinical trial [101], a multicenter prospective randomized study, was able to focus the attention again on mitral valve surgery in patients with dilated heart (diastolic dimension at least 60 mm or ≥30 mm/m^2) and LVEF ≤35%. Only 6.2% of the patients had ischemic MR. However, the trial also enrolled patients with 2+ MR (23.3%), 1+ MR (10.6%), and NYHA class II (23.3%), whereas only 5.2% were in NYHA class IV. Some patients with LVEF of up to 45% were also enrolled. Globally, 184 patients underwent mitral valve surgery (29, 15.8%, mitral valve replacement and 155, 84.2%, mitral valve repair; a band was used in 35% of the cases). Thirty-day mortality was 1.6% and, at 24 months, cumulative survival was 85.2%. Mitral surgery was associated with progressive reductions in LV end-diastolic volume, LV end-systolic volume, and LV mass, and increases in LVEF and sphericity index, all consistent with reverse remodeling. Quality of life, exercise performance, and NYHA class were all improved. Our group [102] showed similar results in patients with dilated cardiomyopathy (end-diastolic left ventricular volume ≥110 ml/m^2 and LVEF ≤35%), with a 5-year survival of 78%.

In patients with mainly non-ischemic MR, the results of surgery over the past decade are encouraging, with low early mortality, good survival, and evident functional improvement.

On the other hand, in patients with ischemic MR, results have been more contradictory. Chronic ischemic MR (CIMR) is more diffused than non-ischemic MR and results have been affected by a lack of comprehension of the mechanisms of MR and of the echocardiographic changes of the mitral valve. Most of the aspects related to the mitral valve have only recently been better understood, and surgical strategies have been adapted to different mechanisms of regurgitation.

CIMR is present in many patients after acute MI, and adversely affects their outcome. The presence of CIMR after acute MI was demonstrated to be related to lower survival, in particular if EROA was ≥20 mm^2 [103]. The excess in mortality was independent from LVEF (risk ratio [RR] 1.84, $P = 0.0065$ if <40%; RR 4.40, $P < 0.001$, if ≥40%) and the functional status (RR 2.15, $P = 0.005$, if NYHA class III/IV; RR 2.19, $P = 0.007$, if NYHA class I/II]. However, any grade of CIMR, measured by EROA, was related, at 5 years, to a higher incidence of congestive heart failure (RR 3.45, $P < 0.002$, if EROA was from 1 to 19 mm^2; RR 4.42, $P < 0.001$, if EROA ≥20 mm^2) and of combined endpoints of congestive heart failure and cardiac death (RR 2.8, $P <0.001$, if EROA was from 1 to 19 mm^2; RR 3.42, $P = 0.0006$, if EROA ≥20 mm^2) [104]. These studies emphasize that the clinical severity of CIMR does not follow conventional MR gradation, but, if EROA is used, a value of ≥20 mm^2 is the cut-off point to define severe grade of CIMR.

Untreated CIMR when CABG is performed is also known to be followed by a worse long-term outcome. Aronson et al [105] found that, in patients with previous acute MI and mild CIMR, the possibility of heart failure was significantly higher than in patients with acute MI without CIMR (RR 2.9, $P = 0.001$).

Other studies demonstrated that any CIMR grade, even mild, detected during perioperative transesophageal echocardiogram, was related to poor outcome [106].

Amigoni et al [107] also showed that any MR grade detected after 5 days from acute MI was related to lower survival and a higher hospitalization rate for heart failure. In patients who survived and underwent a 20-month echocardiogram, MR progression was greater in those with one or more episodes of hospitalization for heart failure during that period than in patients who were event-free (MR jet/LA area ratio 7.8 ± 11.3 versus 1.5 ± 7.7, $P<0.001$). There were no differences in MR progression based on treatment assignment. Our group demonstrated that results of CABG alone on patients with CIMR 2+ were poor if LVEF is $\leq30\%$ [108], and freedom from cardiac death and cardiac events was reduced in patients with LVEF between 31% and 40% and CIMR 1+ or 2+ [109]. Ultimately, there is plenty of evidence in the literature on worse outcome in any subset of patients with any grade of CIMR that follows acute MI.

These data open the debate on surgical indication, as, although there is clear evidence that the presence of CIMR worsens the outcome of patients who had acute MI, there is no evidence that the correction of CIMR can improve outcome. However, even if survival has not changed, in recent years there has been general agreement that functional status is improved after correction of CIMR, as Fattouch et al [110] recently demonstrated in a prospective randomized trial.

Downsizing annuloplasty is the most valid tool to treat patients with functional MR, and still remains the basic strategy to correct CIMR. However, annuloplasty alone, when indicated, is not the only option for surgical treatment of CIMR, as patients can need additional solutions.

When the anterior leaflet length is shorter than 25 mm, augmentation of the leaflet can be obtained by means of a pericardial patch, as suggested by many authors [111–113]. The purpose of augmentation is to increase the coaptation length when it is predicted to be shorter than usual. Other authors [114] have proposed partial posterior leaflet extension to correct severe MR. In the presence of increased tethering of the second-order chords of the anterior leaflet, the second order can be cut, to increase the mobility of the leaflet.

Even if there are different experiences in favor of or against chordal cutting [115–118], clinical results are satisfying. Perioperative ventricular resynchronization is useful in the case of asynchronous ventricular contractility. Some studies have emphasized the need to add ventricular procedures in cases of enlarged cardiac dimensions [119]. In our opinion, ventricular restoration should be performed whenever it is possible. Srichai et al [120] demonstrated that ventricular scarring significantly increased in patients with severe CIMR. Our personal experience shows that, when end-systolic volume index is ≥ 50 ml/m^2, close to 50% of the patients need ventricular surgery. Results are satisfying in terms of survival and functional improvement. We believe that, in the presence of increased LV volumes, ventricular restoration is part of the surgical strategy for CIMR treatment and for preventing MR recurrence.

Other techniques have been proposed by other authors, addressing approximation [121, 122] or relocation [123–126] of the papillary muscles. It is very likely that some could be helpful to stabilize mitral valve repair over time. Their role, however, is yet to be defined.

Nowadays, results of surgical correction of CIMR are completely different from the previous experiences, with low early mortality and good long-term survival and functional results.

Nevertheless, the main problem of surgical treatment of functional MR is recurrent (or residual) MR. This negatively affects survival, especially in patients with 3+ or 4+ MR recurrence [127]. The reason why observational studies do not answer the question of whether functional MR influences outcome in patients with LV dysfunction, is that mitral surgery has demonstrated limitations related to the recurrence of functional MR due to ongoing LV remodeling with reappearance of valve tenting after annuloplasty [87, 128]. The uncertainty regarding functional MR is further complicated by the fact that patients with functional MR also have, in general, worse LV function, remodeling, and clinical presentation [103, 129]. Even after matching patients with and without functional MR for LVEF, one might wonder whether lower intrinsic left ventricular function (undetected by standard methods) is not the main driver for excess risk [103]. Lack of reverse remodeling is surely a cause of poor outcome [130]; unfortunately, it is not clear how to identify patients with a continuous trend to remodel after surgery.

In the Acorn study, 25 out of 117 patients with idiopathic MR had, after 6 months, residual MR $\geq 2+$ [131]. On the other hand, MR recurrence was present, with different percentages, in all the reports regarding CIMR [119, 127,132–136]. Surgery for MR in idiopathic cardiomyopathy is relatively rare and is performed systematically only by a few teams. On the other hand, surgery for CIMR is a common aspect of daily surgical life. The consequent reduction of efficacy of mitral surgery for CIMR has induced surgeons to mistrust any proposal for an aggressive strategy in CIMR treatment. The incidence of $\geq 3+$ MR recurrence (or residual MR) varies from 7% [106] at 1 year, to 9% [135] at 6 months, to 28% [127] at 20 months, and 44% at 5 years [136]. The incidence of $\geq 2+$ MR varies from 11% [133] at 1.4 years, to 20.8% [134] at 1.5 years, to 16% [119] at 3.8 years, and 72% [136] at 60 months.

To reduce the incidence of MR recurrence, our group has proposed a coaptation depth of 10 mm or less as the cut-off point to separate cases where mitral valve repair can be performed from cases where chordal-sparing implantation of a prosthesis is the preferable solution [102]. In fact, to change a bileaflet valve into a unileaflet one, based completely on the anterior leaflet, it is necessary that the anterior leaflet is mobile enough to reach the posterior leaflet. When the papillary muscles are so displaced that anterior leaflet movement is compromised, the result of annular reshaping will be poor. This happens more frequently when both papillary muscles are displaced, as in functional MR, idiopathic cardiomyopathy, and CIMR following anterior acute MI.

As the primary goal of surgery is to eliminate MR, insertion of a prosthesis can be the best solution, if the entire mitral apparatus is preserved, particularly because these patients are those with the largest hearts that will not tolerate MR recurrence. This solution needs to be applied in roughly 10% of cases, with optimal results. How to measure the coaptation depth can influence the surgical strategy. It needs to be emphasized that the mitral annular plane does not start at the level of the insertion of the aortic valve, as often shown [120, 131, 136], but where the anterior leaflet hinges; this reduces the coaptation depth by a few millimeters and can improve decision-making.

Long-term survival in patients who had undergone mitral valve repair or replacement was found to be similar by Al-Radi et al [137] and by Magne et al [138], 9 and 12 years after surgery, respectively.

Different cut-off points have been identified in the literature. Predictors of poor outcome after restrictive annuloplasty were identified in posterior leaflet angle ≥45° [139]; anterior leaflet tethering angle of 39.5° [140]; distal mitral anterior leaflet angle >25° [131]; and in an interpapillary distance >20 mm [141].

We believe that chordal-sparing insertion of a prosthesis has to be considered the most durable way to correct functional MR [142] and not a surgical failure.

Recently, an unfavorable aspect of undersized annuloplasty was underscored by Magne et al [143], who found that patients who underwent such a procedure were at risk of functional mitral stenosis, showing higher pulmonary pressure and worse functional capacity. Gradients seem to be higher when a complete ring is used [90]. These findings were not confirmed by other studies [144], but the discussion is still open.

The outcome after mitral valve surgery for functional MR is nowadays far better than in previous experiences, when the results were dominated by a lack of correct understanding of mitral valve pathophysiology and of proper surgical strategies. Reduction of 30-day mortality is the key point to justify a more aggressive approach to this disease (the most widespread criticism was: why do we have to expose our patients to a perioperative risk twice the normal if the benefit is not evident?). The most recent reports are encouraging, and our knowledge is continuously increasing: mitral valve surgery for functional MR is still a work in progress.

6.3
Treatment of Aortic Stenosis

The most common cause of aortic stenosis (AS) is degenerative calcification of the valve. Although previously considered to be the result of years of mechanical stress on an otherwise normal valve, the evolving concept is that the degenerative process leads to proliferative and inflammatory changes, with lipid accumulation, upregulation of angiotensin-converting enzyme (ACE) activity, and infiltration of macrophages and T lymphocytes, ultimately leading to calcification of the aortic valve. Progressive calcification, initially along the flexion lines at their bases, leads to immobilization of the cusps. The characteristic pathologic findings are discrete, focal lesions on the aortic side of the leaflets that can extend deep into the aortic annulus. The deposits may involve the sinuses of Valsalva and the ascending aorta. The risk factors for the development of calcified AS are similar to those for atherosclerosis, and include elevated serum levels of low-density lipoprotein cholesterol and lipoprotein (a), diabetes, smoking, and hypertension. Age-related aortic valve sclerosis is associated with an increased risk of cardiovascular death and MI.

AS is also observed in a number of other conditions including Paget's disease and end-stage renal disease. Ochronosis with alkaptonuria is another rare cause of AS, which can also cause a rare greenish discoloration of the aortic valve.

Bicuspid aortic valves are the most common congenital cause of AS, and rheumatic heart disease is also an important cause, especially in developing countries.

6.3.1
Surgical Indications

There is no effective medical therapy for AS. Diuretics and digitalis may improve the symptoms of congestive heart failure. ACE inhibitors are relatively contraindicated in patients with AS. Afterload-reduction therapy is contraindicated in patients with AS because it can reduce coronary perfusion pressure.

Aortic valve replacement is indicated for severe symptomatic AS [145]. The classical symptoms of AS are angina, syncope, and heart failure. However, some patients have more subtle symptoms, typically decreased exercise tolerance, or dyspnea on exertion. It is not uncommon for patients to decrease their activity level below their symptom threshold; these patients, in fact, are symptomatic. As the risk of sudden death is high once any symptom is present, valve surgery is appropriate with even mild symptoms. When symptoms are present, valve area is ≤ 1 cm^2, and Doppler velocity is ≥ 4 m/s. In this case the decision to proceed with valve replacement is straightforward.

However, some patients have symptoms with a valve area between 1 and 1.5 cm^2 or a velocity between 3 and 4 m/s. In these patients, careful evaluation, including coronary angiography, for other causes of the symptoms is needed. It is also appropriate to seek objective evidence of clinical decompensation, such as pulmonary congestion on chest radiography, or reduced exercise tolerance, to ensure that symptoms are truly present. With clear symptoms that have no other explanation, valve-replacement surgery should be considered if the valve shows significant calcification, even with "moderate" stenosis only [146].

Aortic valve replacement in asymptomatic patients is currently controversial. Considering the high rate of cardiac events and sudden death in previous reports, early elective surgery can be indicated in a high-risk subset of patients, such as those with an aortic valve area (AVA) of <0.75 cm^2, abnormal exercise test, or increase in transaortic gradient during exercise. Other patients with a poor prognosis are those with moderate or severe valvular calcification and rapid increase in aortic jet velocity between two echocardiographic studies. Moreover, any evidence of impaired left ventricular function, as demonstrated by depressed LVEF, left ventricular dilation, or significantly elevated left ventricular diastolic pressure (LVDP) at rest or during exercise, is an indication for aortic valve replacement.

On the other hand, survival in asymptomatic patients and severe AS seems to be poor: 38% in unoperated patients versus 90% in patients who have undergone aortic valve replacement [147].

Combined CABG and aortic valve replacement (AVR) is generally indicated in patients with coronary artery disease and at least moderate AS and calcified valves. In patients with low LVEF and a small transvalvular gradient, AVR results in improvement in only 50% of patients, the other 50% being complicated by perioperative death or congestive heart failure. Controversy currently exists as to whether asymptomatic patients with mild AS should also undergo AVR at the time of CABG.

6.3.2
Specific Issues

6.3.2.1
Mechanical or Tissue Valves

The aortic valve can be replaced by a mechanical or a tissue valve. Generally, the indication for the prosthesis type is dictated by age, with a prevalence of mechanical valves in younger patients (less than 50 year old) and tissue valves in the elderly (over 70 year old). Between 50 and 70 years of age, the patient's choice is determinant. Undoubtedly, the quality of life is superior with a tissue valve. Therefore, active life and an awareness of the low risk of re-operation, together with the risk of anticoagulation, often lead patients to choose a tissue valve. Furthermore, the more recent generations of tissue valve seem to have a longer life, up to 20 years.

6.3.2.2
Prosthesis–Patient Mismatch

The effect of prosthesis–patient mismatch (PPM) on long-term survival after aortic valve replacement has received considerable attention, but it is still not clear. It is defined by the presence of an in vivo effective orifice area (EOA) of the prosthetic valve that is less than that of the native, non-diseased, human valve.

Controversy still exists regarding the long-term effects of PPM. Jamieson et al. [148] reviewed their results in 3,343 patients with aortic valve replacement, with a mean follow-up of 6.18 ± 4.96 years. Patients were grouped according EOA index categories: normal (>0.85 cm^2/m^2), 1,547 (46.3%); mild-to-moderate (>0.65 cm^2/m^2 to ≤0.85 cm^2/m^2], 1,584 (47.4%); and severe (<0.65 cm^2/m^2), 212 (6.3%). Significant findings of the study are related to significantly reduced long-term survival at 15 years for the severe PPM group, but not related to PPM. There was no influence of mild-to-moderate or severe PPM on early mortality.

It is, however, important to know that the new generation of valvular prostheses, whether mechanical or tissue, have improved the design in such a way that it is possible to accommodate a small prosthesis (#17 or #19) with high EOA. PPM can be considered a solved problem.

6.3.2.3
The Role of Transfemoral or Transapical Aortic Valve Replacement

In the cardiology literature, two papers are often quoted that demonstrate that 33–48% of patients with severe AS are denied surgery, in both the elderly [148] or general [149] population, reinforcing the need for an alternative to conventional surgery. Looking carefully at these studies, it is clear that the decision to refuse surgery was taken not by a cardiac surgeon, but by the "attending practitioner" (cardiologist?) [148]. Moreover, symptomatic patients who were denied surgery were infrequently evaluated by cardiac surgeons and most of them had a logistic EuroSCORE (European System for Cariac Operative Risk Evaluation) of less than 20 [150]. The rationale behind surgery refusal is not clear. It is very likely that a lack of familiarity with current operative risk may have led non-surgeons to overestimate the risk, potentially denying patients access to surgery that was feasible.

The use of non-surgical AVR is spreading, sometimes rationally, sometimes in an uncontrolled way. The use of logistic EuroSCORE is inappropriate, as it overpredicts mortality. Cooperation between cardiologists and surgeons, common sense, selection of patients according to real surgical risk, life expectancy, and recovery of reasonable quality of life, and appropriate choice between the transfemoral and transapical route, are the basis of a successful global strategy for AVR in the modern era.

References

1. Savage DD, Garrison RJ, Devereux RB et al. Mitral valve prolapse in the general population. Epidemiologic features: the Framingham Study. Am Heart J 1983;106:571–576.
2. Freed LA, Levy D, Levine RA et al. Prevalence and clinical outcome of mitral-valve prolapse. N Engl J Med 1999;341:1–7.
3. The changing spectrum of valvular heart disease pathology. In: Braunwald E (ed) Harrison's advances in cardiology. New York: McGraw-Hill, 2002; pp 317–323.
4. Hayek E, Gring CN, Griffin BP. Mitral valve prolapse. Lancet 2005;365:507–518.
5. Enriquez-Sarano M, Akins CW, Vahanian A. Mitral regurgitation. Lancet 2009; 373:1382–1394.
6. Barlow JB, Pocock WA. Mitral valve prolapse, the specific billowing mitral leaflet syndrome, or an insignificant non-ejection systolic click. Am Heart J 1979;97:277–285.
7. Abrams J. Mitral valve prolapse: a plea for unanimity. Am Heart J 1976;92:413–415.
8. Ling LH, Enriquez-Sarano M, Seward JB et al. Clinical outcome of mitral regurgitation due to flail leaflet. N Engl J Med 1996;335:1417–1423.
9. Rosen SE, Borer JS, Hochreiter C et al. Natural history of the asymptomatic/minimally symptomatic patient with severe mitral regurgitation secondary to mitral valve prolapse and normal right and left ventricular performance. Am J Cardiol 1994;74:374–380.
10. Nkomo VT, Gardin JM, Skelton TN et al. Burden of valvular heart diseases: a population-based study. Lancet 2006;368:1005–1011.
11. Iung B, Baron G, Butchart EG et al. A prospective survey of patients with valvular heart disease in Europe: the Euro Heart Survey on Valvular Heart Disease. Eur Heart J 2003;24:1231–1243.
12. Mirabel M, Iung B, Baron G et al. What are the characteristics of patients with severe, symptomatic, mitral regurgitation who are denied surgery? Eur Heart J 2007;28:1358–1365.
13. Bach DS, Awais M, Gurm HS, Kohnstamm S. Failure of guideline adherence for intervention in patients with severe mitral regurgitation. J Am Coll Cardiol 2009;54:860–865.
14. David TE, Ivanov J, Armstrong S, Rakowski H. Late outcomes of mitral valve repair for floppy valves: implications for asymptomatic patients. J Thorac Cardiovasc Surg 2003;125:1143–1152.
15. Adams DH, Anyanwu AC, Rahmanian PB, Filsoufi F. Current concepts in mitral valve repair for degenerative disease. Heart Fail Rev 2006;11:241–257.
16. Enriquez-Sarano M, Tajik AJ. Natural history of mitral regurgitation due to flail leaflets. Eur Heart J 1997;18:705–707.
17. St John Sutton M, Weyman AE. Mitral valve prolapse prevalence and complications: an ongoing dialogue. Circulation 2002;106:1305–1307.
18. Enriquez-Sarano M, Avierinos JF, Messika-Zeitoun D et al. Quantitative determinants of the outcome of asymptomatic mitral regurgitation. N Engl J Med 2005;352:875–883.

19. Chenot F, Montant P, Vancraeynest D et al. Long-term clinical outcome of mitral valve repair in asymptomatic severe mitral regurgitation. Eur J Cardiothorac Surg 2009;36:539–545.
20. Montant P, Chenot F, Robert A et al. Long-term survival in asymptomatic patients with severe degenerative mitral regurgitation: a propensity score-based comparison between an early surgical strategy and a conservative treatment approach. J Thorac Cardiovasc Surg 2009;138:1339–1348.
21. Zoghbi WA, Enriquez-Sarano M, Foster E et al. American Society of Echocardiography. Recommendations for evaluation of the severity of native valvular regurgitation with two-dimensional and Doppler echocardiography. J Am Soc Echocardiogr 2003;16:777–802.
22. Enriquez-Sarano M, Schaff HV, Orszulak TA et al. Valve repair improves the outcome of surgery for mitral regurgitation. A multivariate analysis. Circulation 1995;91:1022–1028.
23. David TE. Outcomes of mitral valve repair for mitral regurgitation due to degenerative disease. Semin Thorac Cardiovasc Surg 2007;19:116–120.
24. Savage EB, Ferguson TB Jr, DiSesa VJ. Use of mitral valve repair: analysis of contemporary United States experience reported to the Society of Thoracic Surgeons National Cardiac Database. Ann Thorac Surg 2003;75:820–825.
25. Braunberger E, Deloche A, Berrebi A et al. Very long-term results (more than 20 years) of valve repair with Carpentier's techniques in nonrheumatic mitral valve insufficiency. Circulation 2001;104(12 Suppl 1):I8–11.
26. David TE, Ivanov J, Armstrong S et al. A comparison of outcomes of mitral valve repair for degenerative disease with posterior, anterior, and bileaflet prolapse. J Thorac Cardiovasc Surg 2005;130:1242–1249.
27. Frater RW. Chordal sparing mitral valve replacement. J Heart Valve Dis 1999;8:42–43.
28. Yun KL, Sintek CF, Miller DC et al. Randomized trial comparing partial versus complete chordal-sparing mitral valve replacement: effects on left ventricular volume and function. J Thorac Cardiovasc Surg 2002;123:707–714.
29. Moss RR, Humphries KH, Gao M et al. Outcome of mitral valve repair or replacement: a comparison by propensity score analysis. Circulation 2003;108(Suppl 1);1:II90–97.
30. Rosenhek R, Rader F, Klaar U et al. Outcome of watchful waiting in asymptomatic severe mitral regurgitation. Circulation 2006;113:2238–2244.
31. American College of Cardiology/American Heart Association Task Force on Practice Guidelines; Society of Cardiovascular Anesthesiologists; Society for Cardiovascular Angiography and Interventions; Society of Thoracic Surgeons, Bonow RO, Carabello BA, Kanu C et al. ACC/AHA 2006 guidelines for the management of patients with valvular heart disease: a report of the American College of Cardiology/American Heart Association Task Force on Practice Guidelines (writing committee to revise the 1998 Guidelines for the Management of Patients With Valvular Heart Disease): developed in collaboration with the Society of Cardiovascular Anesthesiologists: endorsed by the Society for Cardiovascular Angiography and Interventions and the Society of Thoracic Surgeons. Circulation 2006;114:e84–231.
32. Vahanian A, Baumgartner H, Bax J et al, Task Force on the Management of Valvular Heart Disease of the European Society of Cardiology; ESC Committee for Practice Guidelines. Guidelines on the management of valvular heart disease: The Task Force on the Management of Valvular Heart Disease of the European Society of Cardiology. Eur Heart J 2007;28:230–268.
33. Carpentier A, Deloche A, Dauptain J et al. A new reconstructive operation for correction of mitral and tricuspid insufficiency. J Thorac Cardiovasc Surg 1971;61:1–13.
34. Carpentier A. Cardiac valve surgery – the "French correction". J Thorac Cardiovasc Surg 1983;86:323–337.
35. Jebara VA, Mihaileanu S, Acar C et al. Left ventricular outflow tract obstruction after mitral valve repair. Results of the sliding leaflet technique. Circulation 1993;88:II30–34.
36. Saunders PC, Grossi EA, Schwartz CF et al. Anterior leaflet resection of the mitral valve. Semin Thorac Cardiovasc Surg 2004;16:188–193.

37. Galloway AC, Grossi EA, Bizekis CS et al. Evolving techniques for mitral valve reconstruction. Ann Surg 2002;236:288–293.
38. Grossi A, La Pietra A, Galloway AC, Colvin SB. History of mitral valve anterior leaflet repair with triangular resection. Ann Thorac Surg 2001;72:1794–1795.
39. Grossi EA, Galloway AC, LeBoutillier M 3rd et al. Anterior leaflet procedures during mitral valve repair do not adversely influence long–term outcome. J Am Coll Cardiol 1995;25:134–136.
40. Grossi EA, Steinberg BM, LeBoutillier M 3rd et al. Decreasing incidence of systolic anterior motion after mitral valve reconstruction. Circulation 1994;90:II195–197.
41. Smedira NG, Selman R, Cosgrove DM et al. Repair of anterior leaflet prolapse: chordal transfer is superior to chordal shortening. J Thorac Cardiovasc Surg 1996;112:287–291.
42. Salati M, Moriggia S, Scrofani R, Santoli C. Chordal transposition for anterior mitral prolapse: early and long–term results. Eur J Cardiothorac Surg 1997;11:268–273.
43. Salati M, Scrofani R, Fundaró P et al. Correction of anterior mitral prolapse. Results of chordal transposition. J Thorac Cardiovasc Surg 1992;104:1268–1273.
44. Gillinov AM, Cosgrove DM. Chordal transfer for repair of anterior leaflet prolapse. Semin Thorac Cardiovasc Surg 2004;16:169–173.
45. David TE. Artificial chordae. Semin Thorac Cardiovasc Surg 2004;16:161–168.
46. David TE, Omran A, Armstrong S et al. Long-term results of mitral valve repair for myxomatous disease with and without chordal replacement with expanded polytetrafluoroethylene sutures. J Thorac Cardiovasc Surg 1998;115:1279–1285.
47. Phillips MR, Daly RC, Schaff HV et al. Repair of anterior leaflet mitral valve prolapse: chordal replacement versus chordal shortening. Ann Thorac Surg 2000;69:25–29.
48. von Oppell UO, Mohr FW. Chordal replacement for both minimally invasive and conventional mitral valve surgery using premeasured Gore-Tex loops. Ann Thorac Surg 2000;70:2166–2168.
49. Kuntze T, Borger MA, Falk V et al. Early and mid-term results of mitral valve repair using premeasured Gore-Tex loops ("loop technique"). Eur J Cardiothorac Surg 2008;33:566–572.
50. Perier P, Hohenberger W, Lakew F et al. Toward a new paradigm for the reconstruction of posterior leaflet prolapse: midterm results of the "respect rather than resect" approach. Ann Thorac Surg 2008;86:718–725.
51. Maisano F, Torracca L, Oppizzi M et al. The edge-to-edge technique: a simplified method to correct mitral insufficiency. Eur J Cardiothorac Surg 1998;13:240–245; discussion 245–246.
52. Maisano F, Schreuder JJ, Oppizzi M et al. The double-orifice technique as a standardized approach to treat mitral regurgitation due to severe myxomatous disease: surgical technique. Eur J Cardiothorac Surg 2000;17:201–205.
53. Alfieri O, Maisano F, De Bonis M et al. The double-orifice technique in mitral valve repair: a simple solution for complex problems. J Thorac Cardiovasc Surg 2001;122:674–681.
54. Alfieri O, De Bonis M, Lapenna E et al. "Edge-to-edge" repair for anterior mitral leaflet prolapse. Semin Thorac Cardiovasc Surg 2004;16:182–187.
55. Alfieri O, Maisano F. An effective technique to correct anterior mitral leaflet prolapse. J Card Surg 1999;14:468–470.
56. Dreyfus GD, Bahrami T, Alayle N et al. Repair of anterior leaflet prolapse by papillary muscle repositioning: a new surgical option. Ann Thorac Surg 2001;71:1464–1470.
57. Dreyfus G, Al Aylé N, Dubois C, Lentdecker P. Long term results of mitral valve repair: posterior papillary muscle repositioning versus chordal shortening. Eur J Cardiothorac Surg 1999;16:81–87.
58. Adams DH, Anyanwu AC, Rahmanian PB, Filsoufi F. Current concepts in mitral valve repair for degenerative disease. Heart Fail Rev 2006;11:241–257.
59. Chen FY, Cohn LH. Mitral valve repair. In: Cohn LH (ed) Cardiac surgery in the adult. New York: McGraw-Hill, 2008; pp 1013–1030.

60. Fedak PW, McCarthy PM, Bonow RO. Evolving concepts and technologies in mitral valve repair. Circulation 2008;117:963–974.
61. De Bonis M, Lorusso R, Lapenna E et al. Similar long–term results of mitral valve repair for anterior compared with posterior leaflet prolapse. J Thorac Cardiovasc Surg 2006;131:364–370.
62. Gillinov AM, Cosgrove DM, Blackstone EH et al. Durability of mitral valve repair for degenerative disease. J Thorac Cardiovasc Surg 1998;116:734–743.
63. Mohty D, Orszulak TA, Schaff HV et al. Very long-term survival and durability of mitral valve repair for mitral valve prolapse. Circulation 2001;104:I1–I7.
64. Deloche A, Jebara VA, Relland JY et al. Valve repair with Carpentier techniques. The second decade. J Thorac Cardiovasc Surg 1990;99:990–1001.
65. Perier P, Stumpf J, Götz C et al. Valve repair for mitral regurgitation caused by isolated prolapse of the posterior leaflet. Ann Thorac Surg 1997;64:445–450.
66. Tribouilloy CM, Enriquez–Sarano M, Schaff HV et al. Impact of preoperative symptoms on survival after surgical correction of organic mitral regurgitation: rationale for optimizing surgical indications. Circulation 1999;99:400–405.
67. Enriquez-Sarano M, Tajik AJ, Schaff HV et al. Echocardiographic prediction of survival after surgical correction of organic mitral regurgitation. Circulation 1994;90:830–837.
68. O'Brien SM, Shahian DM, Filardo G et al, Society of Thoracic Surgeons Quality Measurement Task Force. The Society of Thoracic Surgeons 2008 cardiac surgery risk models: part 2 – isolated valve surgery. Ann Thorac Surg 2009;88:S23–42.
69. Adams DH, Anyanwu AC, Rahmanian PB et al. Large annuloplasty rings facilitate mitral valve repair in Barlow's disease. Ann Thorac Surg 2006;82:2096–2100.
70. Flameng W, Meuris B, Herijgers P, Herregods MC. Durability of mitral valve repair in Barlow disease versus fibroelastic deficiency. J Thorac Cardiovasc Surg 2008;135:274–282.
71. Flameng W, Herijgers P, Bogaerts K. Recurrence of mitral valve regurgitation after mitral valve repair in degenerative valve disease. Circulation 2003;107:1609–1613.
72. Grande Allen KJ, Borowski AG, Troughton RW et al. Apparently normal mitral valves in patients with heart failure demonstrate biochemical and structural derangements. An extracellular matrix and echocardiographic study. J Am Coll Cardiol 2005;45:54–61.
73. Grande Allen KJ, Barber JA, Klatka KM et al. Mitral valve stiffening in end–stage heart failure: Evidence of an organic contribution to functional mitral regurgitation. J Thorac Cardiovasc Surg 2005;130:783–790.
74. Chaput M, Handschumacher MD, Tournoux F et al. Mitral leaflet adaptation to ventricular remodeling: occurrence and adequacy in patients with functional mitral regurgitation. Circulation 2008;118;845–852.
75. Dal Bianco JP, Aikawa E, Bischoff J et al. Active adaptation of the tethered mitral valve. Insights into a compensatory mechanism for functional mitral regurgitation. Circulation 2009;120:334–342
76. Carabello BA, Nakano K, Corin W et al. Left ventricular function in experimental volume overload hypertrophy. Am J Physiol Heart Circ Physiol 1989;256:H974–981.
77. Urabe Y, Mann DL, Kent RL et al. Cellular and ventricular contractile dysfunction in experimental canine mitral regurgitation. Circ Res 1992;70:131–147.
78. Ishihara K, Zile MR, Kanazawa S et al. Left ventricular mechanics and myocyte function after correction of experimental chronic mitral regurgitation by combined mitral valve replacement and preservation of the native mitral valve apparatus. Circulation 1992;86:16 –25.
79. Spinale FG, Ishihra K, Zile MR et al. Structural basis for changes in left ventricular function and geometry because of chronic mitral regurgitation and after correction of volume overload. J Thorac Cardiovasc Surg 1993;106:1147–1157.
80. Corin WJ, Monrad ES, Murakami T et al. The relationship of afterload to ejection performance in chronic mitral regurgitation. Circulation 1987;76:59–67.

81. Zile MR, Gaasch WH, Levine HT. Left ventricular stress-dimension shortening relations before and after correction of chronic aortic and mitral regurgitation. Am J Cardiol 1985;56:99.
82. Dell'Italia LJ, Meng QC, Balcells E et al. Increased ACE and chymase–like activity in cardiac tissue of dogs with chronic mitral regurgitation. Am J Physiol Heart Circ Physiol 1995;269:H2065–2073.
83. Kapadia SR, Yakoob K, Nader S et al. Elevated circulating levels of serum tumor necrosis factor-alpha in patients with hemodynamically significant pressure and volume overload. J Am Coll Cardiol 2000;36:208–212.
84. Talwar S, Squire IB, Davies JE, Ng LL. The effect of valvular regurgitation on plasma cardiotrophin-1 in patients with normal left ventricular systolic function. Eur J Heart Fail 2000;2:387–391.
85. Otsuji Y, Handschumacher MD, Liel-Cohen N et al. Mechanism of ischemic mitral regurgitation with segmental left ventricular dysfunction: three-dimensional echocardiographic studies in models of acute and chronic progressive regurgitation. J Am Coll Cardiol 2001;37:641–648.
86. Liel-Cohen N, Guerrero JL, Otsuji Y et al. Design of a new surgical approach for ventricular remodeling to relieve ischemic mitral regurgitation. Circulation 2000;101:2756–2763
87. Hung J, Papakostas L, Tahta SA et al. Mechanism of recurrent ischemic mitral regurgitation post–annuloplasty: continued LV remodeling as a moving target. Circulation 2004;110:85–90.
88. Beeri R, Yosefy C, Guerrero JL et al. Early repair of moderate ischemic mitral regurgitation reverses left ventricular remodeling. A functional and molecular study. Circulation 2007;116(Suppl I):I288–293.
89. St. John SM, Pfeffer MA, Plappert T et al. Quantitative twodimensional echocardiographic measurements are major predictors of adverse cardiovascular events after acute myocardial infarction. The protective effects of captopril. Circulation 1994;89:68–75.
90. Caimmi PP, Diterlizzi M, Grossini E et al. Impact of prosthetic mitral rings on aortomitral apparatus function: a cardiac magnetic resonance imaging study. Ann Thorac Surg 2009;88:740–744.
91. Enriquez-Sarano M, Loulmet DF, Burkhoff D. The conundrum of functional mitral regurgitation in chronic heart failure. J Am Coll Cardiol 2008;51;487–489.
92. Vahanian A, Baumgartner H, Bax J et al. Guidelines on the management of valvular heart disease. The Task Force on the Management of Valvular Heart Disease of the European Society of Cardiology. Eur Heart J 2007;28:230–268.
93. Bonow RO, Carabello BA, Chatterjee K et al, American College of Cardiology/American Heart Association Task Force on Practice Guidelines. 2008 focused update incorporated into the ACC/AHA 2006 guidelines for the management of patients with valvular heart disease. A report of the American College of Cardiology/American Heart Association Task Force on Practice Guidelines (Writing Committee to revise the 1998 guidelines for the management of patients with valvular heart disease). Endorsed by the Society of Cardiovascular Anesthesiologists, Society for Cardiovascular Angiography and Interventions, and Society of Thoracic Surgeons. J Am Coll Cardiol 2008;52:e1–142.
94. Otto CM. Evaluation and management of chronic mitral regurgitation. N Engl J Med 2001;345:740–746.
95. Koelling TM, Aaronson KD, Cody RJ et al. Prognostic significance of mitral regurgitation and tricuspid regurgitation in patients with left ventricular systolic dysfunction. Am Heart J 2002;144:524–529.
96. Trichon BH, Felker GM, Shaw LK et al. Relation of frequency and severity of mitral regurgitation to survival among patients with left ventricular systolic dysfunction and heart failure. Am J Cardiol 2003;91:538–543.

97. Robbins JD, Maniar PB, Cotts W et al. Prevalence and severity of mitral regurgitation in chronic systolic heart failure. Am J Cardiol 2003;91:360–362.
98. Bach DS, Awais M, Gurm HS, Kohnstamm S. Failure of guideline adherence for intervention in patients with severe mitral regurgitation. J Am Coll Cardiol 2009;54:860–865.
99. Bolling SF, Pagani FD, Deeb GM, Bach DS. Intermediate–term outcome of mitral reconstruction in cardiomyopathy. J Thorac Cardiovasc Surg 1998;115:381–386.
100. Wu AH, Aaronson KD, Bolling SF et al. Impact of mitral valve annuloplasty on mortality risk in patients with mitral regurgitation and left ventricular systolic dysfunction. J Am Coll Cardiol 2005;45:381–387.
101. Acker MA, Bolling S, Shemin R et al. Mitral valve surgery in heart failure: insights from the Acorn Clinical Trial. J Thorac Cardiovasc Surg 2006;132:568–577.
102. Calafiore AM, Gallina S, Di Mauro M et al. Mitral valve procedure in dilated cardiomyopathy: repair or replacement? Ann Thorac Surg 2001;71:1146–1152.
103. Grigioni F, Enriquez-Sarano M, Zehr KJ et al. Ischemic mitral regurgitation. Long term outcome and prognostic implication with quantitative Doppler assessment. Circulation 2001;103:1759–1764.
104. Grigioni F, Detaint D, Avierinos J-F et al. Contribution of ischemic mitral regurgitation to congestive heart failure after myocardial infarction. J Am Coll Cardiol 2005;45:260–267.
105. Aronson D, Goldsher N, Zukerman R et al. Ischemic mitral regurgitation and risk of heart failure after myocardial infarction. Arch Intern Med 2006;166:2362–2368.
106. Schroder JN, Williams ML, Hata JA et al. Impact of mitral valve regurgitation evaluated by intraoperative transesophageal echocardiography on long–term outcomes after coronary artery bypass grafting. Circulation 2005;112(Suppl I):I293–298.
107. Amigoni M, Meris A,Thune JJ et al. Mitral regurgitation in myocardial infarction complicated by heart failure, left ventricular dysfunction, or both: prognostic significance and relation to ventricular size and function. Eur Heart J 2007;28; 326–333.
108. Di Mauro M, Di Giammarco G, Vitolla G et al. Impact of no-or-moderate mitral regurgitation on late results after isolated coronary artery bypass grafting in patients with ischemic cardiomyopathy. Ann Thorac Surg 2006;81:2128–2134.
109. Calafiore AM, Mazzei V, Iacò AL et al. Impact of ischemic regurgitation on long-term outcome of patients with ejection fraction above 0.30 undergoing first isolated myocardial revascularization. Ann Thorac Surg 2008;86:458–465.
110. Fattouch K, Guccione F, Sampognaro R et al. POINT: efficacy of adding mitral valve restrictive annuloplasty to coronary artery bypass grafting in patients with moderate ischemic mitral valve regurgitation: a randomized trial. J Thorac Cardiovasc Surg 2009;138:278–285.
111. Kinkaid EH, Riley RD, Hines MH et al. Anterior leaflet augmentation for ischemic mitral regurgitation. Ann Thorac Surg 2004;78:564–568.
112. Romano MA, Patel HJ, Pagani FD et al. Anterior leaflet repair with patch augmentation for mitral regurgitation. Ann Thorac Surg 2005;79:1500–1504.
113. Aubert S, Flecher E, Rubin S et al. Anterior mitral leaflet augmentation with autologous pericardium. Ann Thorac Surg 2007;83:1560–1561.
114. De Varennes B, Chaturvedi R, Sidhu S et al. Initial results of posterior leaflet extension for severe type IIIb ischemic mitral regurgitation. Circulation 2009;119:2837–2843.
115. Messas E, Pouzet B, Touchot B et al. Efficacy of chordal cutting to relieve chronic persistent ischemic mitral regurgitation. Circulation 2003;108(Suppl 1):II111–115.
116. Borger MA, Murphy PM, Alam A et al. Initial results of the chordal–cutting operation for ischemic mitral regurgitation. J Thorac Cardiovasc Surg 2007;133:1483–1492.
117. Nielsen SL, Timek TA, Green GR et al. Influence of anterior mitral leaflet second–order *chordae tendineae* on left ventricular systolic function. Circulation 2003;108:486–491.

118. Aazami MH, Salehi M, Satarzadeh R. Whatever the approach, cutting strut chordae would not smell as sweet (letter). J Thorac Cardiovasc Surg 2005;130:1480.
119. Braun J, van der Veire NR, Klautz RJM et al. Restrictive mitral annuloplasty cures ischemic mitral regurgitation and heart failure. Ann Thorac Surg 2008;85:430–437.
120. Srichai MB, Grimm RA, Stillman AE et al. Ischemic mitral regurgitation: impact of left ventricle and mitral valve in patients with left ventricular dysfunction. Ann Thorac Surg 2005;80:170–178.
121. Hvaas U, Tapia M, Baron F et al. Papillary muscle sling: a new functional approach to mitral valve repair in patients with ischemic left ventricular dysfunction and functional mitral regurgitation. Ann Thorac Surg 2003;75:809–811.
122. Fumimoto K, Fukui T, Shimokawa T, Takanashi S. Papillary muscle realignment and mitral annuloplasty in patients with severe ischemic mitral regurgitation and dilated heart. Interact Cardiovasc Thorac Surg 2008;7:368–371.
123. Kron IL, Green GR, Cope JT. Surgical relocation of the posterior papillary muscle in chronic ischemic mitral regurgitation. Ann Thorac Surg 2002;74:600–601.
124. Ueno T, Sakata R, Iguro Y et al. New surgical approach to reduce tethering in ischemic mitral regurgitation by relocation of separate heads of the posterior papillary muscle. Ann Thorac Surg 2006;81:2324–2325.
125. Rama A, Praschker L, Barreda E, Gandjbackhch I. Papillary muscle approximation for functional ischemic mitral regurgitation. Ann Thorac Surg 2007:84:2130–2131.
126. Langer F, Schäfers H-J. RING plus STRING: papillary muscle repositioning as an adjunctive repair technique for ischemic mitral regurgitation. J Thorac Cardiovasc Surg 2007;133:247–249.
127. Crabtree TD, Bailey MS, Moon MR et al. Recurrent mitral regurgitation and risk factors for early and late mortality after mitral valve repair for functional ischemic mitral regurgitation. Ann Thorac Surg 2008;85:1537–1543.
128. Zhu F, Otsuji Y, Yotsumoto G et al. Mechanism of persistent ischemic mitral regurgitation after annuloplasty: importance of augmented posterior mitral leaflet tethering. Circulation 2005;112:I396–1401.
129. Yiu SF, Enriquez-Sarano M, Tribouilloy C et al. Determinants of the degree of functional mitral regurgitation in patients with systolic left ventricular dysfunction: a quantitative clinical study. Circulation 2000;102:1400–1406.
130. De Bonis M, Lapenna E, Verzini A et al. Recurrence of mitral regurgitation parallels the absence of left ventricular reverse remodeling after mitral repair in advanced dilated cardiomyopathy. Ann Thorac Surg 2008;85:932–939.
131. Pui-Wai Lee A, Acker M, Kubo SH et al. Mechanisms of recurrent functional mitral regurgitation after mitral valve repair in non schemic dilated cardiomyopathy. Importance of distal anterior leaflet tethering. Circulation 2009;119:2606–2614.
132. Szalay ZA, Civelek A, Hohe S et al. Mitral annuloplasty in patients with ischemic versus dilated cardiomyopathy. Eur J Cardiothorac Surg 2003:23:567–572.
133. Glower DD, Tuttle RH, Shaw LK et al. Patients survival characteristics after routine mitral valve repair for ischemic mitral regurgitation. J Thorac Cardiovasc Surg 2005;129:860–868.
134. De Bonis M, La Penna E, La Canna G et al. Mitral valve repair for functional mitral regurgitation in end–stage dilated cardiomyopathy. Role of the edge-to-edge technique. Circulation 2005;112(Suppl I):I402–408.
135. Mihaljevic T, Lam B-K, Rajeswaran J et al. Impact of mitral valve annuloplasty combined with revascularization in patients with functional ischemic mitral regurgitation. J Am Coll Cardiol 2007;49:2191–2201.
136. Gelsomino S, Lorusso R, De Cicco G et al. Five-year echocardiographic results of combined undersized mitral ring annuloplasty and coronary artery bypass grafting for chronic ischemic mitral regurgitation. Eur Heart J 2008;29:231–240.

137. Al-Radi OO, Austin PC, Tu JV et al. Mitral repair versus replacement for ischemic mitral rgurgitation. Ann Thorac Surg 2005;79:1260–1267.
138. Magne J, Senechal M, Mathieu P et al. Short- and long-term survival of mitral valve repair versus mitral valve replacement in patients with functional mitral regurgitation. Circulation 2008;118:S698.
139. Magne J, Pibarot P, Dagenais F et al. Preoperative posterior leaflet angle accurately predicts outcome after restrictive mitral valve annuloplasty for ischemic mitral regurgitation. Circulation 2007;115:782–791.
140. Gelsomino S, Lorusso R, Caciolli S et al. Insights on left ventricular mechanisms of recurrent ischemic mitral regurgitation after restrictive annuloplasty and coronary artery bypass grafting. J Thorac Cardiovasc Surg 2008;136:507–518.
141. Roshanali F, Mandegar MH, Yousefnia MA et al. A prospective study of predicting factors in ischemic mitral regurgitation recurrence after ring annuloplasty. Ann Thorac Surg 2007;84:745–749.
142. Bolman III RM. Have we found the surgical solution for ischemic mitral regurgitation? Circulation 2009;119:2755–2757.
143. Magne J, Sénéchal M, Mathieu P et al. Restrictive annuloplasty for ischemic mitral regurgitation may induce functional mitral stenosis. J Am Coll Cardiol 2008;51:1692–1701.
144. Williams ML, Daneshmand MA, Jollis JG et al. Mitral gradients and frequency of recurrence of mitral regurgitation after ring annuloplasty for ischemic mitral regurgitation. Ann Thorac Surg 2009;88:1197–1201.
145. Bonow RO, Carabello BA, Chatterjee K et al. 2008 Focused Update incorporated into the ACC/AHA 2006 Guidelines for the Management of Patients With Valvular Heart Disease: A Report of the American College of Cardiology/American Heart Association Task Force on Practice Guidelines (Writing Committee to Revise the 1998 Guidelines for the Management of Patients With Valvular Heart Disease) Endorsed by the Society of Cardiovascular Anesthesiologists, Society for Cardiovascular Angiography and Interventions, and Society of Thoracic Surgeons. J Am Coll Cardiol 2008;52;e1–e142.
146. Otto CM. Valvular aortic stenosis. Disease severity and timing of intervention. J Am Coll Cardiol 2006;47:2141–2151.
147. Pai RG, Kapoor N, Bansal RC, Varadarajan P. Malignant natural history of asymptomatic severe aortic stenosis: benefit of aortic valve replacement. Ann Thorac Surg 2006;82:2116–2122.
148. Jamieson WRE, Ye J, Higgins J et al. Effects of prosthesis–patient mismatch on long–term survival with aortic valve replacement: assessment to 15 years. Ann Thorac Surg 2010;89:51–59.
149. Iung B, Cachier A, Baron G et al. Decision-making in elderly patients with severe aortic stenosis: why are so many denied surgery? Eur Heart J 2005;26:2714–2720.
150. Bach DS, Cimino N, Deeb GM. Unoperated patients with severe aortic stenosis. J Am Coll Cardiol 2007;50:2018–2019.

Printed in April 2010